Step by Step®
Treatment of Acne Scars

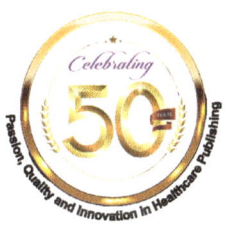

Step by Step® Treatment of Acne Scars

Second Edition

Niti Khunger MD DNB DDV
Consultant Dermatologist
Professor and Head
Department of Dermatology and STD
Vardhman Mahavir Medical College and
Safdarjung Hospital, New Delhi, India

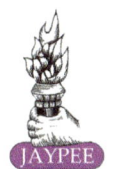

JAYPEE BROTHERS MEDICAL PUBLISHERS
The Health Sciences Publisher
New Delhi | London

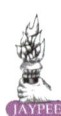

Jaypee Brothers Medical Publishers (P) Ltd

Headquarters
Jaypee Brothers Medical Publishers (P) Ltd
4838/24, Ansari Road, Daryaganj
New Delhi 110 002, India
Phone: +91-11-43574357
Fax: +91-11-43574314
E-mail: jaypee@jaypeebrothers.com

Overseas Office
JP Medical Ltd
83 Victoria Street, London
SW1H 0HW (UK)
Phone: +44 20 3170 8910
Fax: +44 (0)20 3008 6180
E-mail: info@jpmedpub.com

Website: www.jaypeebrothers.com
Website: www.jaypeedigital.com

© 2020, Jaypee Brothers Medical Publishers

The views and opinions expressed in this book are solely those of the original contributor(s)/author(s) and do not necessarily represent those of editor(s) of the book.

All rights reserved. No part of this publication may be reproduced, stored or transmitted in any form or by any means, electronic, mechanical, photocopying, recording or otherwise, without the prior permission in writing of the publishers.

All brand names and product names used in this book are trade names, service marks, trademarks or registered trademarks of their respective owners. The publisher is not associated with any product or vendor mentioned in this book.

Medical knowledge and practice change constantly. This book is designed to provide accurate, authoritative information about the subject matter in question. However, readers are advised to check the most current information available on procedures included and check information from the manufacturer of each product to be administered, to verify the recommended dose, formula, method and duration of administration, adverse effects and contraindications. It is the responsibility of the practitioner to take all appropriate safety precautions. Neither the publisher nor the author(s)/editor(s) assume any liability for any injury and/or damage to persons or property arising from or related to use of material in this book.

This book is sold on the understanding that the publisher is not engaged in providing professional medical services. If such advice or services are required, the services of a competent medical professional should be sought.

Every effort has been made where necessary to contact holders of copyright to obtain permission to reproduce copyright material. If any have been inadvertently overlooked, the publisher will be pleased to make the necessary arrangements at the first opportunity. The **CD/DVD-ROM** (if any) provided in the sealed envelope with this book is complimentary and free of cost. **Not meant for sale.**

Inquiries for bulk sales may be solicited at: jaypee@jaypeebrothers.com

Step by Step® Treatment of Acne Scars

First Edition: 2014

Second Edition: 2020

ISBN: 978-93-89188-36-3

Dedicated to
All my patients who inspire me to,
Innovate, Improvise, Implement,
And to my family
Dr Jitender Mohan, Dr Monica, and Dr Arjun
who encourage me to Aspire, Ascend, Achieve.

Contributors

Aditi Jha MD
Assistant Professor
Department of Dermatology and STD
Adesh Medical College and Hospital
Ambala, Haryana, India

Amit Luthra DNB
Consultant Dermatologist
Ishira Skin Clinic
Panchsheel Park and Ashok Vihar, New Delhi, India

Anil Ganjoo MD
Senior Consultant Dermatologist and Laser Surgeon
Saroj Hospital, New Delhi, India

Anuj Pall MD PHD FISD (USA)
Chief Director
Escallent Institute of Lasers and Aesthetic Medicine (EILAM)
Gurugram, Haryana, India

Apratim Goel
MD DNB FAGE
Dermatologist and Cosmetologist
Goel's Cutis Skin Studio
Mumbai, Maharashtra, India

Ayushi Khandelwal MD
Associate Dermatologist
MS Skin Clinic
Bengaluru, Karnataka, India

Deepali Bhardwaj
MBBS DVDL MPHIL
Dermatologist
Founder
The Skin and Hair Clinic
New Delhi, India

Dhaarna Wadhwa MD DNB
Senior Resident
Department of Dermatology
Vardhman Mahavir Medical College and Safdarjung Hospital, New Delhi, India

Imran Majid MD
Director
Cutis Institute of Dermatology
Srinagar
Jammu and Kashmir, India

Jaishree Sharad
MBBS DDV FAAD Fellowship in Cosmetic Dermatology Fellowship in Lasers
Medical Director and Consultant Cosmetic Dermatologist
Skinfiniti Aesthetic Skin and Laser Clinic
Mumbai, Maharashtra, India

Koushik Lahiri
MBBS DVD (CAL) FIAD FAAD
FFAADV MRCPS (GLASGOW)
Senior Consultant
Dermatologist
Apollo Gleneagles Hospitals
Nightingale Hospitals
WIZDERM
Kolkata, West Bengal, India

Kumar Abhishek
MD DNB MNAMS
Assistant Professor
Department of Dermatology
HiTech Medical College
Bhubaneswar, Odisha, India

Mukta Sachdev
MD DPD (UK) DIP DERM (UK) DD
(UK) Fellow In Cos Derm (USA)
Head and Consultant
Manipal Hospital
Bengaluru, Karnataka, India

Niteen Dhepe MD
Medical Director
Skin City, PG Institute
Pune, Maharashtra, India

Niti Khunger MD DNB DDV
Consultant Dermatologist
Professor and Head
Department of Dermatology
and STD
Vardhman Mahavir Medical
College and Safdarjung
Hospital, New Delhi, India

Ridhima Lakhani MD DNB
Senior Resident
Department of Dermatology
Vardhman Mahavir Medical
College and Safdarjung
Hospital, New Delhi, India

Sanjeev Aurangabadkar MD
Dermatologist
Skin and Laser Clinic
Begumpet
Hyderabad, Telangana, India

Shehnaz Arsiwala MD DDV
Dermatologist
Renewderm Center
Saifee Hospital
Prince Aly Khan Hospital
Mumbai, Maharashtra, India

Shikha Bansal
MD DNB MNAMS
Associate Professor
Department of Dermatology
and STD
Vardhman Mahavir Medical
College and Safdarjung
Hospital, New Delhi, India

Vivek Kumar
MS (Surgery) DNB (Plastic Surgery)
MNAMS MIMSA
Consultant, Plastic and
Cosmetic Surgeon
Sir Ganga Ram Hospital
New Delhi, India

Preface to the Second Edition

Acne is now considered a chronic inflammatory disorder and what was commonly seen in adolescence is persisting in adults right up to the menopause. In spite of advances in the understanding of pathogenesis of acne, the incidence of postacne scarring has not reduced. In fact, more and more patients in the older age group are coming for the treatment of postacne scarring and this poses another challenge. The birth of the second edition was initiated by advances in the field of energy based devices particularly microneedling radiofrequency treatments which are independent of skin color. Innovations in the use of ablative lasers by combining different techniques such as the 5-tier technique are giving better results over a shorter period of time.

This book is intended to be a simple step by step guide for the treatment of acne scars. It can be considered as a comprehensive reference as it not only provides management of individual techniques as well as individual type of scars. An algorithmic approach gives the reader an overall understanding how to plan management of this challenging condition. Each contributor is an expert and they have given practical tips on how best to tackle patients with postacne scars.

I hope this book proves an invaluable resource for dermatologists and plastic surgeons who deal with management of patients with postacne scars.

Niti Khunger

Preface to the First Edition

Acne is a very common disorder in adolescence; and, unfortunately, scarring following acne occurs early and may affect 95% of patients depending on severity of acne and delay in treatment. Acne scars are predominantly seen on the face and can cause profound psychosocial distress in the growing years as well as in adulthood. Treating acne scars is challenging as postacne scars are polymorphic and management involves the use of various modalities depending on the type of scars.

The aim of this book is to give a comprehensive step-by-step guide to the treatment of acne scars, which can be understood and followed by a young physician entering into the world of esthetic surgery as well as older physicians not exposed to newer techniques. This book is unique because individual types of scars have been dealt with in detail so that the physician understands the pathophysiology and principle behind their treatment, as well as approach to the patient as a whole. The book deals with the art and skill of combining various techniques of acne scar revision, their proper application to give optimum results and the unique challenges posed by skin of color. Emphasis has been laid on the possible complications that can occur, particularly in darker skins and their detailed management.

There has been an explosion of newer techniques for treating acne scars and the shift has occurred from invasive technologies requiring a lot of downtime to minimally invasive techniques, requiring lesser downtime, which benefits patients.

Each contributor is an expert in the field with wide experience and has given a practical approach to the management of acne scars. This book will be an invaluable resource to dermatosurgeons, plastic surgeons and esthetic surgeons dealing particularly with facial scars.

Niti Khunger

Acknowledgments

The birth of this book was initiated by young and enthusiastic dermatologists, who showed great interest in my presentations during various scientific meetings. It incubated and took shape when there was an explosion of newer, minimally invasive techniques in dealing with acne scars. I am indebted to my expert contributors who have crystallized their experiences and shared their personal innovative techniques in dealing with the topics.

I am grateful to all my patients for their unwavering support and complete faith reposed in me, which helped to innovate and improvise.

I am thankful to my teachers, particularly, Dr Chetan Oberai and late Dr PN Behl who injected me with academic enthusiasm right from the beginning of my career.

I am also thankful to Shri Jitendar P Vij (Group Chairman), Mr Ankit Vij (Managing Director), Mrs Pooja Bhandari (Head-Production), Ms Chetna Malhotra Vohra (Associate Director—Content Strategy) Dr Rajul Jain (Development Editor), Ms Ruby Sharma (Project Manager) and the entire team of M/s Jaypee Brothers Medical Publishers (P) Ltd, New Delhi, India, for their help in bringing out the book.

My deepest gratitude goes to my family, my spouse Dr JM Khunger and my children, Dr Monica and Dr Arjun, who let me work unhindered in writing this book.

Contents

1. **Current Concepts in the Treatment of Acne**.....................1
   Niti Khunger, Dhaarna Wadhwa
   - Topical Agents 3
   - Systemic Antibiotics 5
   - Hormonal Agents 7
   - Isotretinoin 9
   - Miscellaneous Therapies 10
   - Role of Diet in Acne 11

2. **Pathophysiology of Acne Scars** 16
   Niti Khunger
   - Why does Acne Scar? 17
   - When does Acne Scar? 18
   - Pathogenesis of Acne 19
   - Pathophysiology of Acne Scars 23

3. **Types of Acne Scars and Grading Systems** 31
   Shikha Bansal, Niti Khunger
   - Morphological Types of Acne Scars 33
   - Grading of Acne Scars 42

4. **Prevention of Acne Scars** 48
   Niti Khunger
   - Principles of Prevention of Acne Scars 49
   - Appropriate Treatment of Acne 52

5. **Topical Treatment**.. 59
   Aditi Jha, Niti Khunger
   - Topical Applications 59
   - Silicon Gel and Onion Extract 61
   - Cryotherapy 62
   - Iontophoresis 62

6. **Chemical Peels** 65
   Niti Khunger
   - Principle 66
   - Indications 66
   - Contraindications 66
   - Limitations 71
   - Precautions 72
   - Preprocedure Preparation 72
   - Technique 72
   - Postprocedure Care 73
   - Complications 76

7. **CROSS Technique** 79
   Deepali Bhardwaj, Niti Khunger
   - Principle 80 • Instruments 81
   - Contraindications 81 • Limitations 82
   - Precautions 82 • Preprocedure Preparation 83
   - Technique 85 • Efficacy 86
   - Postprocedure Care 87 • Complications 88

8. **Subcision** 91
   Niti Khunger
   - Principle 92 • Instruments 93
   - Indications 93 • Contraindications 93
   - Precautions 93 • Preprocedure Preparation 94
   - Technique 94 • Postprocedure Care 99
   - Efficacy 99 • Complications 100

9. **Punch Excision Techniques** 103
   Niti Khunger
   - Equipment 103 • Indications 104
   - Relative Contraindications 104
   - Preprocedure Assessment and Preparation 105
   - Procedure 106
   - Postprocedure Care 109 • Complications 111
   - Pros and Cons 114

10. **Microneedling** 115
    Jaishree Sharad
    - Principle of Microneedling 116 • Instruments 116
    - Contraindications 120 • Limitations 120
    - Precautions 121 • Preprocedure Preparation 121
    - Technique 122 • Postprocedure Care 123
    - Complications 127

11. **Microdermabrasion** 130
    Apratim Goel
    - Principle 131 • Instruments 131
    - Indications 138 • Contraindications 138
    - Limitations 139 • Precautions 139
    - Preprocedure Preparation 140 • Technique 140
    - Postprocedure Care 141 • Complications 142

Contents

12. **Lasers and Light Devices** 144
    Sanjeev Aurangabadkar
    - Principle 146 • Ablative CO_2 Laser Resurfacing 148
    - Erbium:YAG Laser Resurfacing 148
    - Ablative Fractional Laser Resurfacing 149
    - Nonablative Lasers 154
    - Intense Pulsed Light Devices 157
    - Patient Selection and Preoperative Care 157
    - Anesthesia 161 • Postoperative Care 161
    - Complications 161
    - Newer Laser Technologies for Acne Scars 165

13. **Fillers** 169
    Amit Luthra
    - Principle 170 • Instruments and Materials 170
    - Indications 173 • Contraindications 174
    - Limitations 175 • Precautions 175
    - Preprocedure Preparation 175 • Technique 176
    - Postprocedure Care 177 • Complications 178
    - Advantages 179 • Disadvantages 180

14. **Autologous Fat Transfer for Acne Scars** 182
    Vivek Kumar, Niti Khunger, Ridhima Lakhani
    - Principle 183 • Instruments 184
    - Indications 186 • Contraindications 186
    - Precautions 186 • Advantages 187
    - Disadvantages 187 • Preprocedure Preparation 187
    - Technique 188 • Postoperative Care 194
    - Follow-up 194 • Efficacy and Survival of Fat 195
    - Complications 196 • Combination Treatments 196
    - Future of Fat 197

15. **Ice Pick Scars** 200
    Niti Khunger
    - Methods of Treatment 201 • Limitations 202
    - Precautions 203 • Preprocedure Preparation 203
    - Technique 204 • Postprocedure Care 207
    - Complications 210

16. Boxcar Scars 212
Niti Khunger, Shikha Bansal
- Sites 213
- Methods of Treatment 213
- Indications 214
- Contraindications 214
- Limitations 215
- Precautions 215
- Preprocedure Preparation 215
- Technique 215
- Postprocedure Care 218
- Complications 218

17. Rolling Scars 221
Niti Khunger
- Methods of Treatment 221
- Instruments 222
- Indications 223
- Contraindications 223
- Limitations 223
- Precautions 224
- Preprocedure Preparation 224
- Technique 224
- Postprocedure Care 226
- Complications 226

18. LInear and Lipoatrophic Acne Scars 228
Niti Khunger
- Methods of Treatment 231
- Limitations 232
- Precautions 232
- Preprocedure Preparation 234
- Technique 234
- Postprocedure Care 236
- Complications 236

19. Papular Scars 238
Niti Khunger
- Methods of Treatment 239
- Instruments 240
- Indications 240
- Contraindications 241
- Limitations 241
- Precautions 241
- Preprocedure Preparation 241
- Technique 242
- Postprocedure Care 243
- Complications 243

20. Keloids, Hypertrophic, and Bridging Scars 246
Niti Khunger
- Pathophysiology and Prevention of Scars 247
- Methods of Treatment 248
- Indications 248
- Contraindications 249
- Limitations 249
- Precautions 249
- Choice of Treatment 249
- Post-treatment Care 249
- Complications 250
- Bridging Scars 251

Contents xix

21. **Acne Scars in Darker Skin Types: Special Precautions**..........................253
    Mukta Sachdev, Ayushi Khandelwal
    - Characteristics 254
    - Clinically Relevant Structural and Functional Differences 255
    - Special Precautions 256
    - Treatment Considerations for Dark Skin Types 257

22. **Acne Scars: Complications of Treatment and their Management**..........................263
    Shehnaz Arsiwala
    - Problems in Darker Skins 264
    - Choice of Treatment Modality 267
    - Basic Precautions and Avoiding Complications 270
    - Intra-treatment Vigilance 273
    - How to Minimize Risks of Complications with Specific Modalities of Treatment? 275
    - Useful Strategies while Conducting Peels 278
    - Management of Complications 289

23. **Imaging Techniques for Acne Scars**..........................304
    Niti Khunger
    - Photography 304
    - High Frequency Ultrasound 305
    - Optical Imaging Devices 306
    - Dermoscopy 308
    - Reflectance Confocal Microscopy 308

24. **Camouflage Techniques for Acne Scars**..........................311
    Niti Khunger, Kumar Abhishek
    - Indications 312
    - Contraindications 312
    - Types of Medical Makeup for Scars 313
    - Makeup Products for Acne Scars 314
    - Tools 314
    - Techniques 315
    - Setting or Fixing the Makeup 317
    - Makeup Removal 318
    - Side Effects 318
    - Brimonidine Gel 318

25. **Newer Techniques: Fractional Microneedle Radiofrequency for the Treatment of Acne Scars** 321
    Anuj Pall
    - Equipment 322
    - Monopolar and Bipolar Radiofrequency 323
    - Combination Treatments 324
    - Newer Advancements 324 • Indications 325
    - Contraindications 325 • Procedure 325
    - Precautions 327 • Post-treatment Care 327
    - Complications 327

26. **Combination Treatments for Acne Scars** 329
    Niti Khunger
    - Advantages of Combination Techniques 330
    - Current Trends 330 • Plan of Treatment 331
    - Combination Triple Laser Technique 336
    - Complications 336

27. **Interesting Case Discussions** 339
    Anil Ganjoo, Shehnaz Arsiwala, Koushik Lahiri,
    Imran Majid, Niteen Dhepe
    - Case 1 339
      Anil Ganjoo
    - Case 2 341
      Anil Ganjoo
    - Case 3 342
      Niteen Dhepe
    - Case 4 344
      Niteen Dhepe
    - Case 5 345
      Niteen Dhepe
    - Case 6 346
      Imran Majid
    - Case 7 348
      Imran Majid
    - Case 8 350
      Koushik Lahiri

Contents

- Case 9 351
  Koushik Lahiri
- Case 10 352
  Koushik Lahiri
- Case 11 353
  Shehnaz Arsiwala
- Case 12 354
  Shehnaz Arsiwala
- Case 13 355
  Shehnaz Arsiwala

28. Algorithmic Approach to Acne Scars..........................357
    Niti Khunger
    - Patient Assessment 357

Index 365

CHAPTER 1

Current Concepts in the Treatment of Acne

Niti Khunger, Dhaarna Wadhwa

IN A NUTSHELL

- ❖ Acne vulgaris is a multifactorial, chronic, inflammatory disorder of the pilosebaceous unit characterized by polymorphic skin lesions that can lead to permanent scarring.
- ❖ Topical treatment is the mainstay of therapy and includes a combination therapy of benzoyl peroxide and retinoid, with or without a topical antibiotic.
- ❖ Systemic antibiotics should be reserved for patients with moderate-to-severe inflammatory acne and given only for 6–12 weeks.
- ❖ Isotretinoin should be reserved for severe or relapsing cases.
- ❖ Women with signs of hyperandrogenism should be investigated and treated accordingly.
- ❖ Treatment should be chosen according to the severity of acne and individualized according to patient skin type.

INTRODUCTION

Acne vulgaris is a multifactorial, chronic, inflammatory disorder of the pilosebaceous unit characterized by polymorphic skin lesions in the form of open or closed comedones (blackheads and whiteheads) and inflammatory lesions, including papules, pustules, nodules, and cysts. The main pathogenic factors are follicular hyperkeratinization, sebum production, microbial colonization with *Cutibacterium acnes* (formerly *Propionibacterium acnes*), and innate and adaptive immune mechanisms. Also implicated are the neuroendocrine factors, genetics, and diet.[1] The implications of acne and acne scarring are often severe causing significant physical and psychological morbidity, poor self-image, anxiety, and depression.[1] Even though no single system for grading of acne has been universally recommended, the commonly used grading classifies acne into four grades:[2]

- *Grade 1*: Comedones, occasional papules
- *Grade 2*: Papules, comedones, and few pustules
- *Grade 3*: Predominant pustules, nodules, and abscesses
- *Grade 4*: Mainly cysts, abscesses, and widespread scarring.

The diagnosis of acne is mainly clinical. Microbiological testing though not routinely indicated may be required in suspicious cases of gram negative or staphylococcal folliculitis.[1] Investigations are required in females to rule out androgen excess and polycystic ovarian syndrome in patients that have concomitant hirsutism, female pattern alopecia, irregular menstrual history, or acanthosis nigricans or are relatively resistant to therapy or relapse quickly after treatment. These patients should be evaluated with total and free testosterone, androstenedione, dehydroepiandrosterone sulfate (DHEAS), follicle-stimulating and luteinizing hormone, in addition to a lipid panel, thyroid panel, fasting and postprandial glucose and insulin levels, and vitamin D level. Obesity is also associated with acne, particularly inflammatory acne due to peripheral hyperandrogenism.[3]

Evaluation of acne to decide treatment includes severity of acne, skin type of the patient (dry, oily, or sensitive), products and medications used, presence of postinflammatory hyperpigmentation, acne scarring, and the psychological impact of acne. Management consists of topical therapy, which is the mainstay of treatment, with systemic therapy when indicated and procedural therapy in selected cases **(Table 1)**.[4,5] Topical therapies include benzoyl peroxide, topical antibiotics, retinoids, azelaic acid, salicylic acid, dapsone, and combinations.

TABLE 1: Treatment algorithm for the management of acne vulgaris in adolescents and young adults.

	Mild	Moderate	Severe
First-line treatment	Benzoyl peroxide (BP) or topical retinoid or topical combination therapy** (BP + Antibiotic or Retinoid + BP or Retinoid + BP + Antibiotic)	Topical combination therapy** or oral antibiotic + Topical retinoid + BP or oral antibiotic + Topical retinoid + BP + Topical antibiotic	Oral antibiotic + Topical combination therapy** or oral isotretinoin
Alternative treatment	Add topical retinoid or BP (if not already) or consider alternate retinoid or consider topical dapsone	Consider alternate combination therapy or consider change in oral antibiotic or add combined oral contraceptive or oral spironolactone (females) or consider oral isotretinoin	Consider change in oral antibiotic or add combined oral contraceptive or oral spironolactone (females) or consider oral isotretinoin
Procedural treatment	Comedone extraction	• Comedone extraction • Chemical peels with salicylic acid, glycolic acid or mandelic acid	• Incision and drainage of cysts • Intralesional steroids

**The drug may be prescribed as a fixed drug combination product or as separate component.

TOPICAL AGENTS

Benzoyl peroxide (BP) is antibacterial and comedolytic. Since no resistance has been reported, it is recommended to be used alone or in combination with topical antibiotics like clindamycin to prevent emergence of resistance. It can also be combined with adapalene for synergistic action. It is available as creams, washes, foams, and gels in strengths from 2.5 to 10%. Adverse effects include irritation which is concentration dependent, bleaching and staining of clothes, and contact allergy. Lesser concentrations and wash-off preparations are better suited for sensitive skin.

Topical antibiotics act as antibacterial and anti-inflammatory agents by accumulating in the hair follicle. Topical clindamycin 1% and nadifloxacin 1% are used as topical agents, but they should not be used as monotherapy due to emergence of resistance. They are recommended in combination with benzoyl peroxide which enhances efficacy and prevents development of resistance.

Topical retinoids are the maintaining in anti-acne therapy. The three main topical agents include—(1) tretinoin (0.025-1% in cream, gel, or microsphere), (2) adapalene (0.1% gel), and (3) tazarotene (0.05%, 0.1% cream and gel). These are vitamin A derivatives which bind to retinoic acid receptors, tretinoin binding to alpha, beta, and gamma and adapalene and tazarotene selectively to beta and gamma with few differences in efficacy and side effects. They are the mainstay of therapy being comedolytic, inhibiting microcomedones and anti-inflammatory. They are recommended as monotherapy for comedonal acne or in combination with topical antibiotics like clindamycin or benzoyl peroxide or systemic antibiotics for severe forms. The most frequent side effects encountered include dryness, irritation, erythema, and burning (retinoid dermatitis) which can be reduced by decreasing the strength, using microsphere formulations, reducing contact time, frequency of application, and liberal use of emollients. Photosensitivity can be decreased by usage at night and coadministration of sunscreens. Tretinoin and benzoyl peroxide should not be used together as benzoyl peroxide may inactivate and oxidize tretinoin. Tretinoin and adapalene are pregnancy category C whereas tazarotene is category X. Retinoids are the Food and Drug Administration (FDA) approved for children ≥12 years. Fixed combination BP 2.5%/adapalene 0.1% gel is approved for patients ≥9 years and tretinoin 0.05% micronized tretinoin gel for patients ≥10 years. Current data show that retinoids in younger patients are effective and are not associated with increased irritation or risk.

Azelaic acid 20% is a pregnancy category B drug that apart from being mildly comedolytic, antibacterial, and anti-inflammatory agent, also has hypopigmenting action, hence is useful to treat postinflammatory hyperpigmentation in pregnant patients, darker skin, Fitzpatrick skin type IV or greater, and in sensitive skin.

Dapsone 5% gel is a sulfone agent having moderate efficacy primarily in reduction of inflammatory lesions through its anti-inflammatory action.[6] It has poor efficacy in comedonal acne and the benefit in women seems to exceed that in men and adolescents.[7] Topical dapsone may be oxidized by coadministration of benzoyl peroxide producing an orange-brown coloration of skin which can be washed off.[1] Topical dapsone is pregnancy category C and can be given to children above 12 years.

Salicylic acid (0.5–2%) is a comedolytic agent available as wash off or gel formulations used as adjunctive therapy.

Topical nicotinamide 2–4% gel is available in combination with clindamycin and has been useful in inflammatory acne.

SYSTEMIC ANTIBIOTICS

Systemic antibiotics have been the mainstay of acne therapy for moderate-to-severe inflammatory acne in combination with topicals.[8] The main classes of drugs include macrolides like azithromycin and erythromycin, tetracyclines like doxycycline and minocycline, and beta-lactams like amoxicillin and cephalexin. The tetracycline class of antibiotics is recommended to be used as first line, acting by inhibiting the protein synthesis by binding to the 30S subunit of bacterial ribosome and having some anti-inflammatory effects like inhibiting chemotaxis and metalloproteinase activity. Minocycline along with tetracycline has been found to be useful in the treatment of acne with equal efficacy.[9] Minocycline is available in the extended release form (at 1 mg/kg) and appears to be safe. Doxycycline is effective at 1.7–2.4 mg/kg and seems to be effective at even low doses of 20 mg twice daily or 40 mg daily.[10] Tetracyclines are contraindicated in pregnancy, ≤8 years, and allergic cases when other classes of antibiotics should be used. Macrolides like azithromycin and erythromycin bind to 50S subunit of ribosome and also exhibit some anti-inflammatory properties. Azithromycin has primarily been used in acne in pulse dosing regimen from three times a week to four times a month given for 2–3 months or till the inflammatory lesions subside.[11] Trimethoprim/sulfamethoxazole by acting on folic acid pathway is bacteriostatic and has been used for treating acne traditionally, but is not routinely used now because of lack of efficacy and high degree of side effects including gastrointestinal disturbances, photosensitivity, blood dyscrasias, fulminant hepatic necrosis, respiratory hypersensitivity, and drug reactions including Stevens-Johnson syndrome and toxic epidermal necrolysis. Similarly, penicillin class of antibiotics (like amoxicillin) and cephalosporins which act by inhibiting cell wall synthesis are sometime used particularly in pregnant patients or patients with allergies to other drugs. Adverse effects mainly include hypersensitivity reactions and gastrointestinal disturbances.[12] Adverse effects to systemic antibiotics though rare include vaginal candidiasis, drug eruptions, inflammatory bowel disease, pharyngitis, and *Clostridium difficile* infection.[13] Specific side effects include photosensitivity secondary to tetracyclines particularly doxycycline and gastrointestinal disturbances. Minocycline has been associated with tinnitus, dizziness, and pigment deposition in skin, mucosae, and teeth more in patients taking higher doses for long durations.[1] Minocycline is associated with a higher risk of serious adverse effects than other tetracyclines including drug reaction with eosinophilia and systemic symptoms (DRESS), drug-induced lupus, pseudotumor cerebri, and other hypersensitivity reactions.[14,15] Macrolide antibiotics are associated with gastrointestinal disturbances (more with erythromycin), cardiac conduction abnormalities, hepatotoxicity, and cutaneous hypersensitivity reactions (more with azithromycin).[1] Antibiotic resistance remains a concern while prescribing systemic antibiotics and the current recommendations are to limit antibiotic use for the shortest possible duration, typically less than 3 months, which can be done by concomitant use of retinoids (topical or oral).[16]

HORMONAL AGENTS

Hormonal therapy includes combined oral contraceptive (COC) pills, spironolactone, and flutamide. COCs contain both an estrogen and progesterone. There are currently four COCs approved by the FDA namely— (1) ethinylestradiol (EE)/norgestimate, (2) EE/norethindrone acetate/ferrous fumarate, (3) EE/drospirenone, and (4) EE/drospirenone/levomefolate. In addition EE (35 μg) with cyproterone acetate (2 mg), a progestin with antiandrogenic properties is available in Europe, India and other countries. They act via their antiandrogenic effects by decreasing androgen production by ovaries, increasing sex hormone-binding globulin (SHBG) which binds to free testosterone and renders it unavailable for binding to androgen receptors and decreasing 5-alpha-reductase activity.[17] COCs should only be used when the benefit outweighs the risk and are particularly helpful in treating acne in women who also desire contraception or have signs of androgen excess. The adverse effect profile includes cardiovascular risk, venous thromboembolic events, risk of myocardial infarction, and breast and cervical cancer.[18,19] It has been recommended that COC should be avoided for acne in girls within first 2 years of menarche and in <14 years unless it is clinically warranted. Drospirenone-containing COCs are FDA approved for 14 years and norgestimate- and norethindrone-containing COCs for 15 years or over.[1] Women with signs of hyperandrogenism such as hirsutism, premenstrual flares of acne, acne along jawline, and female pattern hair loss should be investigated for underlying cause and will benefit with COCs. For acne, they can be used alone or in combination with other treatment like oral antibiotics or spironolactone. Acne reduction with COC use takes time usually up to three cycles, hence it may be recommended to add another medication for the initial few months.

Spironolactone is a potent antiandrogen acting by blocking the androgen receptors. It also inhibits 5-alpha-reductase and increases SHBG. Its use in acne is not FDA approved, but it has been used in doses of 50–200 mg daily and seen to reduce sebum production and acne severity. Side effects include diuresis, menstrual irregularities, breast enlargement, headache, and dizziness. It is a pregnancy category C drug and hence concomitant use of COCs is recommended to regulate pregnancy and for contraception. Hyperkalemia is rare in young healthy females and hence routine monitoring of potassium is not recommended before start of therapy, but should be done if patient is on angiotensin-converting enzyme inhibitors or receptor blockers and nonsteroidal anti-inflammatory drugs or digoxin, with monitoring required at baseline and after dose incrementation.[20] Such patients should also be counseled by low dietary intake of potassium-rich food like coconut water. Spironolactone may safely be used with drospirenone-containing COCs. Spironolactone comes with a black box warning of carcinogenicity (thyroid, testicular, hepatic, and breast adenomas), though case reports of cancer have been rare and no real association has been found.[21]

Flutamide is a nonsteroidal antiandrogen used for prostate cancer and though not the FDA approved for acne, it has shown efficacy in doses 62.5 mg daily to 250 mg twice daily. Side effects include gastrointestinal distress, breast tenderness, hot flashes, headache, xerosis, decreased libido, and idiosyncratic fatal hepatotoxicity (dose and age related). Flutamide use for acne is discouraged, except when benefit outweighs risk.[22]

Low-dose prednisolone in doses ranging from 5 to 15 mg daily with or without COCs has been seen to be beneficial. They are currently indicated in acne fulminans in doses of 0.5–1 mg/kg/day and to prevent isotretinoin-induced acne fulminans-like reaction. They should never be given as monotherapy and should be slowly tapered as oral antibiotics/retinoids start to act.[1]

ISOTRETINOIN

It is FDA approved for severe recalcitrant acne in >30 years and acts by decreasing sebum production, acne lesions, and scarring. It has also been used in moderate acne which is either treatment resistant or relapsing quickly on oral and topical antibiotic therapy.[23,24] It is indicated in severe nodulocystic acne, in moderate acne which is causing severe scarring, is treatment recalcitrant, or causing psychosocial distress. It is given initially at 0.5 mg/kg/day and increased to 1 mg/kg/day after the first month as tolerated with a cumulative dose of 120–150 mg/kg/day with some studies supporting higher doses for lesser relapse.[25] In moderate acne which is treatment resistant or quick relapsing cases, lower doses of 0.25–0.4 mg/kg/day and low cumulative dose are effective and comparable to higher doses preventing the adverse effects and leading to improved tolerability.[26] Isotretinoin is highly lipophilic and is best absorbed with food. Common adverse effects include mucocutaneous, musculoskeletal, and ophthalmic and rarer effects including inflammatory bowel disease, depression, cardiovascular risk factors, bone mineralization, risk of scarring, and *Staphylococcus aureus* (*S. aureus*) colonization. Several conflicting studies exist on association between inflammatory bowel disease and isotretinoin intake, but current evidence is insufficient to prove an association/causality between the two.[27] Similarly, even though depression, anxiety, mood disturbances, and suicidal ideation have been reported in patients taking isotretinoin, no causality has been established in population-based studies with some indicating improvement in mood, memory, and executive function in those on treatment. Short-term increase in serum cholesterol, triglycerides, and transaminases is known with isotretinoin therapy and lipid profile and liver function tests should be assessed before and during therapy.[1] Delayed wound healing and hypertrophic scarring and keloid formation have been previously shown to occur in those on therapy, even though recent studies show safety with chemical peels, dermabrasion, and lasers. Hence, it has been recommended that superficial procedures can be safely performed, but more aggressive procedures such as dermabrasion should be delayed for 6–12 months when possible, but careful consideration may be given on a case-by-case basis.[1,28-30] Higher rates of colonization by *S. aureus* causing minor skin infections like folliculitis, cheilitis, and abscesses while on therapy have been shown. The teratogenic effects in the form of retinoid embryopathy are well known due to which it is imperative for all men and women on isotretinoin to enroll and adhere to iPLEDGE risk management program which requires to abstain from sex or to use two contraceptive methods to prevent pregnancy while on therapy. Patient independent forms of birth control like long-acting reversible contraceptives should be considered whenever appropriate.[1]

MISCELLANEOUS THERAPIES

Chemical peels like salicylic acid and glycolic acid may help noninflammatory comedonal acne when multiple treatments are given, but the results are not long lasting.[31,32] Among laser and light devices, photodynamic therapy (PDT) has the most evidence. In PDT, a photosensitizer such as aminolevulinic acid which is absorbed by sebocytes is applied to skin for 15 minutes to 3 hours followed by laser or light device used to activate it, producing singlet oxygen species damaging the sebaceous glands. This has shown to be beneficial, but studies are needed to develop guidelines for the same.[33] Intralesional triamcinolone acetonide for large nodulocystic lesions has been seen to cause rapid improvement. Side effects include local atrophy and adrenal suppression because of systemic absorption which can be managed by lesser concentration and dosing.[34] Alternative therapies having poor clinical evidence include tea tree oil, oral barberry extract, and gluconolactone solution. Even though they are a part of over-the-counter cosmetic products, there are no guidelines for their use in the management of acne.[35,36]

ROLE OF DIET IN ACNE

Given the current data, no specific dietary changes are recommended in the management of acne, but high glycemic index diet may be associated with higher risk and low glycemic index diet may be associated with therapeutic response.[37] Some association has also been postulated with consumption of dairy products like skimmed milk and ice cream, which may increase acne particularly in women who consumed ≥two glasses of skimmed milk per day.[38,39] No association with consumption of yoghurt and cheese has been found. Similarly, even though some benefit has been seen with antioxidants (including oral zinc), fish oil, and probiotics, there are no current recommendations for the same.[40,41]

CONCLUSION

Acne is a multifactorial chronic inflammatory disease, hence multiple treatment modalities are required for appropriate and adequate treatment. The goal of therapy is resolution of lesions, without scarring. Hence selection of appropriate treatment is essential.

REFERENCES

1. Zaenglein AL, Pathy AL, Schlosser BJ, Alikhan A, Baldwin HE, Berson DS, et al. Guidelines of care for the management of acne vulgaris. J Am Acad Dermatol. 2016;74(5):945-73.e33.
2. Adityan B, Kumari R, Thappa DM. Scoring systems in acne vulgaris. Indian J Dermatol Venereol Leprol. 2009;75:323-6.
3. Tsai MC, Chen W, Cheng YW, Wang CY, Chen GY, Hsu TJ. Higher body mass index is a significant risk factor for acne formation in schoolchildren. Eur J Dermatol. 2006;16:251-3.
4. Sacchidanand SA, Lahiri K, Godse K, Patwardhan NG, Ganjoo A, Kharkar R, et al. Synchronizing pharmacotherapy in acne with review of clinical care. Indian J Dermatol. 2017;62:341-57.
5. Oon HH, Wong SN, Aw DCW, Cheong WK, Goh CL, Tan HH. Acne management guidelines by the dermatological society of Singapore. J Clin Aesthet Dermatol. 2019;12:34-50.
6. Lucky AW, Maloney JM, Roberts J, Taylor S, Jones T, Ling M, et al. Dapsone gel 5% for the treatment of acne vulgaris: safety and efficacy of long-term (1 year) treatment. J Drugs Dermatol. 2007;6:981-7.
7. Tanghetti E, Harper JC, Oefelein MG. The efficacy and tolerability of dapsone 5% gel in female vs male patients with facial acne vulgaris: gender as a clinically relevant outcome variable. J Drugs Dermatol. 2012;11:1417-21.
8. Gold LS, Cruz A, Eichenfield L, Tan J, Jorizzo J, Kerrouche N, et al. Effective and safe combination therapy for severe acne vulgaris: a randomized, vehicle-controlled, double-blind study of adapalene 0.1%-benzoyl peroxide 2.5% fixed-dose combination gel with doxycycline hyclate 100 mg. Cutis. 2010;85:94-104.
9. Garner SE, Eady A, Bennett C, Newton JN, Thomas K, Popescu CM. Minocycline for acne vulgaris: efficacy and safety. Cochrane Database Syst Rev. 2012;(8):CD002086.
10. Leyden JJ, Bruce S, Lee CS, Ling M, Sheth PB, Stewart DM, et al. A randomized, phase 2, dose-ranging study in the treatment of moderate to severe inflammatory facial acne vulgaris with doxycycline calcium. J Drugs Dermatol. 2013;12:658-63.

11. Antonio JR, Pegas JR, Cestari TF, Do Nascimento LV. Azithromycin pulses in the treatment of inflammatory and pustular acne: efficacy, tolerability and safety. J Dermatolog Treat. 2008;19:210-5.
12. Fenner JA, Wiss K, Levin NA. Oral cephalexin for acne vulgaris: clinical experience with 93 patients. Pediatr Dermatol. 2008;25: 179-83.
13. Margolis DJ, Fanelli M, Kupperman E, Papadopoulos M, Metlay JP, Xie SX, et al. Association of pharyngitis with oral antibiotic use for the treatment of acne: A cross-sectional and prospective cohort study. Arch Dermatol. 2012;148:326-32.
14. Shaughnessy KK, Bouchard SM, Mohr MR, Herre JM, Salkey KS. Minocycline-induced drug reaction with eosinophilia and systemic symptoms (DRESS) syndrome with persistent myocarditis. J Am Acad Dermatol. 2010;62:315-8.
15. Tripathi SV, Gustafson CJ, Huang KE, Feldman SR. Side effects of common acne treatments. Exp Opin Drug Saf. 2013;12:39-51.
16. Tan J, Gold LS, Schlessinger J, Brodell R, Jones T, Cruz A, et al. Short-term combination therapy and long-term relapse prevention in the treatment of severe acne vulgaris. J Drugs Dermatol. 2012;11:174-80.
17. Arowojolu AO, Gallo MF, Lopez LM, Grimes DA. Combined oral contraceptive pills for treatment of acne. Cochrane Database Syst Rev. 2012;(6):CD004425.
18. Katsambas AD, Dessinioti C. Hormonal therapy for acne: why not as first line therapy? facts and controversies. Clin Dermatol. 2010;28:17-23.
19. Gierisch JM, Coeytaux RR, Urrutia RP, Havrilesky LJ, Moorman PG, Lowery WJ, et al. Oral contraceptive use and risk of breast, cervical, colorectal, and endometrial cancers: a systematic review. Cancer Epidemiol Biomarkers Prev. 2013;22:1931-43.
20. Plovanich M, Weng QY, Mostaghimi A. Low usefulness of potassium monitoring among healthy young women taking spironolactone for acne. JAMA Dermatol. 2015;151:941-4.
21. Biggar RJ, Andersen EW, Wohlfahrt J, Melbye M. Spironolactone use and the risk of breast and gynecologic cancers. Cancer Epidemiol. 2013;37:870-5.
22. George R, Clarke S, Thiboutot D. Hormonal therapy for acne. Semin Cutan Med Surg. 2008;27:188-96.
23. Agarwal US, Besarwal RK, Bhola K. Oral isotretinoin in different dose regimens for acne vulgaris: a randomized comparative trial. Indian J Dermatol Venereol Leprol. 2011;77:688-94.

24. Lee JW, Yoo KH, Park KY, Han TY, Li K, Seo SJ, et al. Effectiveness of conventional, low-dose and intermittent oral isotretinoin in the treatment of acne: a randomized, controlled comparative study. Br J Dermatol. 2011;164:1369-75.
25. Blasiak RC, Stamey CR, Burkhart CN, Lugo-Somolinos A, Morrell DS. High-dose isotretinoin treatment and the rate of retrial, relapse, and adverse effects in patients with acne vulgaris. JAMA Dermatol. 2013;149:1392-8.
26. Amichai B, Shemer A, Grunwald MH. Low-dose isotretinoin in the treatment of acne vulgaris. J Am Acad Dermatol. 2006;54:644-6.
27. Etminan M, Bird ST, Delaney JA, Bressler B, Brophy JM. Isotretinoin and risk for inflammatory bowel disease: a nested case-control study and meta-analysis of published and unpublished data. JAMA Dermatol. 2013;149:216-20.
28. Chandrashekar BS, Varsha DV, Vasanth V, Jagadish P, Madura C, Rajashekar ML. Safety of performing invasive acne scar treatment and laser hair removal in patients on oral isotretinoin: a retrospective study of 110 patients. Int J Dermatol. 2014;53:1281-5.
29. Kim HW, Chang SE, Kim JE, Ko JY, Ro YS. The safe delivery of fractional ablative carbon dioxide laser treatment for acne scars in Asian patients receiving oral isotretinoin. Dermatol Surg. 2014;40:1361-6.
30. Yoon JH, Park EJ, Kwon IH, Kim CW, Lee GS, Hann SK, et al. Concomitant use of an infrared fractional laser with low-dose isotretinoin for the treatment of acne and acne scars. J Dermatolog Treat. 2014;25:142-6.
31. Dréno B, Fischer TC, Perosino E, Poli F, Viera MS, Rendon MI, et al. Expert opinion: efficacy of superficial chemical peels in active acne management—what can we learn from the literature today? Evidence-based recommendations. J Eur Acad Dermatol Venereol. 2011;25:695-704.
32. Ilknur T, Demirtasoglu M, Bicak MU, Ozkan S. Glycolic acid peels versus amino fruit acid peels for acne. J Cosmet Laser Ther. 2010;12:242-5.
33. Wang XL, Wang HW, Zhang LL, Guo MX, Huang Z. Topical ALA PDT for the treatment of severe acne vulgaris. Photodiagnosis Photodyn Ther. 2010;7:33-8.
34. Lee SJ, Hyun MY, Park KY, Kim BJ. A tip for performing intralesional triamcinolone acetonide injections in acne patients. J Am Acad Dermatol. 2014;71:e127-8.

35. Enshaieh S, Jooya A, Siadat AH, Iraji F. The efficacy of 5% topical tea tree oil gel in mild to moderate acne vulgaris: a randomized, double-blind placebo-controlled study. Indian J Dermatol Venereol Leprol. 2007;73:22-5.
36. Fouladi RF. Aqueous extract of dried fruit of Berberis vulgaris L. in acne vulgaris, a clinical trial. J Diet Suppl. 2012;9:253-61.
37. Smith RN, Mann NJ, Braue A, Makelainen H, Varigos GA. The effect of a high-protein, low glycemic-load diet versus a conventional, high glycemic-load diet on biochemical parameters associated with acne vulgaris: a randomized, investigator-masked, controlled trial. J Am Acad Dermatol. 2007;57:247-56.
38. Kwon HH, Yoon JY, Hong JS, Jung JY, Park MS, Suh DH. Clinical and histological effect of a low glycaemic load diet in treatment of acne vulgaris in Korean patients: a randomized, controlled trial. Acta Derm Venereol. 2012;92:241-6.
39. Sardana K, Garg VK. An observational study of methionine-bound zinc with antioxidants for mild to moderate acne vulgaris. Dermatol Ther. 2010;23:411-8.
40. Jung GW, Tse JE, Guiha I, Rao J. Prospective, randomized, open-label trial comparing the safety, efficacy, and tolerability of an acne treatment regimen with and without a probiotic supplement and minocycline in subjects with mild to moderate acne. J Cutan Med Surg. 2013;17:114-22.
41. Khayef G, Young J, Burns-Whitmore B, Spalding T. Effects of fish oil supplementation on inflammatory acne. Lipids Health Dis. 2012;11:165.

CHAPTER 2

Pathophysiology of Acne Scars

Niti Khunger

IN A NUTSHELL

- ❖ Acne is a chronic inflammatory disease of the pilosebaceous unit.
- ❖ Etiologic factors include excessive sebum production secondary to androgen stimulation, abnormal follicular keratinization resulting in follicular plugging, proliferation of *Cutibacterium acnes*, and inflammation.
- ❖ Scarring occurs due to a severe inflammatory response to *C. acnes* bacteria.
- ❖ The extent and depth of the inflammation, in combination with the host's immunity and response to the inflammation, determines the amount, type, and depth of scarring.

INTRODUCTION

Scars are areas of fibrous tissue that replace normal tissues after any injury or disease. It is a natural process of wound healing. There are two types of healing processes: regeneration and repair. The liver and the epidermis of the skin heal by regeneration, i.e., multiplication of cells to restore original structure. Organs in humans, including the dermis of the skin, heal by repair, i.e., deposition of fibrous tissue, in order to maintain continuity of tissues. This process of repair leads to scar formation. Scar formation can be atrophic with loss of tissue or hypertrophic with excess tissue. In acne, scarring is more commonly atrophic leading to depressions and uncommonly hypertrophic leading to elevated scars.

WHY DOES ACNE SCAR?

Acne is an inflammatory process that extends into the dermis, hence scarring occurs early. In the early microinflammatory phase, when there are only comedones, there is no scarring. Once the microinflammatory lesion evolves into a deeper inflammatory lesion, the mechanisms of wound healing are activated. If the inflammation is extensive and deep, extending into the deep dermis and continues untreated, scarring results. The different types of scars in acne are a result of the extent, depth, and degree of inflammation that is followed by repair. A study compared the histopathological and immunohistochemical features of acne lesions that were prone to scarring versus those that did not scar.[1] It was found that a predominantly specific immune response was present in patients prone to scarring, which was initially smaller and ineffective, but was increased and activated in resolving lesions. Excessive inflammation in healing tissue was conducive to scarring. In contrast, lesions that did not scar showed a large and active nonspecific inflammatory response (few memory T cells) in early lesions, which subsided quickly when the lesion was resolving. Hence, controlling inflammation early is probably the key to prevent or reduce scarring in acne.

Recent studies also point to the role of *Cutibacterium acnes (formerly Propionibacterium acnes)* in the scarring process. Different phylotypes are associated with varying degrees of inflammation and the acne-associated phylotypes IA-2 p+, IB-1, and IC-induced high levels of inflammatory interferon gamma (IFN-γ) and interleukin 17 (IL-17).[2] Of greater interest is that the hyaluronic acid (HA) lyase, a ubiquitous enzyme present in the *C. acnes* population, has two distinct variants. This enzyme, along with other enzymes, secreted by *C. acnes* are capable of destroying proteins, HA, and other glycosaminoglycans which are essential components of the dermal and epidermal extracellular matrix. The enzyme present in type IA induces greater inflammation and can lead to greater destruction and scarring.[3]

WHEN DOES ACNE SCAR?

Scarring in acne begins early and can affect 90% of patients. To understand the pathophysiology of acne scars, it is first essential to understand the pathogenesis of acne (**Figs. 1A to D**).

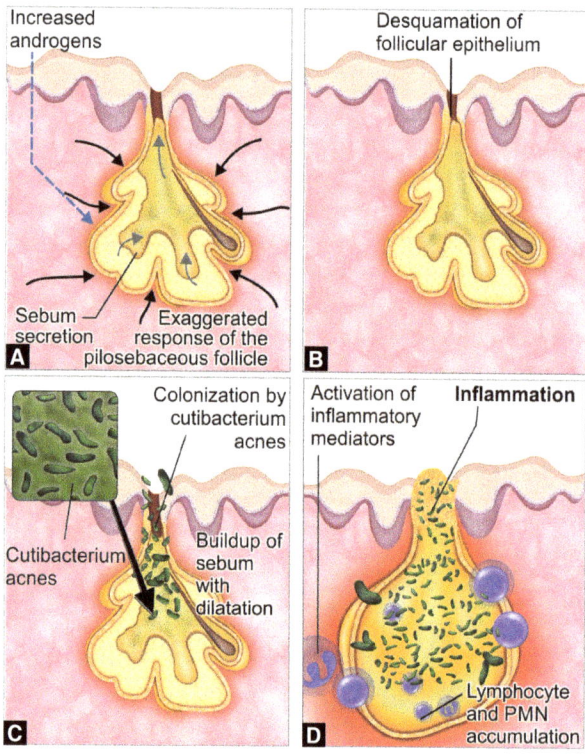

Figs. 1A to D: Pathogenesis of acne. (A) Increased sebaceous secretion; (B) Ductal hyperkeratosis with obstruction of the pilosebaceous follicle; (C) Bacterial colonization by *C. acne*; (D) Secondary inflammation. (PMN: polymorphonucleocyte)

PATHOGENESIS OF ACNE[2-5]

Acne is an extremely complex disease with an interplay of multiple pathogenetic factors that involve abnormalities in epidermal keratinization, androgen secretion, increased sensitivity to circulating androgens, sebaceous function, bacterial growth, inflammation, and immunity. There are four basic mechanisms involved in the pathogenesis of acne vulgaris which are as follows:
1. Hyperkeratinization of the sebaceous duct
2. Colonization with *C. acne*
3. Increased sensitivity to circulating androgens
4. Inflammation.

Acne begins in the pilosebaceous follicle that has a small pilary structure and a large sebaceous gland. The follicular canal is composed of two portions—the superficial upper section, the acroinfundibulum that is structurally similar to the epidermis, and the lower infrainfundibulum. The earliest event is the formation of the microcomedo, which is clinically unapparent, but gives rise to inflammatory acne. Defective desquamation of the infrainfundibular portion of the follicular lining results in the epithelium coming off in sheets instead of shedding as fine particles. These are incapable of exiting through the follicular orifice. This results in a plug of keratinous material which distends the sebaceous follicle, forming a comedone. Comedogenesis is thus the accumulation of corneocytes in the pilosebaceous duct. This could be due to either hyperproliferation of ductal keratinocytes, inadequate separation of the ductal corneocytes (increased stickiness), or a combination of both factors. Androgens also play a role in comedogenesis. The enzyme 5 alpha-reductase (type 1) is present in the infrainfundibulum part of the duct and the sebaceous gland. Antiandrogen therapy results in decreased comedogenesis.[6] The microcomedo may stay as it is, may resolve spontaneously with the hair cycle, enlarge into a closed or open comedone, or it may become an inflamed acne lesion, from which scarring is more likely. The trigger for the inflammation of the microcomedo is the *C. acnes*, which resides in the microcomedo and activates the inflammatory and immune responses. The greater the immunity, the greater is the inflammatory response and the higher the chances of scarring. Inflammation plays a major role in the development of lesions and in acne scarring. In fact, evidence is emerging that subclinical inflammation occurs even before comedo formation and acne is primarily a chronic inflammatory disease. Recent reports have shown that *C. acne* activates the toll-like receptor 2 on monocytes and neutrophils, which leads to the production of multiple proinflammatory cytokines, including IL-12, IL-8, and tumor necrosis factor.[7] The process of inflammation leads to a rupture of the follicular wall, with inflammation extending into the dermis. Acne scar begins when the comedone evolves into an inflammatory lesion and begins the process of wound healing in the dermis.

Phases of Wound Healing

The wound healing process has three primary phases[8] (**Fig. 2**):
1. Phase of inflammation.
2. Phase of proliferation.
3. Phase of maturation or remodeling.

The three phases of wound healing are overlapping. This multistep process is regulated by several cytokines that include epidermal growth factor (EGF), transforming growth factor-beta (TGF-β), basic fibroblast growth factor (bFGF), mitogen-activated protein kinases (MAPs), and matrix metalloproteinases (MMPs). Sato et al.[8] have reported that *C. acnes* not only facilitates sebum production in the sebaceous gland, but also augments the formation of acne scars due to enhanced extracellular matrix degradation by augmenting the expression of proMMPs-1 and -9 in human monocytes and that of proMMP-2 in human dermal fibroblasts.

Pathophysiology of Acne Scars

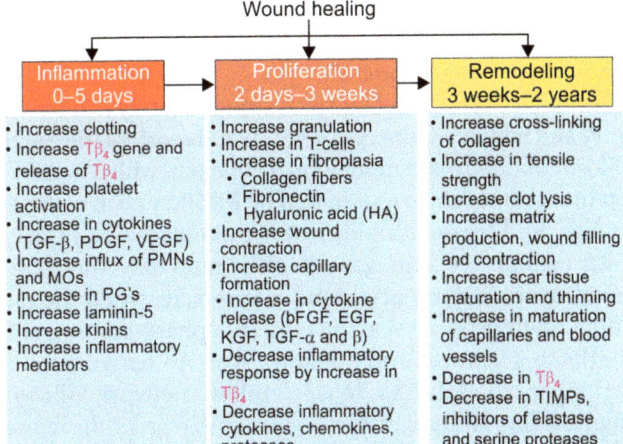

Fig. 2: Phases of wound healing. (bFGF: basic fibroblast growth factor; EGF: epidermal growth factor; KGF: keratinocyte growth factor; MO: monocytes; PDGF: platelet-derived growth factor; PMN: polymorphonucleocyte; TIMP: tissue inhibitor of metalloproteinase; TGF: transforming growth factor-beta; VEGF: vascular endothelial growth factor)

Phase of inflammation lasts from 24 to 48 hours. Platelets, neutrophils, and macrophages release cytokines and control this process.

In the phase of proliferation, there is cellular migration and proliferation, re-epithelialization, angiogenesis, and fibroplasia. Epidermal repair takes place by migration of adjacent keratinocytes into the wound and their proliferation and differentiation in order to restore an intact stratified epidermis. This usually takes 24–48 hours. Dermal repair begins 3–4 days after injury or disease and is characterized by granulation tissue formation which includes new blood vessels (angiogenesis) and accumulation of fibroblasts and ground substance (fibroplasia). The fibroblasts synthesize various proteins such as collagen, proteoglycan, fibronectin, and elastin, which help in forming the extracellular matrix. Collagen synthesis continues at a maximal rate for 2–4 weeks and slows down subsequently.

The phase of remodeling starts approximately 21 days after injury and it involves the degradation and reorientation of the collagen fibers. This remodeling of collagen, which is the last step in tissue repair, is modulated by MMPs, which cause the damage, and tissue inhibitors of metalloproteases (TIMPs), which contain the damage. When the ratio of MMPs/TIMPs is low, atrophic scars occur and, conversely, when the ratio is high, hypertrophic scars occur. This phase continues for months to a year to form a mature scar. An early immature scar appears red due to dense capillary network following inflammation, and as it matures, capillaries regress, the redness reduces, and the actual color of the scar becomes evident. An older or mature scar may be hypopigmented or normal skin colored. In darker skins and patients who have excessive sun exposure, the scars commonly get hyperpigmented and tend to be persistent. Therefore, it is important to protect the early scars from sun exposure to prevent darkening. An inadequate response to tissue repair results in diminished deposition of collagen and formation of an atrophic scar while an exuberant response results in a hypertrophic scar. In acne, atrophic scars are more common as compared to hypertrophic scars.

Insulin-like growth factor 1 (IGF-1) and survivin have also been implicated in the pathogenesis of acne and acne scarring.[9,10] IGF-1 has been shown to increase acne and sebum secretion by increasing androgen synthesis, sebocyte proliferation and lipogenesis, transduction of androgen receptor signaling, and stimulating 5α-reductase. This leads to increased acne lesions. IGF-1 is also implicated in the pathogenesis and progression of postacne scars by stimulating fibroblast proliferation and increasing messenger RNA (ribonucleic acid) levels of procollagen-I.[9] Survivin, a member of the inhibitor of apoptosis (IAP) family, has also been implicated in the pathogenesis of acne by causing abnormal apoptosis and prolonged sebocyte survival, thus altering infundibular keratinocyte differentiation and sebum production.

El-Tahlawi et al. reported increased levels of IGF-1 and survivin in patients with acne and acne scars as compared to controls.[9]

PATHOPHYSIOLOGY OF ACNE SCARS[2-6,11]

The depth and degree of inflammation determines the amount, type, and depth of scarring in acne. Acne lesions are unusual because the inflammation is initiated beneath the epidermis in the infrainfundibular region of the pilosebaceous structure. The enzymatic activity and inflammatory mediators destroy the dermal structures, hence scarring involves the deeper structures first. Contraction leads to an atrophic scar.

Acne scars are classified into various types, depending on the color, depth, contour, and surface texture[12] (**Fig. 3**). In macular scars, the inflammation involves only the superficial

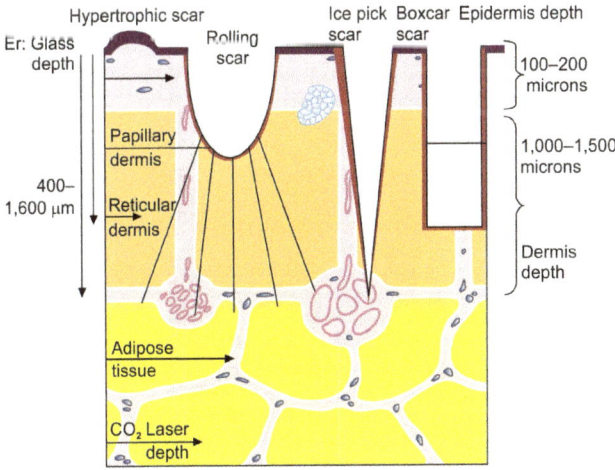

Fig. 3: Depth of various types of acne scars.

dermis and epidermis and gives rise to a persistent change in color. Early scars appear erythematous, whereas older scars appear hyperpigmented due to postinflammatory hyperpigmentation. The inflammatory mediators stimulate melanogenesis and these scars can be persistent, particularly in darker skin individuals. In ice pick scars, severe inflammation of the dermis can lead to total necrosis of the follicle with sloughing of the follicle, producing a focal ice pick scar. Ice pick scars are narrow, punctiform, and deep. They are so named because these scars appear as if the skin has been pierced by an ice pick (**Fig. 4**). They are sharply marginated epithelial tracts that extend vertically into the deep dermis or subcutaneous tissue. Histopathological picture is characterized by reticulate tunnels lined by hyperplastic epithelium. Often there are remnants of inflammation, even in the old scars of this type. In rolling scars, inflammation extends beyond the hair follicle, into the surrounding subcuticular area, the sweat glands and along the vascular channels, it causes wide and deep scarring,

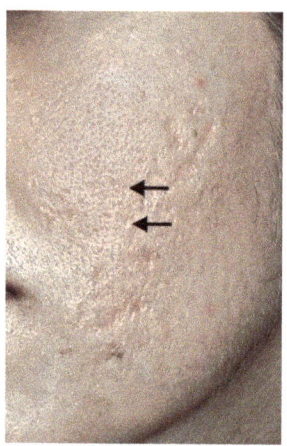

Fig. 4: Ice pick scars.

leading to rolling scars. Rolling scars are due to tethering of the epidermis and dermis to the underlying subcutaneous tissue. The surface often has a normal texture. They are wider than deeper (**Fig. 5**).

Boxcar scars are round, oval, or irregular depressions with sharp vertical edges. They are wider at the surface than ice pick scars and do not taper to a point. They appear punched out and may be shallow or deep (**Fig. 6**). Linear scars occur when there is extensive dermal inflammation. They appear as linear atrophic, hypopigmented lines, with relatively normal skin in between. They may be narrow linear scars, where they appear as thin lines or broad linear scars, appearing as linear dermal depressions (**Fig. 7**). Bridging scars occur when there is recurrent inflammation in a particular area, resulting in multichanneled tracts. Foul-smelling sebum and epithelial debris often collects in the tracts (**Fig. 8**). Perifollicular or papular scars are hypopigmented or skin-colored elevated scars that result from destruction of collagen and elastin fibers in the dermal tissues around the hair follicles. They are most common

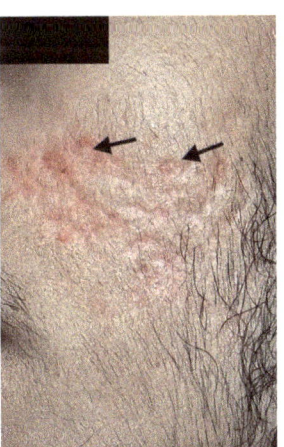

Fig. 5: Rolling scars.

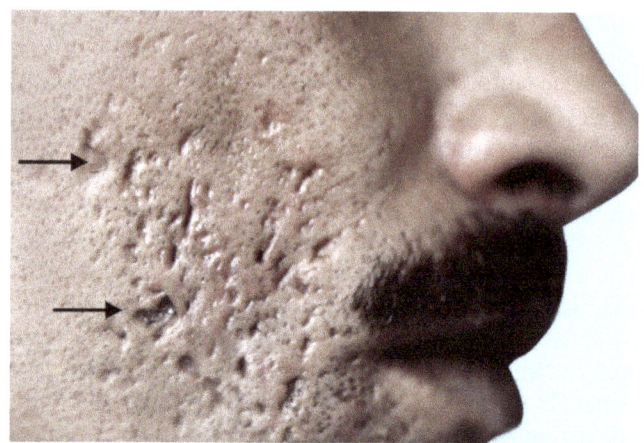

Fig. 6: Boxcar scars.

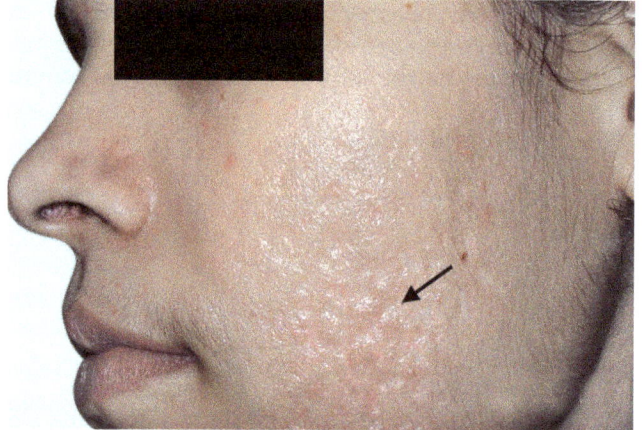

Fig. 7: Linear scars.

on the trunk, chin, and nose (**Figs. 9A and B**). Lipoatrophic scars forms when there is extensive prolonged inflammation as in cystic acne, the inflammatory mediators destroy the facial fat.

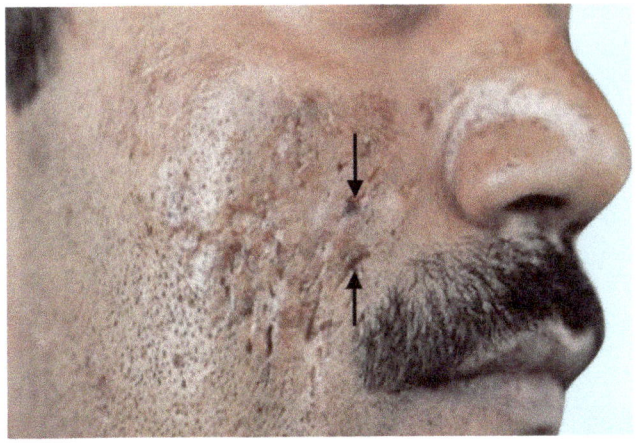

Fig. 8: Bridging scars.

The cystic lesions are also space occupying and their eventual involution leaves an empty space that cannot be filled by the atrophied subcutaneous tissues. Instead the tissues are drawn in from surface layers, leading to severe depression, and this effect is worsened by the contracture of the tissues around these cysts (**Fig. 10**). This cystic involution and maturation followed by fibrosis probably explains the incongruous worsening of a patient's appearance that is occasionally seen after treatment of cystic acne, especially by isotretinoin. This type of scarring becomes worse as the patient ages.[5] Hypertrophic scars occur because of excess collagen deposition and decreased collagenase activity. They appear pink or skin colored, firm and raised, commonly seen on the mandibular area, shoulders, chest, and back (**Fig. 11**). There are thick hyalinized collagen bundles similar to that of other dermal scars. Keloids appear as reddish-purple papules and nodules that extend beyond the borders of the original acne lesion and may be itchy or painful. Histologically, they are characterized by thick bundles of hyalinized acellular collagen arranged in whorls.

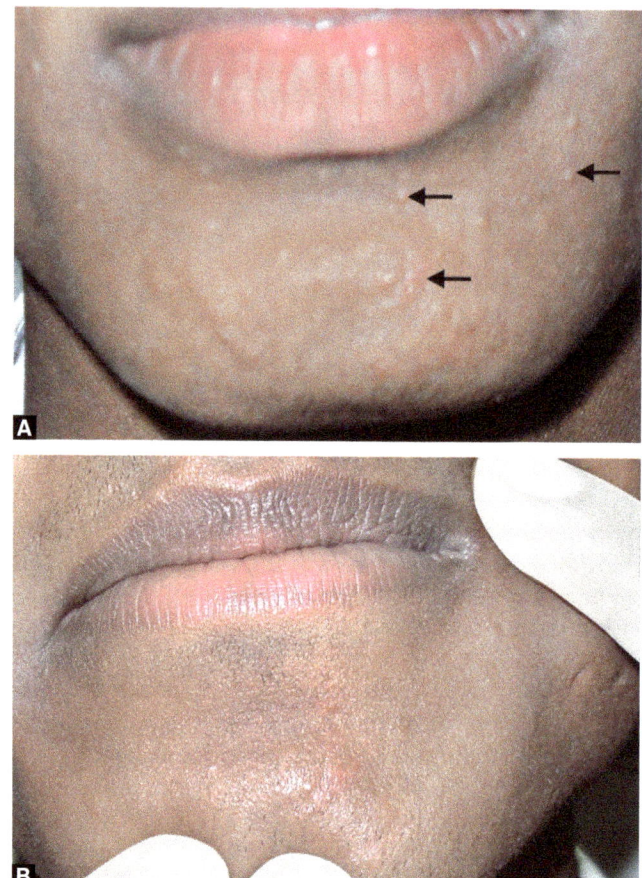

Figs. 9A and B: (A) Papular scars; (B) Disappear on stretching the skin.

CONCLUSION

Scarring in acne occurs due to inflammation. The degree, depth and extent of inflammation determine the type of scars. Controlling inflammation early and adequately is the key to preventing postacne scars.

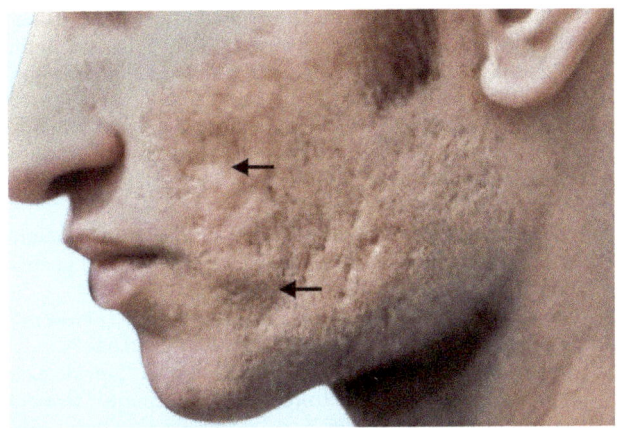

Fig. 10: Lipoatrophic scars.

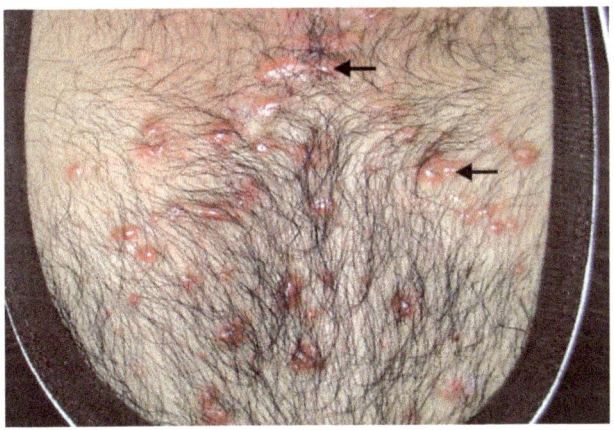

Fig. 11: Hypertrophic scars on the chest.

REFERENCES

1. Holland DB, Jeremy AH, Roberts SG, Seukeran DC, Layton AM, Cunliffe WJ. Inflammation in acne scarring: a comparison of the responses in lesions from patients prone and not prone to scar. Br J Dermatol. 2004;150(1):72-81.

2. Yu Y, Champer J, Agak GW, Kao S, Modlin RL, Kim J. Different propionibacterium acnes phylotypes induce distinct immune responses and express unique surface and secreted proteomes. J Invest Dermatol. 2016;136(11):2221-8.
3. Dréno B, Pécastaings S, Corvec S, Veraldi S, Khammari A, Roques C. Cutibacterium acnes (Propionibacterium acnes) and acne vulgaris: a brief look at the latest updates. J Eur Acad Dermatol Venereol. 2018;32(Suppl 2):5-14.
4. Fabbrocini G, Annunziata MC, D'Arco V, De Vita V, Lodi G, Mauriello MC, et al. Acne scars: pathogenesis, classification and treatment. Dermatol Res Pract. 2010;2010:893080.
5. Goodman GJ. Post-acne scarring: A short review of its pathophysiology. Australas J Dermatol. 2001;42(2):84-90.
6. Cunliffe WJ, Holland DB, Clark SM, Stables GI. Comedogenesis: some new aetiological, clinical and therapeutic strategies. Dermatology. 2003;206:11-6.
7. Kim J, Ochoa MT, Krutzik SR, Takeuchi O, Uematsu S, Legaspi AJ, et al. Activation of toll-like receptor 2 in acne triggers inflammatory cytokine responses. J Immunol. 2002;169(3):1535-41.
8. Sato T, Kurihara H, Akimoto N, Noguchi N, Sasatsu M, Ito A. Augmentation of gene expression and production of promatrix metalloproteinase 2 by Propionibacterium acnes-derived factors in hamster sebocytes and dermal fibroblasts: a possible mechanism for acne scarring. Biol Pharm Bull. 2011;34(2):295-9.
9. El-Tahlawi S, Ezzat Mohammad N, Mohamed El-Amir A, Sayed Mohamed H. Survivin and insulin-like growth factor-I: potential role in the pathogenesis of acne and post-acne scar. Scars Burn Heal. 2019;5:2059513118818031.
10. Assaf HA, Abdel-Maged WM, Elsadek BE, Hassan MH, Adly MA, Ali SA. Survivin as a novel biomarker in the pathogenesis of acne vulgaris and its correlation to insulin-like growth factor-I. Dis Markers. 2016;2016:7040312.
11. Goodman GJ. Postacne scarring: A review of its pathophysiology and treatment. Dermatol Surg. 2000;26(9):857-71.
12. Jacob CI, Dover JS, Kaminer MS. Acne scarring: A classification system and review of treatment options. J Am Acad Dermatol. 2001;45(1):109-17.

CHAPTER 3

Types of Acne Scars and Grading Systems

Shikha Bansal, Niti Khunger

IN A NUTSHELL

- ❖ Acne scars are polymorphic and have different shapes, sizes, depth and surface texture.
- ❖ Multiple types usually coexist in the same patient.
- ❖ There are several scales to grade acne scars in use, but none are ideal.
- ❖ It is also important to assess the psychosocial impact of acne scars when judging severity.

INTRODUCTION

Acne is one of the most common chronic inflammatory disorder occuring in adolescence and young adults that is increasingly persisting in older adults. It affects the pilosebaceous apparatus, characterized by variable morphology and severity with a tendency to scarring. Acne scars are the product of end-stage inflammatory lesions. Mild and adequately treated acne can resolve without any residual scars, while chronic, severe, or inappropriately treated acne results in scarring. Postacne scarring is one of the most common causes of facial scarring that can lead to great psychosocial distress.

Acne scars can be broadly divided into three categories (**Table 1**):
1. Macular
2. Atrophic
3. Hypertrophic.

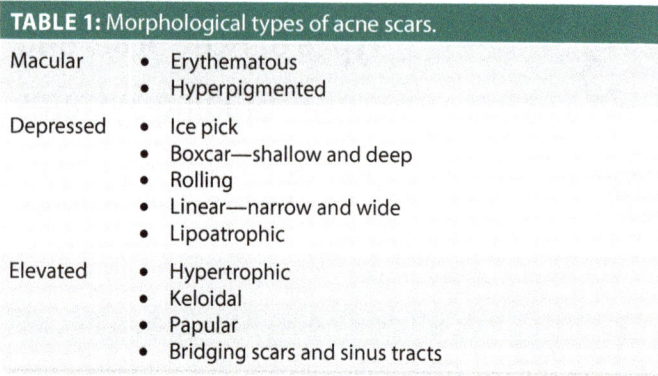

TABLE 1: Morphological types of acne scars.	
Macular	• Erythematous • Hyperpigmented
Depressed	• Ice pick • Boxcar—shallow and deep • Rolling • Linear—narrow and wide • Lipoatrophic
Elevated	• Hypertrophic • Keloidal • Papular • Bridging scars and sinus tracts

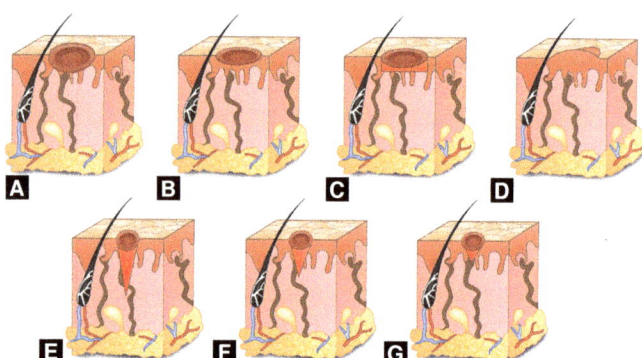

Figs. 1A to G: Types of acne scars: (A) Deep rolling scar; (B) Shallow rolling scar; (C) Boxcar scar; (D) Raised papules; (E) Deep ice pick scar; (F) Ice pick scar; (G) Enlarged pore.

Atrophic scars are due to loss of collagen, whereas increase in collagen tissue causes hypertrophic scars. The atrophic scars are the most common followed by the macular, the least common being hypertrophic scars. Each type of scar has its own unique characteristics and features. Because of these differences, it is important to know the type of scar to choose the optimal treatment (**Figs. 1A to G**). Multiple types usually coexist in the same patient and thus there is no single ideal procedure for all types of acne scars.

The incidence of various types of scars has not been well studied. In one of the early studies, it was found that ice pick scars were the most common, representing 60–70% of total scars, the boxcar scars represented 20–30%, and rolling scars 15–25% among the different types of acne scars.[1]

MORPHOLOGICAL TYPES OF ACNE SCARS

There have been various classifications of acne scars, with often confusing and descriptive nomenclature.[1-3]

Macular Scars

Though these lesions are macules and not strictly scars, they are so-called because they tend to persist for months together. They can be further subdivided into erythematous and hyperpigmented macules. Hypopigmented macules following acne are rare. The hypopigmented lesions seen are true atrophic acne scars rather than macules (**Fig. 2**).

Erythematous

Erythematous macules are seen following resolution of inflammatory acne lesions. They are more common in lighter skins and tend to persist in patients that have sensitive skins, photosensitivity, or rosacea-like skin. They give the impression of active acne lesions and are prone to permanent scarring (**Fig. 3**).

Hyperpigmented

Hyperpigmented macules occur due to postinflammatory hyperpigmentation. They can be very persistent and are more common in darker skinned patients and in those patients who constantly pick at their lesions (acne excoriée) (**Fig. 4**).

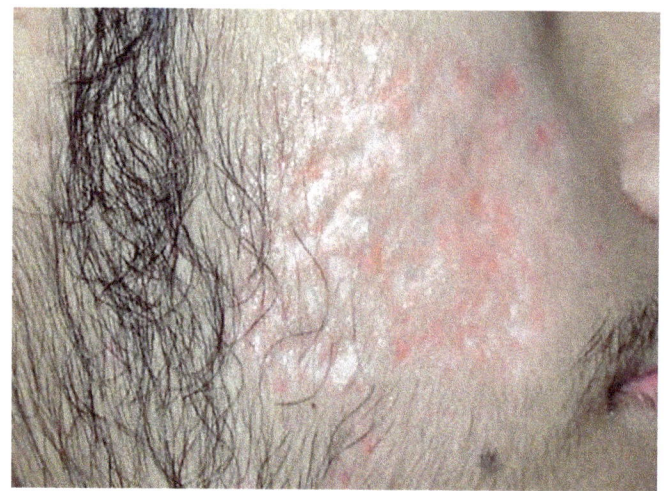

Fig. 2: Depigmented macules.

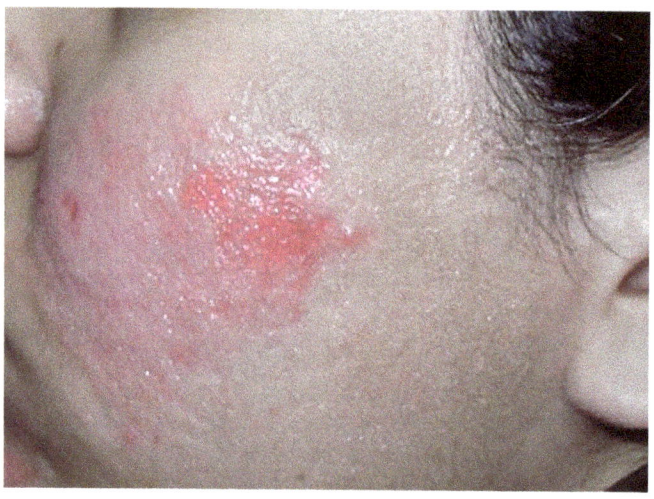

Fig. 3: Persistent erythematous macules.

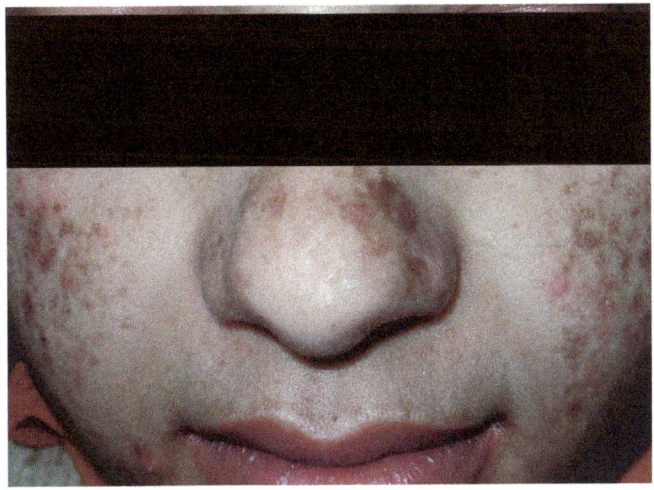

Fig. 4: Persistent hyperpigmented macules.

Depressed Scars

Depressed atrophic scars are the most common type of scars seen following acne. They can be further subdivided according to the shape, depth, and size.

Ice Pick Scars

These are one of the most common scars seen in acne and also the most difficult to treat. Ice pick scars are deep, narrow, sharply defined epithelial tracts that extend vertically to the deep dermis or subcutaneous tissue. The surface opening is wider than the deeper portion as it tapers into a "V" shape. They appear as if the skin has been pricked with an ice pick, which is an instrument with a tapering sharp point (**Figs. 5A and B**). They tend to worsen with age as the skin becomes loose and appear as open pores giving a mature look to the patient's skin.

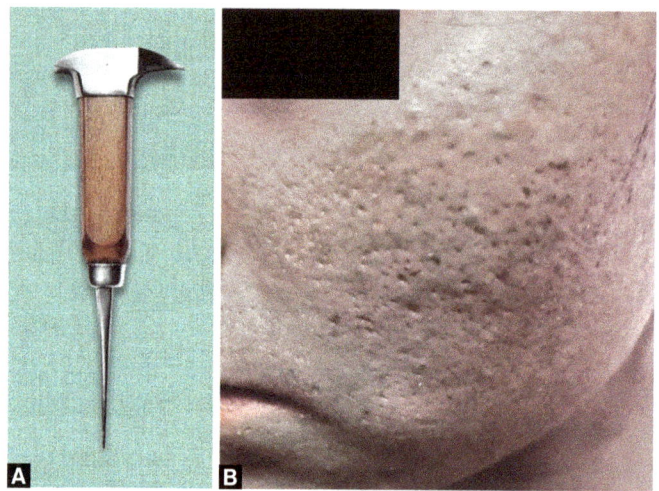

Figs. 5A and B: (A) Ice pick; (B) Typical ice pick scars.

These scars are more commonly seen on the cheeks, glabellar region, and nose.

Boxcar Scars

Boxcar scars are round, oval, or irregular sharply defined scars with vertical edges, similar to varicella scars. They are called boxcar scars because on cross-section, they appear sharply punched out like a boxcar which is a wagon of a goods train (**Figs. 6A and B**). They are wider at the surface than ice pick scars, appear punched out and do not taper to a point at the base. They may be shallow (0.1–0.5 mm) or deep (>0.5 mm) and are most often 1.5–4.0 mm in diameter. They are most common on the temples and cheeks.

Rolling Scars

Rolling scars are wide distensible undulating scars, with relatively normal-appearing overlying skin (**Fig. 7**). They virtually disappear on stretching the skin. They occur due to

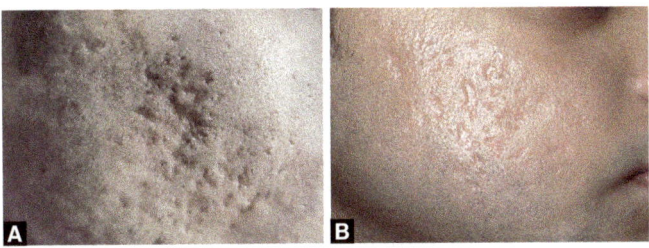

Figs. 6A and B: Boxcar scars: (A) Shallow; (B) Deep.

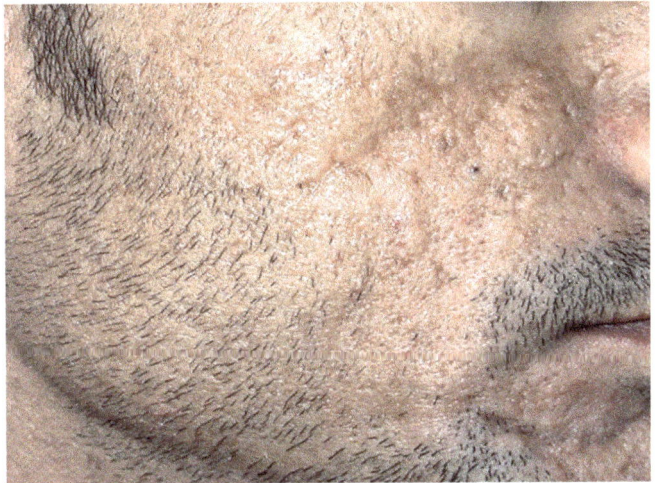

Fig. 7: Rolling scars.

dermal tethering of the epidermis and dermis to the underlying subcutis leading to superficial shadowing and a rolling or undulating appearance. They appear most common on the lower cheeks and mandibular area and worsen with age.

Linear Scars

These scars have not been commonly described in reported literature, though they are often observed. They appear as linear atrophic lines that are commonly hypopigmented with relatively normal skin in between. They may be narrow linear scars, where they appear as thin lines connecting each other or broad linear scars appearing as wider linear dermal depressions (**Fig. 8**).

Lipoatrophic Scars

These scars occur following resolution of cystic acne, which destroys the fat. They are more common in males with a thin asthenic face, giving the face a gaunt appearance (**Fig. 9**).

Elevated Scars

Elevated scars are less common following acne. These may be of different types as described here.

Hypertrophic Scars

They are elevated, dome-shaped fibrotic scars, skin-colored or hyperpigmented, frequently seen in the mandibular area of the

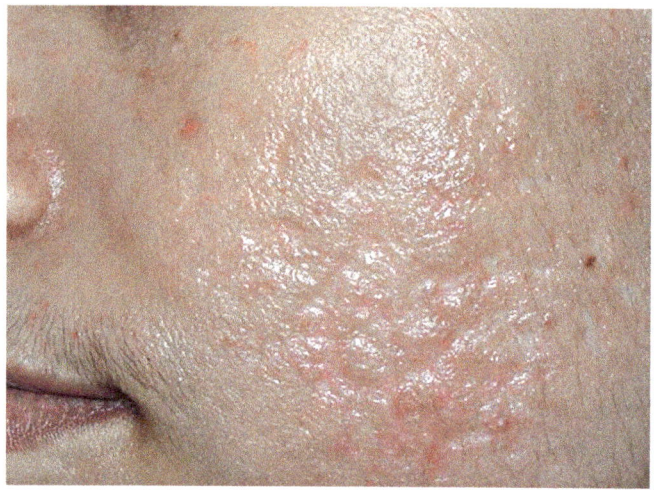

Fig. 8: Linear scars—wide and narrow.

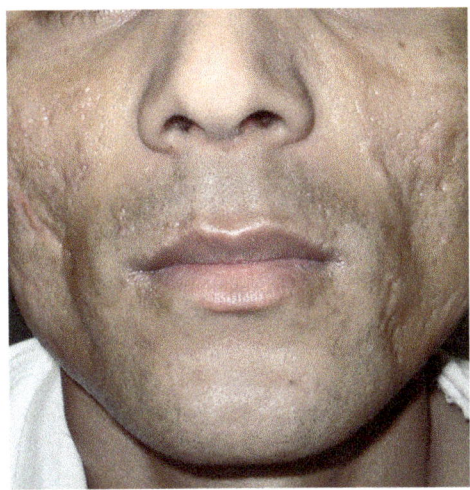

Fig. 9: Lipoatrophic scars—more common in males and in lower cheeks.

face and back (**Fig. 10**). They are more common in males and in darker skin types. They remain localized and do not extend beyond the surface of the acne lesions.

Keloidal Scars

These are keloids developing in acne lesions, which extend beyond the original acne lesions. They have irregular borders and are often symptomatic causing itching or pain. They are seen more often in males on the back, shoulders, and chest (**Fig. 11**).

Papular Scars

These scars appear as raised, hypopigmented, and papular lesions, most commonly seen on the back, chin, and nose (**Figs. 12A and B**). They occur due to destruction of the perifollicular dermis and are in fact outpouchings of the epidermis due to loss of support of the underlying dermis.

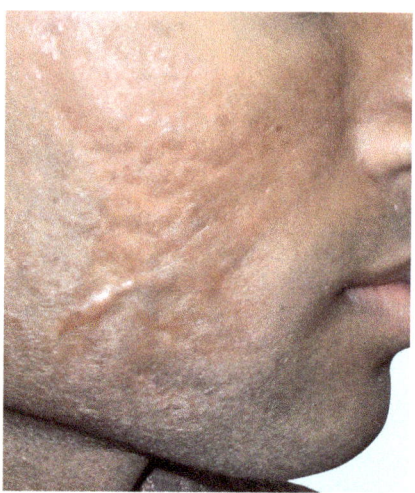

Fig. 10: Hypertrophic scars.

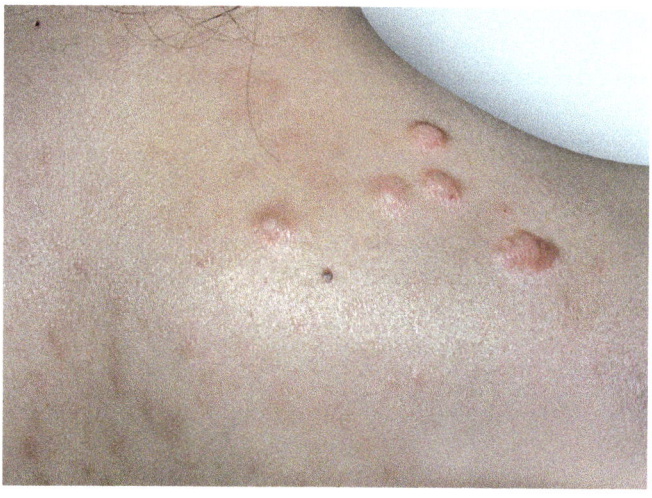

Fig. 11: Keloidal scars on the back and shoulder in a young female.

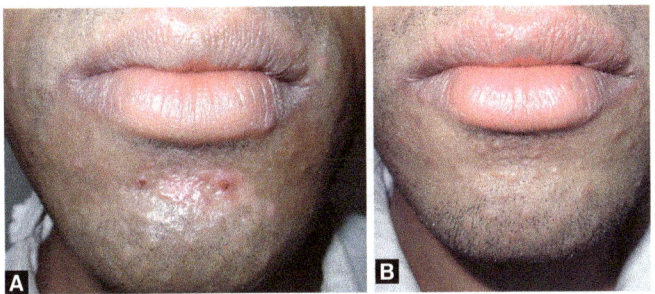

Figs. 12A and B: Evolving and established papular scars on the chin.

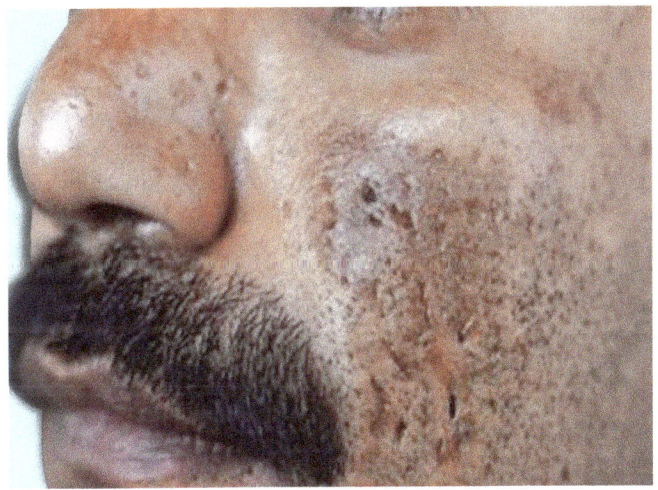

Fig. 13: Bridging scars on the cheeks.

Bridging Scars and Sinus Tracts

These are channels joined together by epithelial tracts overlying normal or atrophic skin (**Fig. 13**). They often contain foul-smelling products of sebum and cause great distress.

GRADING OF ACNE SCARS

Grading of acne scars helps in assessing the severity of scars and response to treatment in an objective manner. This is also necessary for communication to others for teaching and research. There are several grading scales in use, but none are ideal. Grading of acne scars can be based on different evaluation methods. These can be: (1) scar counting, (2) physician evaluation, (3) patient self-evaluation, and (4) imaging-based evaluation.

Scar Counting

The Leeds system was the earliest reported by Layton.[3]

Leeds Acne Scar System

According to this system, the severity of acne scarring is evaluated by a simple lesion count of the various types of acne scars. Atrophic scars are defined morphologically as ice pick, macular atrophic, or follicular macular atrophic—these translated into scores ranging from 1 to 6 representing number of scars.

No. of scar	Score
1–5	Score 1
6–10	Score 2
11–25	Score 3
26–50	Score 4
51–100	Score 5
>100	Score 6

Ice pick scars are described as those with an irregular border, jagged edges, and sharp margins with steep sides leading to a fibrotic base. Macular atrophic scars are described as soft and distensible. Follicular macular atrophic scars are described as small white perifollicular papules or macules.

Keloidal and hypertrophic scars are separately quantified owing to their greater level of disfigurement.

No. of scar	Score
1–3	Score 2
4–7	Score 4
>7	Score 6

Keloidal scars are described as those that are indurated and extending beyond the boundaries of the initiating inflammatory acne lesion, while hypertrophic scars are defined as less raised and limited to the area of the primary acne lesion. A total scar score is then obtained by adding the scores from both atrophic and hypertrophic categories. Total scores can then be calculated separately for the face, chest, and back to provide a comprehensive system for scar evaluation. A potential limitation of this system is the time required for calculation of the relevant scar scores. In addition, it may not be able to track improvement as scars may remain the same with improvement in color and depth.

Physician Evaluation

Goodman and Baron proposed two scales—a qualitative scale and a quantitative scale.

Global Acne Qualitative Scale[4] (Goodman and Baron)

This scale is based on scar morphology and ease of masking by makeup or normal hair patterns. According to this scale, acne scarring is classified into four grades:

- *Grade 1*: Macular scarring.
- *Grade 2*: Mild atrophy or hypertrophic scarring that may not be evident at 50 cm or greater and may be adequately masked by makeup or hair patterns.
- *Grade 3*: Moderate atrophic or hypertrophic scarring obvious at social distances and not easily masked.
- *Grade 4*: Severe atrophic or hypertrophic scarring.

The extent of involvement can also be indicated by the number of cosmetic units involved with each severity grade of scarring. It is a simple scale, especially useful with mild acne, but not in severe cases as it is not comprehensive.

Quantitative Scale[5] (Goodman and Baron)

This scale assigns fewer points to macular and mild atrophic scars than to moderate and severe atrophic scars according to this scale.
- Macular or mildly atrophic—1 point
- Moderately atrophic—2 points
- Punched out or linear-troughed severe scars—3 points
- Hyperplastic papular scars—4 points.

The multiplication factor for these lesion types is based on the numerical range whereby, for 1-10 scars, the multiplier is 1; for 11-20, it is 2; for more than 20, it is 3.

For hypertrophic and keloidal scars, scores are allocated dependent on the size of these lesions.
- An area of less than 5 cm^2—6 points
- 5-120 cm^2—12 points
- More than 20 cm^2—18 points.

The upper limit of this system has a score of 84. This system is time-intensive and acknowledged by the authors to be cumbersome.

ECCA Scale[6]

The ECCA (Echelle d'Evaluation Clinique des Cicatrices d'Acne) scale for facial acne scarring is also a quantitative scale based on the sum of individual types of scars and their numerical extent. Scar types considered to be more visibly disfiguring are weighted more heavily. Specific scar types and their associated weighting factors are the as follows:
- Atrophic scars with diameter less than 2 mm—15
- U-shaped atrophic scars with a diameter of 2-4 mm—20

- M-shaped atrophic scars with diameter greater than 4 mm—25
- Superficial elastolysis—30
- Hypertrophic scars with a less than 2-year duration—40
- Hypertrophic scars of greater than 2-year duration—50.

A semiquantitative assessment of the number of each of these scar types is then determined with a four-point scale, in which 0 indicates no scars, 1 indicates <5 scars, 2 indicates between 5 and 20 scars, and 3 indicates >20 scars.

Using this scale, the qualitative aspects of scars define the type of scar, which is then associated with a quantitative score (0-4) determined semiquantitatively and multiplied by a weighting factor (15-50) of clinical severity, leading to possible totals of 0-540. It was found to have good interinvestigator reliability, although it did not focus on ice pick, rolling, or boxcar specifically but rather variations of atrophic and hypertrophic scar. The potential advantages of this system include independent accounting of specific scar types. Potential shortcomings include restriction to facial involvement, time required, and undetermined clinical relevance of score.

Another scale has been published called the Shamban scale[7] **(Table 2)**. This scale combines the severity of acne with the severity of scarring and pigmentation.

However, there is still a lack of a true consensus scale which hinders standardization of diagnosis and treatment of acne scarring.

TABLE 2: Shamban acne scale.

Acne	Scarring	Pigmentation
0. None	0. None	0. None
1. Mild	1. Mild	1. Mild
2. Moderate	2. Moderate	2. Moderate
3. Severe	3. Severe	3. Severe

Patient Self-evaluation

Acne Scars and the Quality of Life

There is often a discrepancy between the severity of acne scars and their psychosocial impact affecting the quality of life. This is because of variation between patient assessment of scars and a dermatologist's assessment. Specific quality of life scores should also be included when judging severity of acne scars. Two such scores are in use for assessment in acne scars. One is the self-assessment of clinical acne-related scars (SCARS) and the other is facial acne scar quality of life (FASQoL).[8] These are questionnaire based where patients quantify the severity of their atrophic acne scars and assess the impact of the scars on their quality of life. Though these are useful from the patients' point of view, they are not very reliable for objective assessment of acne scars.

Image-based Evaluation

There is a need for developing objective methods such as specialized software that can accurately judge the severity of acne scars. Silicon molds have been used but are cumbersome. Ultrasound imaging has also been used but needs validation.

CONCLUSION

Currently, there is a lack of a comprehensive ideal acne scar scoring system. Common problems associated with developing a grading scale for postacne scars include the wide variety of scars present, how to quantify the lesions, the three-dimensional nature of the scar, which may not be appreciable in a photograph, how to document the change in scars over time, and the wide range of treatment results depending on scar type.

REFERENCES

1. Jacob CI, Dover JS, Kaminer MS. Acne scarring: A classification system and review of treatment options. J Am Acad Dermatol. 2001;45(1):109-17.
2. Goodman GJ. Postacne scarring: A review of its pathophysiology and treatment. Dermatol Surg. 2000;26(9):857-71.
3. Layton AM, Henderson CA, Cunliffe WJ. A clinical evaluation of acne scarring and its incidence. Clin Exper Dermatol. 1994;19(4):303-8.
4. Goodman GJ, Baron JA. Postacne scarring: a qualitative global scarring grading system. Dermatol Surg. 2006;32(12):1458-66.
5. Goodman GJ, Baron JA. Postacne scarring—a quantitative global scarring grading system. J Cosmet Dermatol. 2006;5(1):48-52.
6. Dreno B, Khammari A, Orain N, Noray C, Mérial-Kieny C, Méry S, et al. ECCA grading scale: an original validated acne scar grading scale for clinical practice in dermatology. Dermatology. 2007;214(1):46-51.
7. Shamban AT, Narurkar VA. Multimedial treatment of acne, acne scars and pigmentation. Dermatol Clin. 2009;27(4):459-71.
8. Layton A, Dréno B, Finlay AY, Thiboutot D, Kang S, Lozada VT, et al. New patient-oriented tools for assessing atrophic acne scarring. Dermatol Ther (Heidelb). 2016;6(2):219-33.

CHAPTER 4

Prevention of Acne Scars

Niti Khunger

IN A NUTSHELL

- ❖ Acne scar prevention is important.
- ❖ Treat acne early as soon as it develops.
- ❖ Choose the correct treatment according to the severity of acne.
- ❖ Decreasing inflammation is most important.
- ❖ Severe cases of acne, particularly cystic acne, should be promptly and adequately managed and never be left untreated.
- ❖ Isotretinoin initially may aggravate acne. Severe flares can cause severe scars.
- ❖ Use hormonal therapy judiciously when required.
- ❖ Repeated patient counseling to avoid picking, scrubbing, and squeezing is important.
- ❖ Discuss way to improve compliance and reduce side effects of therapy.

INTRODUCTION

Acne is temporary, but unfortunately acne scarring is permanent. Scarring in acne occurs early, depending on severity of acne and delay in treatment. Treating acne *early*, *appropriately*, and *adequately* is important to minimize scarring.

PRINCIPLES OF PREVENTION OF ACNE SCARS[1] (BOX 1)

Treat Acne as Soon as it Develops

The most effective way to avoid postacne scarring is by preventing acne from developing into a more severe form. Treatment should be started right away as soon as acne begins in the comedonal or papular stage. Parents of adolescents should be counseled to start treatment in the early stages and not wait till it becomes severe. Most parents delay treatment in the belief that acne is a part of the growing phase and will go away spontaneously when the child grows up. Many teenagers start over-the-counter treatments or medications advised by their friends, chemists, or over the net. Often they apply topical steroids in order to get instant relief from erythema, which further aggravates acne. Steroid-induced acne is a very common and unfortunate dermatoses, particularly in countries where steroids are available without prescription (**Fig. 1**). A large prospective multicenter study reported that 433 of 2,926 patients with facial dermatoses were found to be inappropriately using topical steroids.[2] Unfortunately, out of these, 104 (24%) were using it for acne. Acne was also the most common side effect seen. Thus, this is a vicious cycle and can lead to severe debilitating fulminant acne followed by scarring (**Fig. 2**).

Avoid Inflammation and Treat Early

Inflamed acne lesions are much more likely to cause scars than noninflamed lesions. Hence, special attention should be paid

> **Box 1:** Principles of prevention of acne scars.
> - Treat acne as soon as it develops
> - Avoid inflammation
> - Treat inflammatory lesions early
> - Treat severe acne aggressively
> - Treat patients prone to hyperpigmentation carefully
> - Advise patient not to squeeze or pick acne lesions

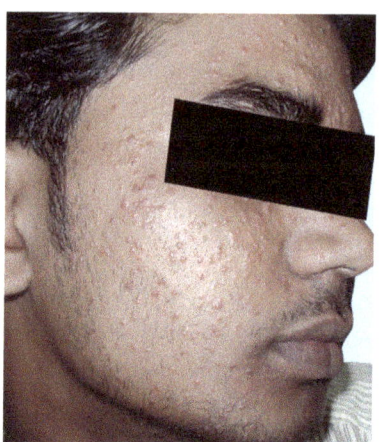

Fig. 1: Steroid-induced acne.

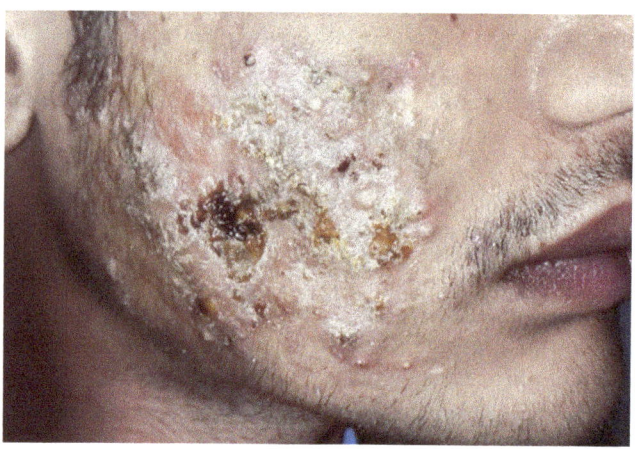

Fig. 2: Fulminant acne following application of superpotent steroid, clobetasol.

to inflamed lesions. Anything that irritates the skin such as aggressive scrubbing, facials, and irritant skin care products, which can aggravate inflammation, should be avoided.

Severe Acne should be Treated Aggressively

Patient with severe forms of acne such as nodules and cysts invariably leave scars. Deep nodules or cysts often leave deep and permanent atrophic scars as the infection destroys skin tissue. Quick and effective treatment can help lessen the chance of developing deep scars.

Patients Who are Prone to Hyperpigmentation and Scarring should be Treated Carefully

Patients who are prone to postinflammatory hyperpigmentation, hypertrophic and keloidal scarring should be treated cautiously particularly with procedures. Good history taking and examination of sites of injury will give a clue to patients with poor scarring potential. Darker skin types are particularly prone to these complications and aggressive procedures without proper priming should be avoided.

Patient Counseling is Important

Patients, particularly teenagers, should be repeatedly told not to squeeze, pop, or pick at pimples. This is a very common habit. They often stand in front of the mirror and squeeze the pimple to hasten resolution, particularly before important social events. Squeezing can force inflammation deeper into the follicle and in the dermis, spread infection, and lead to scar formation. Acne excoriée is an example of extreme picking that can lead to persistent hyperpigmented scars, particularly in dark-skinned patients. Staying free of scarring often comes down to the habits of the patient. Emphasis should be laid on avoiding pinching or squeezing, and regular treatment and hygiene. They can be counseled by saying a whitehead or blackhead can only bother you for a day or two, but acne scarring can plague you for a lifetime (**Figs. 3A and B**).

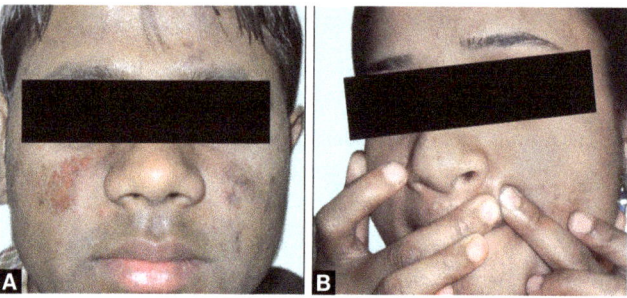

Figs. 3A and B: (A) Typical teenager with acne excoriée; (B) Squeezing habit of teenager.

APPROPRIATE TREATMENT OF ACNE[3,4]

Medical Therapy

In mild comedonal acne (Grade 1), start with comedolytics such as topical retinoids or benzoyl peroxide. The correct usage of retinoids should be clearly explained to avoid irritant reactions or dermatitis (**Box 2**), e.g., in a patient with dry and sensitive skin, start application with adapalene 0.1% every other day, initially for 15 minutes only. Some patients cannot tolerate the gel base as adapalene is not available in cream base. Such patients can be started with tretinoin 0.025% in a cream base for short periods. As tolerance improves, the duration is gradually increased by an hour till they are able to apply it overnight. They can then be switched to daily applications. Strict instructions should be given to stop application if they show hot spots or undergo any procedure and should strictly follow physician's advice.

In moderate acne (Grade 2), use topical anti-inflammatory agents or topical antibiotics such as clindamycin along with sunscreen in gel base in the day time. These should be combined with topical retinoids or benzoyl peroxide at night. In pustular and inflammatory acne (Grade 3), combine topical and systemic therapy with systemic antibiotics. Topical steroid

> **Box 2:** Tips to avoid retinoid dermatitis.
>
> - Start with the lowest concentration
> - Use cream base for patients with dry and sensitive skin
> - Use gel base for patients with oily skin
> - In places with extreme climates, gel base in summer and monsoon and cream base in winter is a better option
> - Begin application for a short duration initially, 1 hour or every alternate day
> - Increase duration of application gradually over a period of 1 week
> - Give strict instructions to patient to withhold application if there is excessive dryness, scaling, or redness
> - Avoid daytime applications
> - Avoid topical retinoids immediately after a resurfacing procedure such as chemical peels and laser resurfacing.

applications should be avoided at all costs because patients tend to use these unsupervised and develop worsening of their acne, along with skin thinning, telangiectasia, and hypertrichosis. It is better to use topical or systemic anti-inflammatory agents instead of topical steroids.

Salicylic acid, nicotinamide, mandelic acid, benzoyl peroxide, adapalene, azelaic acid, clindamycin, and dapsone all have anti-inflammatory effects and are safer alternatives. Salicylic acid is the best because it has a strong anti-inflammatory effect, is lipophilic and can penetrate the pilosebaceous follicle easily, and is safe for all skin types. Salicylic acid 20% as a peeling agent used once a week or once a fortnight is very effective for active inflammatory lesions as well as comedones (**Figs. 4A and B**).

In severe pustular, inflammatory, or nodulocystic acne (Grade 4), isotretinoin should be used. This type of acne should be treated aggressively as it leaves prominent severe scars, which are disfiguring and difficult to treat. Retinoids have been shown to reduce inflammation in acne through inhibition of migration of leukocytes in the skin.[5] Isotretinoin also reduces the expression of matrix metalloproteinases 9 (MMP-9) and

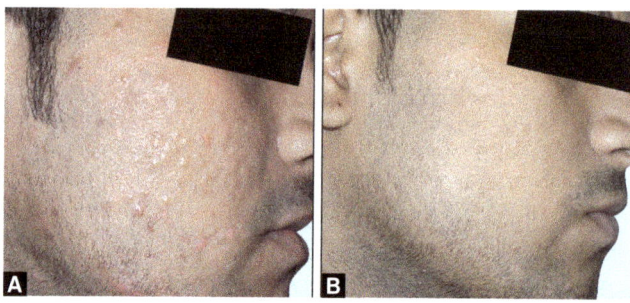

Figs. 4A and B: Improvement of acne following comedone extraction followed immediately by salicylic acid peels 20% at 2 weekly intervals following four peels.

MMP-13 in the sebum of acne patients.[6] Therefore, these agents may be useful in reducing the risk of subsequent scar formation by shifting the balance of MMPs and tissue inhibitors toward normal.[7]

Flare of Acne with Isotretinoin

Isotretinoin initially may aggravate acne and cause a sudden flare up. It is usually mild and common, but a severe flare is rare and is reported in less than 6% of patients.[8] A severe flare can lead to severe inflammation, crusting, and even ulceration followed by extensive scarring. Predictive factors for severe flare following isotretinoin include presence of multiple large macrocomedones, truncal nodules, male gender, and young patients.[9] It is safer to use systemic antibiotics such as doxycycline or azithromycin for the first 2-3 weeks before starting isotretinoin. If the flare is severe, isotretinoin should be stopped or the dose should be reduced to 0.1 mg/kg and systemic prednisolone 0.5-1.0 mg/kg should be given for 2-4 weeks. The prednisolone should be tapered gradually and dose of isotretinoin increased slowly.

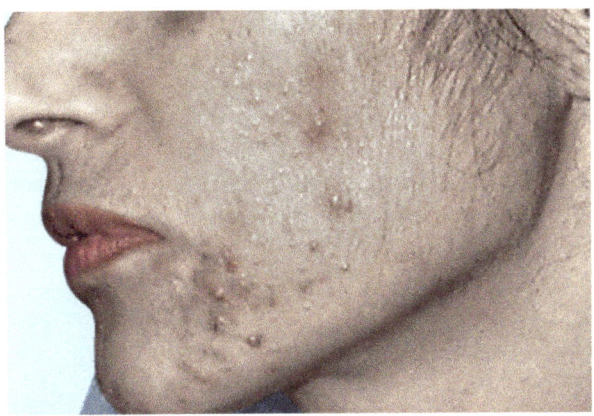

Fig. 5: Adult acne with predominant inflammatory lesions in the lower face.

Hormonal Therapy

Hormonal acne is highly influenced by androgens, chiefly testosterone. It is suspected when there are distinct premenstrual flares of acne or associated menstrual irregularities, obesity, hirsutism, female pattern alopecia, hypothyroidism, or infertility. It is mainly observed in adult women (**Fig. 5**) and teenagers with polycystic ovarian syndrome. Appropriate investigations for hormonal imbalance should be done and hormonal therapy instituted according to the investigations.[10] Hormonal treatment should be continued for at least 6–12 months or longer, depending on severity and response. Spironolactone combined with an oral contraceptive such as ethinyl estradiol and cyproterone acetate or drospirenone gives good results.

Surgical Therapy

Surgical treatment is a useful adjunct to hasten response in active acne.[1] It leads to quicker resolution of lesions, reduces inflammation, and hence has the potential to reduce scarring.[11]

In predominantly comedonal acne (Grade 1), comedone extraction combined with or without superficial chemical peels offers an advantage to prevent inflammation and thus minimize the incidence of scars (**Figs. 6A to C**). Salicylic acid 20–30% and mandelic acid 40–50% used as single agents or as combination peels are particularly beneficial. Peels in alcoholic base should be selected in oily skins and gel base in normal, dry, or sensitive skins.

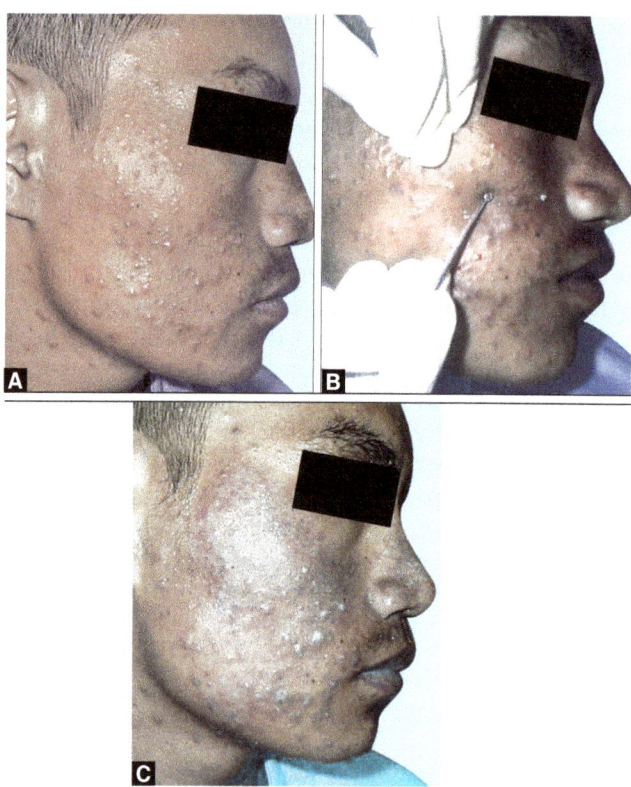

Figs. 6A to C: Comedone extraction followed immediately with salicylic acid peels 20%.

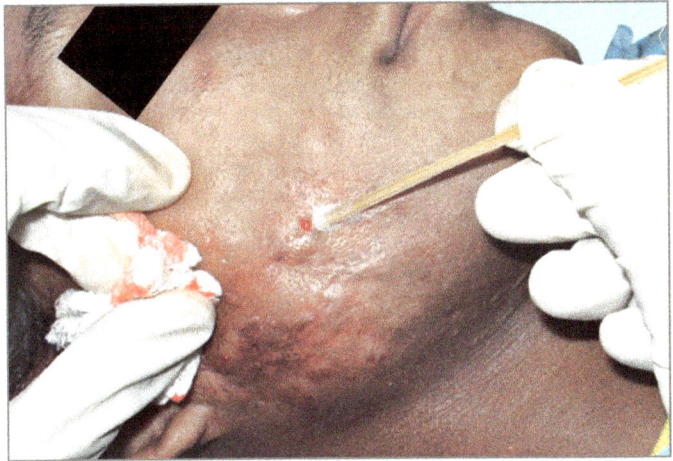

Fig. 7: Treatment of cystic acne with drain eye of cyst followed by phenolization.

In the presence of predominantly inflammatory papules (Grade 2 and Grade 3) chemical peels, cryotherapy or lasers, light therapy, and photodynamic therapy may be beneficial along with systemic antibiotics. These are particularly useful in resistant cases or if a quick response is desired.

When there are predominantly nodulocystic lesions (Grade 4), incision/drainage of cysts with phenolization, intralesional corticosteroids, and cryotherapy helps in quicker resolution of lesions, thus reducing the severity of scars (**Fig. 7**).

CONCLUSION

Preventing acne scars is an important goal of acne therapy. The key to prevention is timely and adequate treatment of acne and reducing side effects of therapy and counseling patients to improve compliance with treatment.

REFERENCES

1. Khunger N. Acne. In: Khunger N, Sachdev M (Eds). Practical Manual of Cosmetic Dermatology and Surgery, 1st edition. Pune: Mehta Publishers India; 2010. pp. 22-42.
2. Saraswat A, Lahiri K, Chatterjee M, Barua S, Coondoo A, Mittal A, et al. Topical corticosteroid abuse on the face: a prospective, multicenter study of dermatology outpatients. Indian J Dermatol Venereol Leprol. 2011;77(2):160-6.
3. Nast A, Dréno B, Bettoli V, Degitz K, Erdmann R, Finlay AY, et al. European Dermatology Forum. J Eur Acad Dermatol Venereol. 2012;26(Suppl 1):1-29.
4. Kubba R, Bajaj AK, Thappa DM, Sharma R, Vedamurthy M, Dhar S, et al. Acne in India: guidelines for management - IAA consensus document. Indian J Dermatol Venereol Leprol. 2009;75(Suppl 1):1-2.
5. Zouboulis CC. Isotretinoin revisited: pluripotent effects on human sebaceous gland cells. J Invest Dermatol. 2006;126(10):2154-6.
6. Papakonstantinou E, Aletras AJ, Glass E, Tsogas P, Dionyssopoulos A, Adjaye J, et al. Matrix metalloproteinases of epithelial origin in facial sebum of patients with acne and their regulation by isotretinoin. J Invest Dermatol. 2005;125(4):673-84.
7. Thiboutot D, Gollnick H, Bettoli V, Dréno B, Kang S, Leyden JJ, et al. New insights into the management of acne: an update from the Global Alliance to Improve Outcomes in Acne group. J Am Acad Dermatol. 2009;60(Suppl 5):S1-50.
8. Clark SM, Cunliffe WJ. Acne flare and isotretinoin-incidence and treatment (abstract). Br J Dermatol. 1995;133:26.
9. Demircay Z, Kus S, Sur H. Predictive factors for acne flare during isotretinoin treatment. Eur J Dermatol. 2008;18(4):452-6.
10. Ebede TL, Arch EL, Berson D. Hormonal treatment of acne in women. J Clin Aesthet Dermatol. 2009;2(12):16-22.
11. Khunger N; IADVL Task Force. Standard guidelines of care for acne surgery. Ind J Dermatol Venereol Leprol. 2008;74(Suppl):S28-36.

CHAPTER 5

Topical Treatment

Aditi Jha, Niti Khunger

IN A NUTSHELL

- Sunscreens should be noncomedogenic and gel based.
- Topical creams containing retinoids and alpha hydroxy acids, particularly glycolic acid and mandelic acid, are useful.
- Silicon gels may be useful in hypertrophic scars. There have been no reported studies on the use of these gels, specifically for acne scars.
- Cryotherapy is helpful, but should be judiciously used to prevent pigmentary complications.
- Iontophoresis has not been widely used and warrants further study.

INTRODUCTION

Acne scars can cause tremendous psychological distress. Though the treatment of scars is mainly surgical, topical treatment can play a role in the treatment of mild scarring. It also acts as an adjuvant therapy in the ongoing treatment with surgical methods to enhance results and minimize complications.

TOPICAL APPLICATIONS

Sunscreens

Broad-spectrum sunscreens are recommended after any procedure done for acne scar treatment to prevent postinflammatory hyperpigmentation, particularly in darker skins. They should also be used as a part of the priming regimens before doing the peel or laser therapy for acne scars.[1] The sunscreen should be noncomedogenic and preferably be gel based.

Retinoids

Topical retinoic acid is useful in the treatment of keloids and hypertrophic scars. The daily application of topical retinoic acid to intractable hypertrophic scars has been shown to cause scar softening, decrease in pruritus, and reduction in the size of scars. Topical retinoic acid also has a proven role in the treatment of fine acne scarring.[2]

Alpha Hydroxy Acids

Glycolic acid is an alpha hydroxy acid, soluble in alcohol, derived from fruit and milk sugars. It acts by thinning the stratum corneum, promoting epidermolysis, and dispersing basal layer melanin. It increases dermal hyaluronic acid and collagen gene expression by increasing secretion of interleukin 6 (IL-6).[3] Topical preparations containing 6% and 12% glycolic acid as well as formulations combined with kojic acid and hydroquinone are available. Topical application alone is helpful for the treatment of hyperpigmented scars. They can be used between chemical peels or with any resurfacing modality to reduce the incidence of postinflammatory hyperpigmentation. They are also useful as maintenance therapy between and after procedures. Mandelic acid is another alpha hydroxy acid that is available as a topical formulation. It is useful if the patient also has active acne lesions. It is well tolerated as an adjunctive treatment and patient compliance is excellent. Contraindications include contact dermatitis, pregnancy, and glycolate hypersensitivity. Side effects, such as temporary hyperpigmentation or irritation, are not very significant.[4]

Pyruvic acid is an alpha-keto acid, with strong antimicrobial effect. It seems to promote collagen synthesis and formation of elastic fibers. The use of 40–70% pyruvic acid has been proposed for the treatment of moderate acne scars, but its effects are better in active papulopustular acne and rosacea. Side effects include desquamation, crusting, intense stinging, and a burning sensation during treatment. Pyruvic acid has stinging and irritating vapors for the upper respiratory mucosa, and adequate ventilation during application is required.[5,6]

SILICON GEL AND ONION EXTRACT

Silicon gel is a topical formulation used for hypertrophic scars and, although less effective, also for keloids. The effects are however variable with results more likely attributable to occlusion or hydration.[7] Pressure is also one supported mechanism along with other mechanisms that include raised temperature, increased oxygen tension, electrostatic properties, or immunologic effects. There are conflicting reports of its efficacy. One study noted improved pruritus, pain, and pliability, but found no improvement in pigmentation or elevation of scars.[8] A separate review of effects, efficacy, and safety of silicone elastomer sheeting on hypertrophic scars elucidated that it was effective in the treatment of hypertrophic scars and keloids with little risk of adverse effects.[9] Rare side effects include pruritus, contact dermatitis, maceration, skin breakdown, xerosis, and odors.

Allium cepa or onion extract is an ingredient in several products marketed for scar treatment. It has been shown to suggest a role in extracellular matrix remodeling by reducing fibroblast proliferation and inducing matrix metalloproteinase-1 (MMP-1) expression.[10] Commonly used preparations include a combination of 10% onion extract, 50 U of sodium heparin per 1 g of gel, 1% allantoin (Contractubex®) or 10% aqueous onion extract, and 1% allantoin (Mederma®). Most studies on onion extract preparations are available for postsurgical scars with paucity of data on their effectiveness on acne scars.[11,12] Onion extract creams are effective mainly in improving color, reducing erythema, pruritus, and consistency of hypertrophic scars as compared to topical corticosteroid treatment with fewer side effects.[13,14] One study showed significant improvement in scar characteristics with reduction of the increase of scar width in the Contractubex® treated group as compared with the untreated group.[15]

CRYOTHERAPY

Cryotherapy is the controlled destruction of tissue by the application of a freezing agent called cryogen that causes cell death. Liquid nitrogen is the most widely used cryogen. The others are solid carbon dioxide and nitrous oxide. Cryopeeling is preferred for acne and superficial postacne scars. In this method, a cryoroller dipped in liquid nitrogen is rapidly rolled over the face for 2–4 seconds after cleaning the face with acetone. One cosmetic area is covered at one time starting from the forehead. Alternatively, gauze is dipped and rolled lightly on the skin. The base of the scar can also be pressed lightly with a cotton swab dipped in liquid nitrogen. Crushed solid carbon dioxide mixed with acetone may also be used, if liquid nitrogen is not available. Erythema and light edema of the skin is seen which may last for 24 hours. Mild topical steroids may be used after the procedure. The process has to be repeated every 2–3 weeks till a satisfactory response is seen. It should be done lightly as hypo- or hyperpigmentation may occur.

IONTOPHORESIS

Stratum corneum is the main barrier for transdermal delivery of drugs. Iontophoresis is a noninvasive method to enhance transdermal drug delivery using small electric current applied by an iontophoretic chamber containing similarly charged active agent and its vehicle. Tretinoin iontophoresis has been used as a noninvasive treatment for atrophic acne scars.[16,17]

Studies have been done with tretinoin 0.025% gel used for 20 minutes twice a week over a period of 3 months. Clinical improvement in the form of reduction in scar depth was seen in around 94% of the patients. Collagenogenesis induced by tretinoin may explain the clinical efficacy in these patients. Side effects of this technique are minimal in the form of erythema, stinging, and flaring of acne lesions.

A technique using estriol iontophoresis is a safe, noninvasive treatment of atrophic acne scars. Schimdt et al.[18] performed estriol iontophoresis in 18 women twice weekly for 3 months. Photographic and clinical follow-up of the skin was obtained monthly and venous blood samples for serum levels of prolactin and estradiol were obtained. After the treatment, improvement of acne scars was observed in 100% of women treated with estriol iontophoresis. No side effects or hormonal changes were noted with estriol treatment.

CONCLUSION

Topical therapy can play a crucial role in the management of acne scars. It is useful as an initial treatment in mild scars, as priming agents to reduce incidence of complications, and as maintenance therapy between surgical techniques.

REFERENCES

1. Khunger N; IADVL Task Force. Standard guidelines of care for chemical peels. Indian J Dermatol Venereol Leprol. 2008;74(Suppl):S5-12.
2. Harris DW, Buckley CC, Ostlere LS, Rustin MH. Topical retinoic acid in the treatment of fine acne scarring. Br J Dermatol. 1991;125(1):81-2.
3. Bernstein EF, Lee L, Brown DB, Yu R, Van Scott E. Glycolic acid treatment increases type I collagen mRNA and hyaluronic acid content of human skin. Dermatol Surg. 2001;27(5):429-33.
4. Javaheri SM, Handa S, Kaur I, Kumar B. Safety and efficacy of glycolic acid facial peel in Indian women with melasma. Int J Dermatol. 2008;40(5):354-7.

5. Griffin TD, Vanscott EJ, Maddin S. The use of pyruvic acid as a chemical peeling agent. J Dermatol Surg Oncol. 1989;15:131-6.
6. Berardesca E, Cameli N, Primavera G, Carrera M. Clinical and instrumental evaluation of skin improvement after treatment with a new 50 percent pyruvic acid peel. Dermatol Surg. 2006;32(4):526-31.
7. Chang CC, Kuo YF, Chiu HC, Lee JL, Wong TW, Jee SH. Hydration, not silicone, modulates the effects of keratinocytes on fibroblasts. J Surg Res. 1995; 59(6):705-11.
8. Phillips TJ, Gerstein AD, Lordan V. A randomized controlled trial of hydrocolloid dressing in the treatment of hypertrophic scars and keloids. Dermatol Surg. 1996;22(9):775-8.
9. Signorini M, Clementoni M. Clinical evaluation of a new self-drying silicone gel in the treatment of scars: a preliminary report. Aesthetic Plast Surg. 2007;31(2):183-7.
10. Cho JW, Cho SY, Lee SR, Lee KS. Onion extract and quercetin induce matrix metalloproteinase-1 in vitro and in vivo. Int J Mol Med. 2010;25(3):347-52.
11. Campanati A, Savelli A, Sandroni L, Marconi B, Giuliano A, Giuliodori K, et al. Effect of allium cepa-allantoin-pentaglycan gel on skin hypertrophic scars: clinical and video-capillaroscopic results of an open-label, controlled, nonrandomized clinical trial. Dermatol Surg. 2010;36(9):1439-44.
12. Willital GH, Simon J. Efficacy of early initiation of a gel containing extractum cepae, heparin, and allantoin for scar treatment: an observational, noninterventional study of daily practice. J Drugs Dermatol. 2013;12(1):38-42.
13. Draelos Z. The ability of onion extract gel to improve the cosmetic appearance of postsurgical scars. J Cosmet Dermatol. 2008;7(2):101-4.
14. Chung VQ, Kelley L, Marra D, Jiang SB. Onion extract gel versus petrolatum emollient on new surgical scars: prospective double-blinded study. Dermatol Surg. 2006;32(2):193-7.
15. Willital GH, Heine H. Efficacy of Contractubex gel in the treatment of fresh scars after thoracic surgery in children and adolescents. Int J Clin Pharmacol Res. 1994;14(5-6):193-202.
16. Schmidt JB, Donath P, Hannes J, Perl S, Neumayer R, Reiner A. Tretinoin-iontophoresis in atrophic acne scars. Int J Dermatol. 1999;38(2):149-53.
17. Knor T. Flattening of atrophic acne scars by using tretinoin by iontophoresis. Acta Dermatovenerol Croat. 2004;12(2):84-91.
18. Schmidt JB, Binder M, Macheiner W, Bieglmayer C. New treatment of atrophic acne scars by iontophoresis with estriol and tretinoin. Int J Dermatol. 1999;34(1):53-7.

CHAPTER 6

Chemical Peels

Niti Khunger

IN A NUTSHELL

- ❖ Chemical peels are useful for erythematous and hyperpigmented macular acne scars, acne excoriée, and atrophic mild superficial scars.
- ❖ Additive improvement occurs when they are combined with other procedures such as subcision, microneedling, and chemical reconstruction of skin scars technique.
- ❖ They are a useful adjunct when patient has active acne, photodamage, and postinflammatory hyperpigmentation.
- ❖ Salicylic acid, mandelic acid, glycolic acid, Jessner's solution, and trichloroacetic acid are most frequently used, singly or as combination peels.

INTRODUCTION

Traditionally, medium-depth and deep peels were carried out for the treatment of acne scars. Trichloroacetic acid (TCA) and phenol were the common agents used.[1] However, medium-depth and deep peels carry a higher risk of complications, particularly in darker skins, and they have been largely supplanted by fractional lasers. Still, repeated superficial chemical peels can play an active role in the treatment of persistent macular hyperpigmented and erythematous lesions and superficial acne scars, particularly in darker skin types. An advantage is that superficial peels can be utilized for mild acne scars and additionally help to improve pigmentary dyschromias, photoaging, and the texture of the skin.

PRINCIPLE

Superficial chemical peels ablate the epidermis only. This is followed by epidermal regeneration and collagen formation in the dermis. The exfoliating effects and the increased epidermal turnover explain their efficacy on macular scars. Because they are mildly potent, repeated treatments are required to obtain the desired effects. They are predominantly useful in hyperpigmented and erythematous macular lesions and mild atrophic rolling and boxcar scars. Medium-depth chemical peels extend to the papillary dermis. The inflammatory reaction has stimulatory effects on fibroblasts resulting in new collagen formation. This explains their efficacy on atrophic scars.

INDICATIONS

- Macular erythematous acne scars
- Hyperpigmented acne scars
- Acne excoriée
- Atrophic mild superficial scars.

For atrophic scars, better results are obtained if they are combined with subcision. The subcision is done first, followed by the chemical peel. An advantage of chemical peeling is that it can be used when patient has active acne, particularly comedones and inflammatory papules, and pustules. It also leads to improvement of skin texture and pigmentation **(Figs. 1 and 2)**.

CONTRAINDICATIONS

- *Active herpes simplex*: It is safer to treat the herpes simplex with antivirals and then do the peels under the cover of prophylactic antivirals starting 2 days prior to the procedure and continuing for a week after the peel **(Fig. 3)**.

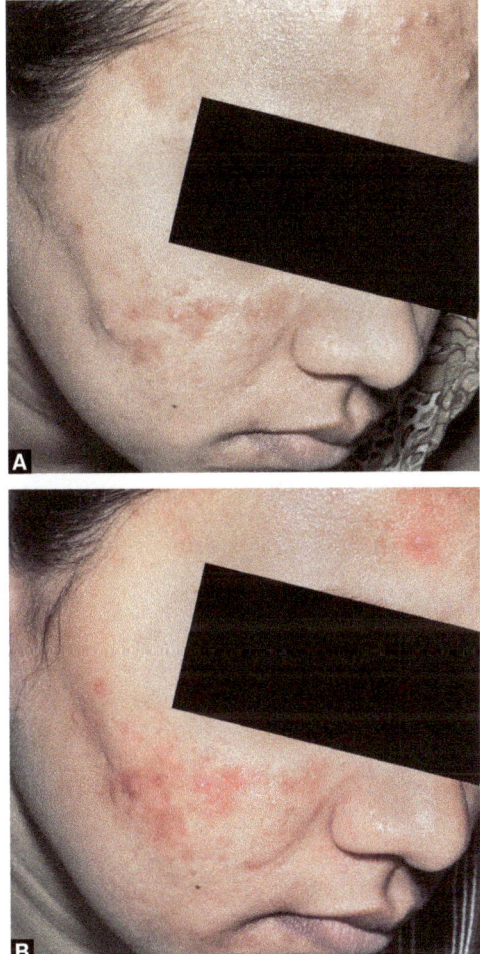

Figs. 1A and B: Improvement of active acne and macular acne scars. (A) Using a combination; (B) Peel containing acetic acid, salicylic acid, jasmonic acid, citric acid, and lactic acid as monotherapy at weekly intervals after three peels (Black peel® Theraderm, Korea).

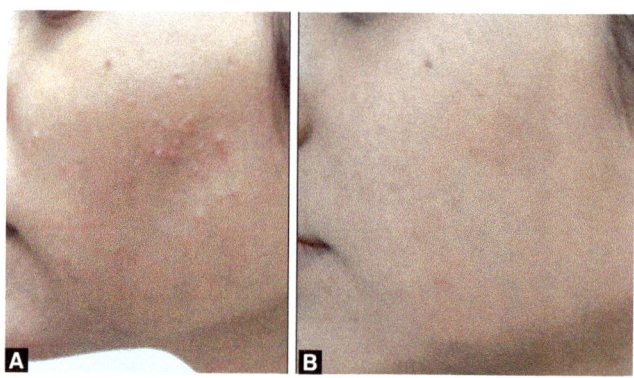

Figs. 2A and B: Improvement of active acne and improvement in pigmentation and texture following mandelic acid peels 50% at weekly intervals after six peels.

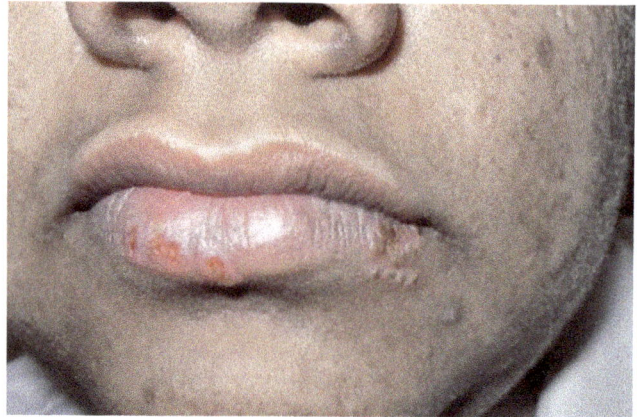

Fig. 3: Active herpes simplex with acne. Peeling should be postponed.

- *Viral warts or molluscum contagiosum* on the area to be peeled. These should first be treated.
- *Open wounds on the peeling area*: These can lead to increased penetration of the peel followed by scarring.

- *History of taking photosensitive drugs*: Chemical peels should be performed with caution in patients on photosensitive drugs, particularly doxycycline and minocycline, as they can lead to greater and persistent erythema, followed by postinflammatory hyperpigmentation (PIH).
- *History of hypertrophic scars and keloids*: Medium-depth and deep peels should be avoided, while superficial peels may be performed with caution.
- *Isotretinoin use in the last 6 months*: This is a contraindication only in patients who require deep peels. Superficial peels can be safely done.
- *Uncooperative patient*: Patients who do not apply the sunscreen and medications as frequently as prescribed or are careless about sun exposure should be cautiously taken up for chemical peels. They have higher chances of pigmentary complications, which can worsen the clinical condition.
- *Timing of the peel*: Peeling should not be done immediately before an important event as an unexpected reaction can lead to a very angry patient.
- *Patient with unrealistic expectations*: Superficial chemical peels are useful only for macular and mild superficial atrophic acne scars. They are not useful for deeper ice pick and boxcar scars or in a patient with extensive atrophy.

All these are relative contraindications and it implies that peels may be done following all precautions and the patients must be warned of the higher risk of complications. Adequate instructions should be given to patients to follow all the instructions provided.

Choosing the Peeling Agents

A wide variety of peeling agents have been used for acne scars:
- Salicylic acid—20-30%
- Mandelic acid—40-50%

- Lactic acid—90%
- Glycolic acid—35-70%
- Modified Jessner's solution—14% salicylic, 14% lactic, and 14% citric acid
- TCA—15-35%
- Pyruvic acid—40-60%
- Combination peels.

Salicylic and mandelic acid are the peeling agents of choice in macular and superficial acne scars.[2] The advantage of these two peeling agents is that they can also be used in the presence of active acne lesions. They are particularly useful for hyperpigmented scars and are safe for darker skin types. A combination peel, salicylic and mandelic acid peel (SMP), is widely used for active acne and superficial acne scars. A study that compared glycolic acid 70% with the combination SMP reported a modest 13.2% improvement in ice pick scars with SMP versus 10.4% with glycolic acid. The boxcar scars improved by approximately 20%, while the rolling scars showed no improvement.[3] There was no statistically significant difference between the two peels, but SMP had fewer adverse effects and was better for treating acne and hyperpigmentation.

Lactic acid is safe during pregnancy and low concentrations are safer for sensitive skins. A study utilizing full strength 92% lactic acid in seven patients with Fitzpatrick skin type IV-V reported significant improvement (>75% clearance of lesions) in one patient (14.28%), good improvement (51-75% clearance) in three patients (42.84%), moderate improvement (26-50% clearance) in two patients (28.57%), and mild improvement (1-25% clearance) in one patient (14.28%).[4]

Glycolic acid, TCA, and pyruvic acid are more aggressive peeling agents and can reach a greater depth in the dermis. A study comparing serial glycolic acid peels with increasing concentration from 20 to 70% with topical glycolic acid cream 15% reported significantly better results with glycolic acid peels as compared to the home regimen.[5] At least six peeling sessions were required to obtain a significant response. Glycolic acid is a good peeling agent if there are many comedones. However, there may be an initial flare due to comedolysis. Patient should be counseled regarding this.

Sequential peels increase the depth of peels, and are reported to be safe in darker skins. A study utilized a sequential peel with Jessner's solution followed by 35% TCA.[6] The Jessner's solution was applied in 2-3 coats first till frosting occurred.[6] Following this, 35% TCA was applied over the same areas in three consecutive layers, 2 minutes apart, till a complete frost occurred, which took about 3-4 minutes.[6] The uniform frost indicates an upper reticular dermis peel. From the second peeling session onward, 50% TCA was used to treat the edges of deeper scars, followed by the standard 35% TCA application to the remainder of the treatment areas. Significant improvement was seen only in one patient (6.6%), moderate improvement in six patients (50%), mild improvement in three patients (25%), minimal improvement in one patient (8.3%), and no response in one patient. Hence, chemical peels are not very effective for deeper acne scars, and also carry a higher risk of pigmentary changes. A modified phenol peel, Exoderm®, has also been used in Asian patients with acne scars.[7] Though an improvement was observed in 7 out of 11 patients (64%), PIH was observed in 74%, and 1 patient developed persistent hypopigmentation. Hence, phenol peels are better avoided in darker skin types, besides the risk of cardiac arrhythmias. The newer combination peels have multiple modes of action and have a wide margin of safety, though they may require more sessions and may be only moderately effective.

LIMITATIONS

Superficial chemical peels cannot be utilized for deep scarring that extends beyond the papillary dermis, such as ice pick scars and deep boxcar scars. Medium-depth and deep peels that were previously extensively used for deep acne scars are now best avoided in darker skins. Microneedling and fractional lasers are better alternatives.

The chemical reconstruction of skin scars (CROSS) technique using 65–100% TCA is a modified form of a chemical peel used for ice pick scars. It is a focal deep chemical peel and is effective in all skin types. For details, see Chapter 7.

PRECAUTIONS

The patient should be primed with skin lightening agents such as hydroquinone 2–4%, tretinoin 0.025%, or adapalene at least 2–4 weeks before the procedure. Triple combination creams containing steroids should be strictly avoided as it can lead to aggravation of acne. The peeling agent should be chosen with care as there can be aggravation of acne and PIH with aggressive treatments. Sun exposure should be avoided and sunscreens should be regularly applied. A gel-based noncomedogenic or aqueous sunscreen is preferred.

PREPROCEDURE PREPARATION

Priming is very important and should be done at least 2 weeks before peeling. Photoprotection along with sunscreens and skin lightening agents containing hydroquinone, azelaic acid, kojic acid, and tretinoin or adapalene should be used. Antivirals should be given 2 days prior in patients with history of herpes simplex.

TECHNIQUE

- Ensure that the patient has been adequately counseled and primed.
- Take informed consent and adequate photographs.
- Contact lenses should be removed before the peel.

- Ask the patient to wash the face with soap and water and remove all makeup, dirt, and grime.
- The hair is pulled back with a hair band or cap.
- The patient is either sitting or at 45°.
- First inspect the skin to see that there are no abrasions or inflammation.
- Using 2" × 2" gauze pieces, clean the skin with alcohol and then degrease with acetone or a prepeel cleanser.
- Check the label carefully and pour the peeling agent of required strength in a glass beaker and keep the neutralizing agent ready.
- Apply the agent with a cotton-tipped applicator or gauze piece quickly on the entire face going along the cosmetic units. There should be no dripping of the agent. Begin from the forehead in an upward direction, then the right cheek, nose, left cheek, and chin in that order. The perioral, upper, and lower eyelids, if required, are treated last. Feathering strokes are applied at the edges, to blend with surrounding skin and prevent demarcation lines. Do not leave the room and closely watch out for increasing redness, hot spots, and epidermolysis. The peel is neutralized as required according to the peeling agent. The skin is gently dried with gauze and the patient is asked to wash with cold water till the burning subsides. The patient then applies a sunscreen, before leaving the clinic.

POSTPROCEDURE CARE

Patients may feel tightness of the skin after a peel or may show frank desquamation, especially after the first peel (**Fig. 4**).

They should be prepared for this. A sunscreen in aqueous base should be used. If required, a noncomedogenic moisturizer may be used postpeel if the patient is uncomfortable. Healing may be delayed in older skins and in patients with many atrophic scars. A mild soap or nonsoap cleanser may be used.

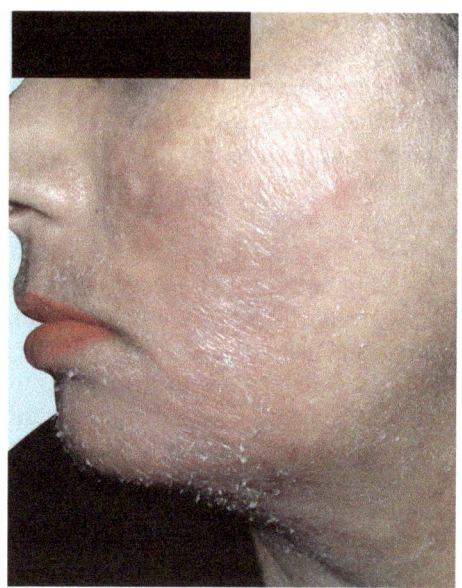

Fig. 4: Erythema, scaling, and desquamation following 30% salicylic acid peeling.

If there is crusting, topical antibacterial ointment should be used to prevent bacterial infection as older patients are much more prone to infection. Patients should be emphatically told to avoid peeling or scratching the skin. Hypopigmenting agents are restarted after the peel. Superficial peels can be repeated every 2 weeks. If performed, medium-depth peels may be repeated after 6–9 months, while deep peels should not be repeated before 1 year.

Combination Treatments

The advantage of chemical peels is that they can be combined with other treatments such as subcision, microneedling, and lasers for an additive effect. While subcision and microneedling take care of the atrophy in the dermis, chemical peels improve the texture of the skin. The author uses the two modalities alternatively, every 2 weeks. When combining chemical peels with subcision, the subcision is done first, followed by the peel. This can be done in the same session. The two modalities can be used alternatively, every 2 weeks (**Figs. 5A to C**). Superficial chemical peeling can also be combined between two laser sessions. It has an additive effect and reduces the risk of PIH. In a review of different nonenergy-based modalities for acne scars, chemical peeling was found to be more effective with clinical improvement occurring in more than 70% of patients.[8]

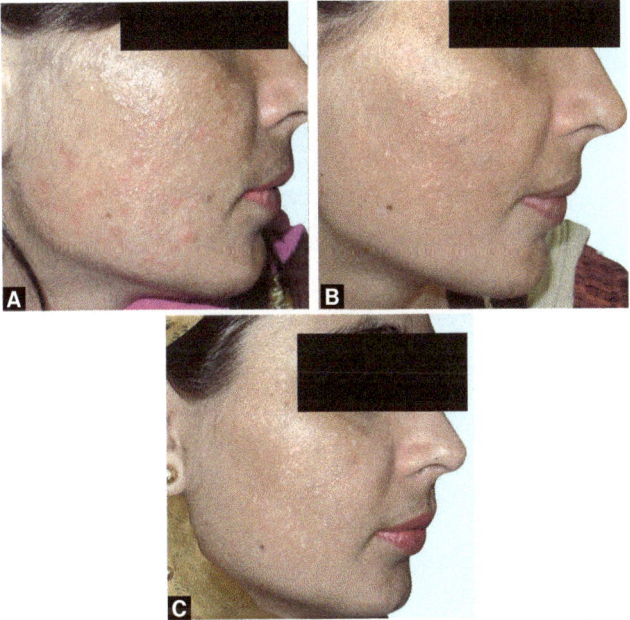

Figs. 5A to C: Improvement of acne, texture, and superficial scars following subcision combined with combination salicylic–mandelic acid peels.

COMPLICATIONS

The best way to avoid complications during peeling, particularly in patients with acne, is to use combination peels. A well-primed skin will heal faster with fewer complications. Strict sun protection and good postpeel care are important. Severe burning may be experienced postpeel, especially over active lesions. This can be reduced by frequent applications of ice cold saline and sunscreen. Complications with superficial peels are uncommon. PIH is most frequently seen, particularly if the patient has not been primed with skin lightening agents **(Fig. 6)**. Skin irritation, infection, aggravation of acne, flare up of herpes, and pigmentary abnormalities are complications

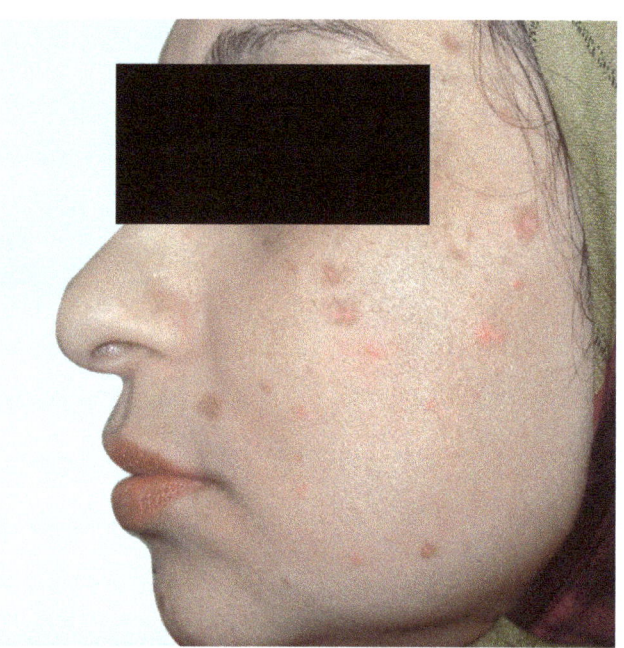

Fig. 6: Postinflammatory hyperpigmentation following spot.

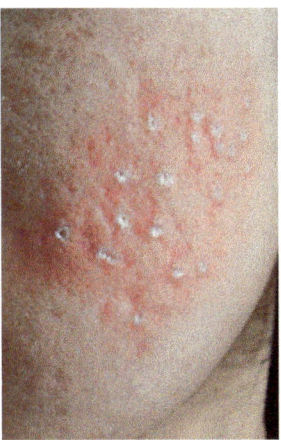

Fig. 7: Excessive erythema following CROSS technique.

that can occur following medium-depth chemical peels. Excessive crusting, desquamation, inflammation, and erythema can occur with all peels **(Fig. 7)**. These should be treated aggressively to prevent PIH, particularly in skins of color. Short course of mild topical steroid, like fluticasone, can be prescribed for 2-4 days to tide over the inflammatory phase, only if it is very severe. The skin returns to normal in superficial peels in 2-5 days and in 7-10 days in medium peels.

CONCLUSION

Superficial chemical peels can be a useful adjunct to therapy of acne scars. The advantages they offer are that they can be used in the presence of active acne and they improve the pigmentary changes and texture of the skin. They can also be combined with other procedures such as subcision, CROSS technique, and microneedling for additive effects. In addition, if used judiciously, they can help to minimize risk of PIH when used between laser sessions.

REFERENCES

1. Landau M. Cardiac complications in deep chemical peels. Dermatol Surg. 2007;33(2):190-3; discussion 193.
2. Khunger N; IADVL Task Force. Standard guidelines of care for chemical peels. Indian J Dermatol Venereol Leprol. 2008;74(Suppl):S5-12.
3. Garg VK, Sinha S, Sarkar R. Glycolic acid peels versus salicylic-mandelic acid peels in active acne vulgaris and postacne scarring and hyper pigmentation: A comparative study. Dermatol Surg. 2009;35(1):59-65.
4. Sachdeva S. Lactic acid peeling in superficial acne scarring in Indian skin. J Cosmet Dermatol. 2010;9(3):246-8.
5. Erbağci Z, Akçali C. Biweekly serial glycolic acid peels vs. long-term daily use of topical low-strength glycolic acid in the treatment of atrophic acne scars. Int J Dermatol. 2000;39(10):789-94.
6. Al-Waiz MM, Al-Sharqi AI. Medium-depth chemical peels in the treatment of acne scars in dark-skinned individuals. Dermatol Surg. 2002;28(5):383-7.
7. Park JH, Choi YD, Kim SW, Kim YC, Park SW. Effectiveness of modified phenol peel (Exoderm) on facial wrinkles, acne scars and other skin problems of Asian patients. J Dermatol. 2007;34(1):17-24.
8. Kravvas G, Al-Niaimi F. A systematic review of treatments for acne scarring. Part 1: Non-energy-based techniques. Scars Burn Heal. 2017;3:2059513117695312.

CHAPTER 7

CROSS Technique

Deepali Bhardwaj, Niti Khunger

IN A NUTSHELL

- ❖ Trichloroacetic acid chemical reconstruction of skin scars technique is an excellent treatment strategy for ice pick acne scars.
- ❖ It can be combined with fractional laser skin resurfacing using 1,550 nm Erbium Glass laser or fractional CO_2 laser or percutaneous collagen induction technique with dermaroller to enhance results and improve other type of scars.
- ❖ Acne scars still remain a therapeutic challenge and hence, combination treatments are the only key to treating them well.

INTRODUCTION

Severe scarring caused by acne is associated with substantial cosmetic and psychological distress, particularly in adolescents.[1] Atrophic acne scars are more common than keloids and hypertrophic scars with a ratio 3:1. They have been subclassified into ice pick, boxcar, and rolling scars. With atrophic scars, the ice pick type represents 60-70% of total scars, the boxcar 20-30%, and rolling scars 15-25%. Chemical reconstruction of skin scars (CROSS) is a technique using high concentrations of trichloroacetic acid (TCA) focally on the atrophic acne scars to induce collagenization leading to their cosmetic improvement.[2]

Trichloroacetic acid is well known as a peeling agent that was first used by Unna, a German dermatologist, in 1882. It is a versatile peeling agent since the peel depth varies according to its concentration. Since it is a self-neutralizing agent and not absorbed in the systemic circulation, it is safe if used even in high concentration with precautions. In order to maximize the effects of TCA and to overcome the complications such as scarring, hyperpigmentation, and hypopigmentation that can occur when applied over large areas, the technique of applying it precisely to the scars, CROSS is becoming increasingly popular. It was first described by Lee et al.,[2] where a high concentration of TCA was applied focally to ice pick acne scars by pressing hard on the entire depressed area using a sharpened wooden applicator to produce frosted white spots on each scar. The advantage is that dermal thickening and collagen production increases with higher TCA concentration.[3] Healing is more rapid and associated with a lower complication rate as the adjacent normal tissue and adnexal structures are spared which makes it a better tool than ablative laser skin resurfacing.

PRINCIPLE

Application of the caustic agent, TCA, focally into the depth of the acne scar causes precipitation of proteins and coagulative necrosis of cells in the epidermis and necrosis of collagen in the papillary to upper reticular dermis. An increase in dermal volume as a result of an increased collagen production, glycosaminoglycan and elastin fragmentation and reorganization are seen. It has been shown that dermal collagen remodeling may continue for several months. Hence, a continuous collagen remodeling with increased volumes will definitely help in scar remodeling and help fill up the scar tissue after TCA CROSS technique **(Fig. 1)**.

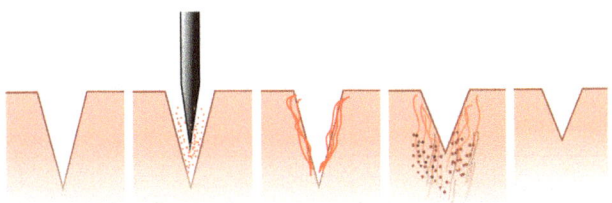

Ice pick scar Focal application Inflammation Collagenization Improvement
of high concentration
of TCA-65–100%

Fig. 1: Principle of chemical reconstruction of skin scar (CROSS) technique. (TCA: trichloroacetic acid)

INSTRUMENTS

- TCA 50–100% **(Fig. 2A)**
- Sharpened wooden applicator or toothpick **(Fig. 2B)**. Alternatively, 30 G needle mounted on an insulin syringe **(Fig. 2C)** can also be used.
- Methyl alcohol (spirit) and acetone for cleansing.

Indications

Ice pick scars—narrow, deep, sharply demarcated tracts that extend vertically into deep dermis or subcutaneous layer.

CONTRAINDICATIONS

- No absolute contraindication
- *Relative*:
    - Active inflammatory lesions or infections such as herpes labialis
    - Patient with keloidal tendency
    - Immediately postablative laser skin resurfacing or dermabrasion
    - Large or wide atrophic boxcar scars.

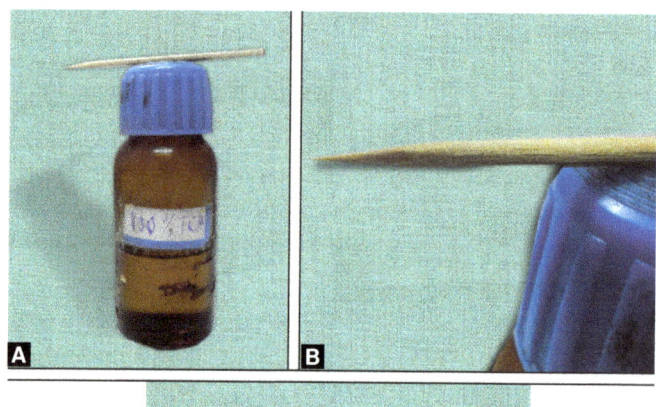

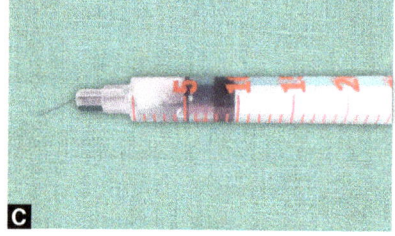

Figs. 2A to C: (A) Simple tools for TCA CROSS technique; (B) Sharpened wooden toothpick; (C) Bent insulin syringe.

LIMITATIONS

- Downtime of 3–6 days is always there, as there is a crust formation due to precipitation of proteins **(Fig. 3)**.
- Boxcar-type sharp shouldered, broad atrophic, and undulated or rolling scars show lesser improvement as compared to ice pick acne scars.

PRECAUTIONS

- Proper priming of skin for at least 2 weeks before the procedure helps in increased efficacy of the treatment and prevents the complications of hyperpigmentation. This is important in darker skins.

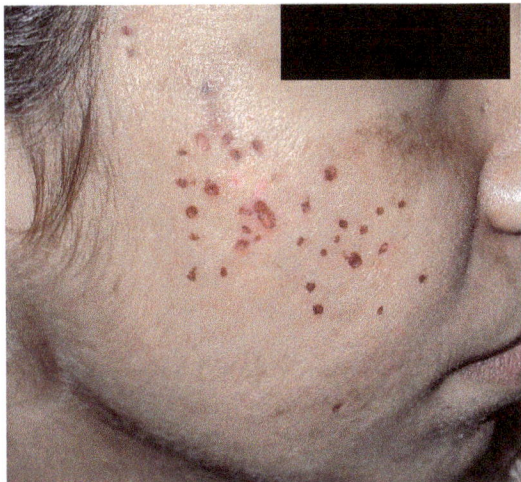

Fig. 3: Crusting on the third day following the CROSS technique.

- During the technique, skin should be stretched to reach the bottom of the scar and then 50 or 100% TCA should be focally applied by pressing hard on the entire depressed area of the scars taking care to avoid spillage to the surrounding skin **(Fig. 4)**. The spread of TCA to surrounding normal skin should not happen at all as it can lead to increased size of the scar **(Figs. 5A and B)**.
- Patient should be aligned well regarding the procedure. Scratching/scrubbing off of the crusts is to be strictly avoided.

PREPROCEDURE PREPARATION

- Priming for 2 weeks with tretinoin 0.025% cream at night and a sunscreen containing avobenzone and octinoxate, and 2% hydroquinone in morning is most ideal.
- No anesthesia is required during the procedure.
- Photography should be done before each session in three views of the treatment area—front, right, and left oblique.

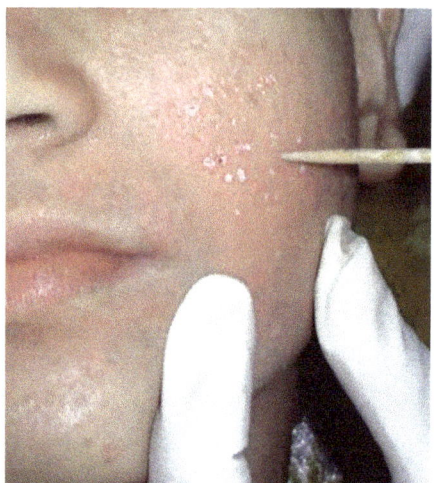

Fig. 4: Correct technique pinpoint frosting.

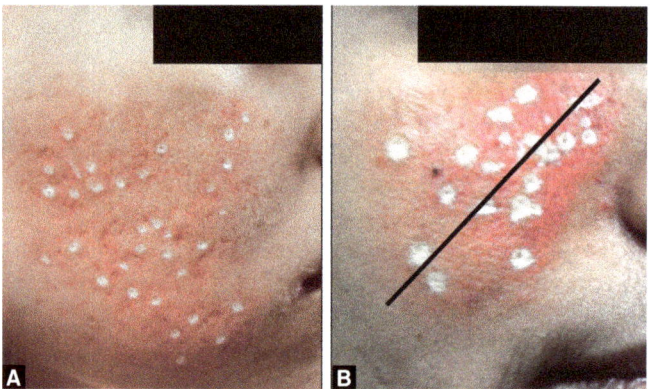

Figs. 5A and B: (A) Typical deep frosting following 100% TCA indicating deep dermis depth and erythema; (B) Spillage of TCA outside the scar—incorrect technique.

- Patient should be explained in detail regarding the downtime involved. All precautions before starting the

procedure and a duly signed consent form should be taken before the first session from every patient.
- There should be good focused preferably oblique lighting on the skin and the patient should be either standing or sitting during the session.
- All the ice pick acne scars should be marked with a pen and counted before each session to assess the efficacy of this treatment effectively.
- Skin should be properly cleaned and disinfected by using methylated spirit before starting the procedure and degreasing with acetone should be performed.

TECHNIQUE[4]

- Ensure informed consent and photographs are taken.
- The patient is sitting up or lying at 45° with hair tied behind the face and a headband is used.
- No anesthesia is required.
- Degrease with acetone.
- Sharpen a wooden toothpick till it is fine and pointed at the tip.
- The skin is stretched to reach the bottom of the scar and 100% TCA is then focally applied by pressing hard on the entire depressed area of the atrophic scar taking care to avoid spillage to the surrounding skin **(Fig. 4)**. The skin is kept stretched and monitored carefully until a refrigerated "frosted" appearance after a single application is seen. Frosting is seen generally in 10–15 seconds and is a result of coagulation of epidermal and dermal proteins and is used mainly to monitor the peel depth **(Figs. 5A and B)**. It is important to keep the skin stretched till frosting is complete before moving on to another area.
- When cheeks are being treated, it is advisable to start from lateral to medial side on the left cheek and from medial to lateral side on the right cheek for a right-handed person.

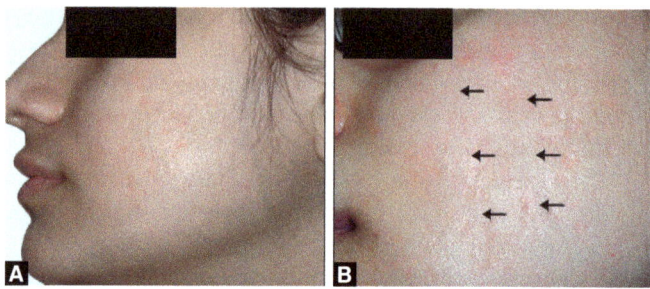

Figs. 6A and B: Improvement of ice pick scars following a single session of CROSS with 100% TCA and direction of application from lateral to medial side on the left cheek and medial to lateral side on the right cheek to avoid spread of free acid.

This is to avoid spread of TCA from the stretching hand to adjacent normal skin **(Figs. 6A and B)**.
- Once a thick white frost has appeared and the sensation of burning has reduced, the process is completed.
- The face is washed and the patient is sent from the clinic with application of sunscreen.
- The procedure has to be repeated at every 2-4 weeks till satisfactory improvement. Experiences have shown that, compared with other procedures, this technique can avoid scarring and reduce the risk of hypopigmentation by sparing the adjacent normal skin and adnexal structures.
- If it is combined with subcision in the same sitting, the subcision is done first. It can also be combined with chemical peels, microneedling, and fractional lasers at different sittings for greater efficacy and reduction of total time taken to achieve a satisfactory response.

EFFICACY

Improvement Expected

Lee et al.[2] reported that 82% of patients improved with 65% TCA and 94% patients improved with 100% TCA. The degree

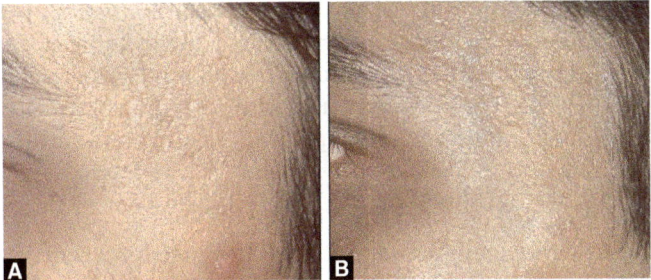

Figs. 7A and B: Improvement of scars following three sessions of subcision combined with 100% TCA CROSS technique.

of improvement was greater in patients who underwent more number of procedures. We have also observed that 100% pure TCA is better in efficacy than 50% TCA for CROSS technique and induces better collagenization **(Figs. 7A and B)**. In our study of 30 patients, more than 70% improvement was observed in the majority of patients (73.3%), while 50–70% improvement was seen in 20% patients, and 6.7% patients had fair results (30–49%) at the end of four sessions.[4] However, Fabbrocini et al.[5] reported that 50% TCA was also effective in their study of five patients. Leheta et al.[6] compared the CROSS technique using 100% TCA with microneedling using the dermaroller and reported that both the procedures were equally effective. CROSS was more effective in treating ice pick and boxcar scars and microneedling was more efficacious for rolling scars.

POSTPROCEDURE CARE

Patient should be well informed regarding the crusting. These should not be peeled but allowed to fall of spontaneously. Sunscreens and antibiotic creams should be continued till the crusts are detached which takes almost 2–4 days. No oral antibiotics are required unless an ablative laser resurfacing or some other procedure is done on the same day. Also, 1 week after CROSS, a moisturizer along with a cream consisting of 4% hydroquinone and a tretinoin cream at night can be given. The application of makeup for camouflage is allowed 24 hours after CROSS. When CROSS is combined with other procedures such as subcision or laser resurfacing, CROSS should be done first.

COMPLICATIONS

The CROSS technique is a relatively safe procedure. Transient side effects include postinflammatory hyperpigmentation (PIH) and hypopigmentation. Hyperpigmentation is more common, particularly in darker skin types **(Fig. 8)**. Persistent erythema can occur if the crusts are forcibly and prematurely removed. Scar extension is a feared complication as it is permanent and difficult to treat **(Fig. 9)**. It occurs due to improper technique, when there is spillage of the TCA on surrounding normal skin. Depending on the area of the scar, it has to be treated with subcision and excision or punch elevation.

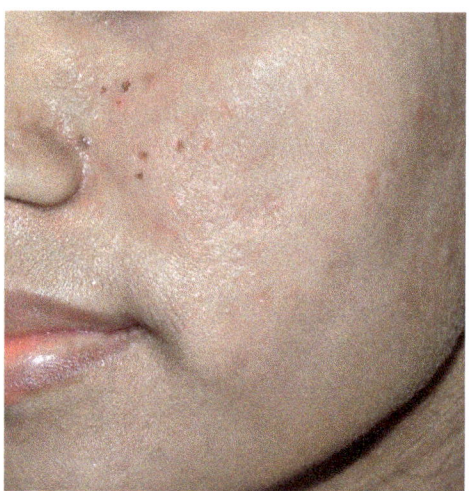

Fig. 8: Postinflammatory hyperpigmentation following CROSS.

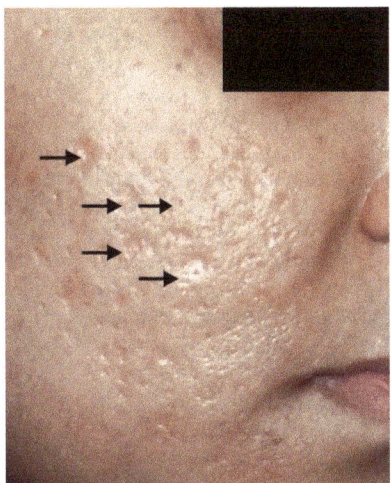

Fig. 9: Worsening of scar following incorrect technique and spillage of TCA to surrounding normal skin.

CONCLUSION

Chemical reconstruction of skin scars with 50 or 100% TCA is a cost-effective, minimally invasive technique with a good efficacy for ice pick scars, which are difficult to treat even with lasers. The advantage is that it can be used safely in the cosmetic management of ice pick acne scarring in dark skin type individuals with proper priming.

REFERENCES

1. Ghodsi SZ, Orawa H, Zouboulis CC. Prevalence, severity, and severity risk factors of acne in high school pupils: a community-based study. J Invest Dermatol. 2009;129(9):2136-41.
2. Lee JB, Chung WG, Kwahck H, Lee KH. Focal treatment of acne scars with trichloroacetic acid: Chemical reconstruction of skin scars method. Dermatologic Surgery. 2002;28(11):1017-21.

3. Yug A, Lane JE, Howard MS, Kent DE. Histologic study of depressed acne scars treated with serial high-concentration (95%) trichloroacetic acid. Dermatol Surg. 2006;32(8):985-90.
4. Khunger N, Bhardwaj D, Khunger M. Evaluation of CROSS technique with 100% TCA in the management of ice pick acne scars in darker skin types. J Cosmet Dermatol. 2011;10(1):51-7.
5. Fabbrocini G, Cacciapuoti S, Fardella N, Pastore F, Monfrecola G. CROSS technique: chemical reconstruction of skin scars method. Dermatol Ther. 2008;21(Suppl 3):S29-32.
6. Leheta T, El Tawdy A, Hay RA, Farid S. Percutaneous collagen induction versus full-concentration trichloroacetic acid in the treatment of atrophic acne scars. Dermatol Surg. 2011;37(2):207-16.

CHAPTER 8

Subcision

Niti Khunger

IN A NUTSHELL

- Subcision is a process of elevation of depressed scars by the introduction of a sharp needle beneath the scar that breaks the fibrous adhesions tethering the scar.
- A simple modification by bending the needle at a right angle makes the procedure safe and easy.
- The advantage is that it is a simple cost-effective office procedure with a low incidence of complications in all skin types.
- The disadvantage is that improvement is slow, and it cannot improve the texture of the skin overlying the scar.
- Combining subcision with a resurfacing procedure such as fractional laser resurfacing leads to greater improvement than either technique alone.

INTRODUCTION

There are various types of acne scars, all of which require individualized treatment and multiple modalities.[1] Subcision is a simple surgical technique for the treatment of depressed scars that can be carried out as an office procedure. Though the first report of subcision was described by Spangler[2] who reported the use of a Bowman iris needle to cut the fibrous strands beneath the deeply depressed facial scar in 1957, the technique was given the name "subcutaneous incision less surgery" or subcision by Orentreich and Orentreich in 1995.[3]

PRINCIPLE

In this technique, a sharp needle is introduced into the skin just beneath the scar. It has a scalpel-like effect, causing incision of the fibrous bands that depress the scar. As a result of breakage of these adhesions, the scar surface is released from the underlying fibrous attachments, which lifts up the scar. There is organization of blood in the induced dermal pocket **(Figs. 1A to C)**. This injury induces connective tissue formation beneath the scar, without injury to the skin surface. In atrophic

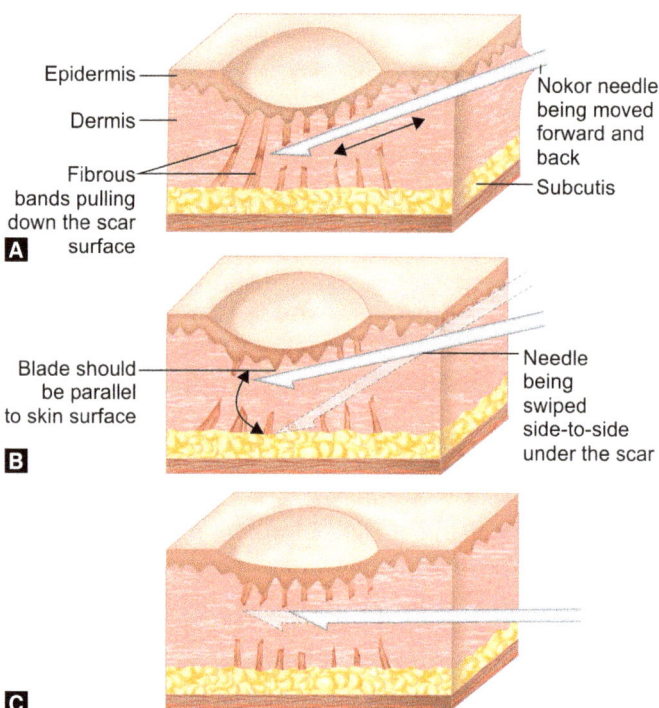

Figs. 1A to C: (A and B) Principle of subcision—traditional; (C) Modified subcision.

acne scars, subcision is mainly useful for rolling scars that are distensible with gentle sloping edges.[3] It is partially effective for ice pick or boxcar scars, where it has to be combined with other modalities.

INSTRUMENTS

- Spirit swab, povidone-iodine for surgical cleansing, and gauze pieces
- Surgical marking pen
- Nokor needle or sterile hypodermic needle of different gauges; 18–24 gauge
- Topical anesthetic.

INDICATIONS

Subcision is basically indicated for depressed scars:
- Depressed linear traumatic or surgical scars
- Depressed rolling scars with distensible edges
- All depressed postacne scars, including boxcar scars
- Ice pick scars
- Chickenpox scars.

CONTRAINDICATIONS

- Patients with bleeding diathesis. These patients are more prone to hematoma collection, which can get organized, forming persistent nodules.
- History of keloid formation and patients on isotretinoin therapy are partial contraindications, though subcision can be performed, with careful monitoring.

PRECAUTIONS

If medically feasible, any drugs (e.g. aspirin and vitamin E) that could prolong bleeding should be avoided or stopped 1 week prior. If there is an active infection in the surrounding area, it should be treated before subcision.

PREPROCEDURE PREPARATION

There is no active preparation that is required. Patients should stop aspirin or vitamin E 7 days before the procedure to avoid prolonged bleeding.

TECHNIQUE[4-6]

- The area is first surgically cleaned with spirit and povidone-iodine.
- The scars are marked with a surgical marking pen with the patient upright in the sitting or standing position. Lying down will efface many scars, particularly the rolling scars.
- *Anesthesia*—if there are few scars, anesthesia may not be essential. If there are multiple scars, anesthesia is required. Topical anesthesia with eutectic mixture of lignocaine and prilocaine (Toplap®) applied 1 hour prior or tetracaine 7% and lignocaine 7% (Tetralid®) may be used. Often anesthesia is not complete and in anxious patients with multiple scars, infiltration anesthesia with 1% lignocaine is useful. But infiltration should be done only after marking the scars. Alternatively, an infraorbital nerve block may be given.
- *Needle selection*—a Nokor needle that is sharp and has a triangular tip or a hypodermic needle can be used **(Fig. 2)**. The gauge depends on the size of the scar. Routinely, Nokor needle no. 18 or hypodermic needle 18G is used. For finer, smaller scars 23 or 24 gauge needle may be used.
- The skin is stretched and the needle is introduced in the dermis at the edge of the scar, with the bevel pointing upward and forwarded beneath the scar. It is then moved back and forth in a lancing motion to cover the entire scar and then moved in a fanning motion to break all adhesions that tether the scar to the underlying tissues **(Fig. 3)**.

Subcision

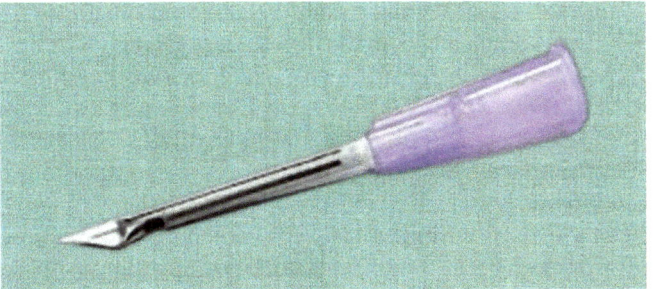

Fig. 2: Nokor needle.

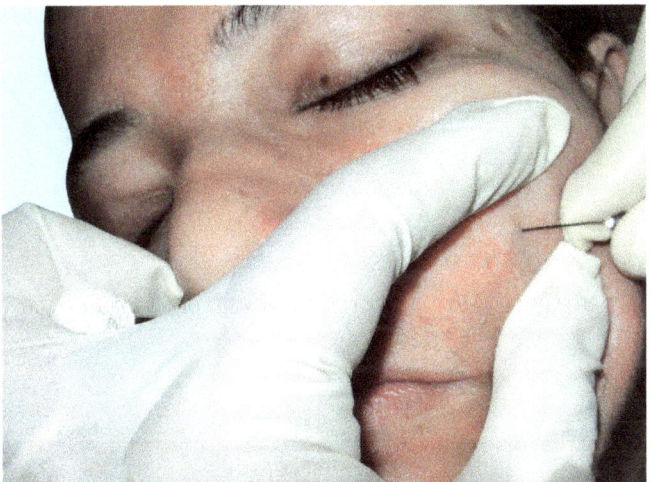

Fig. 3: Traditional subcision.

- The needle should remain parallel to the skin surface.
- The depth of insertion should be superficial to mid dermis. A grating sound will be heard as the fibrous strands are cut.
- *Modification*—when the needle is introduced straight in the manner described above, there is a risk of going deeper or penetrating the skin superficially. To obviate this, a modification has been described by the author that

prevents these complications.[7] Before insertion, the needle is bent at right angles at the bevel or slightly higher with the help of a sterile artery forceps, and then introduced in the skin **(Figs. 4A to F)**. In this way, insertion is quick and the same plane is preserved in the dermis, parallel to the skin surface. This reduces the chances of complications of piercing the skin superficially or going deeper.

- In a further modification, if the needle is again bent at a right angle and mounted on a syringe, the procedure becomes more comfortable **(Figs. 5A to D)**.
- The endpoint of the procedure is a visible lifting up of the scar surface and absence of resistance when the needle is moved in a sweeping or rotatory motion.

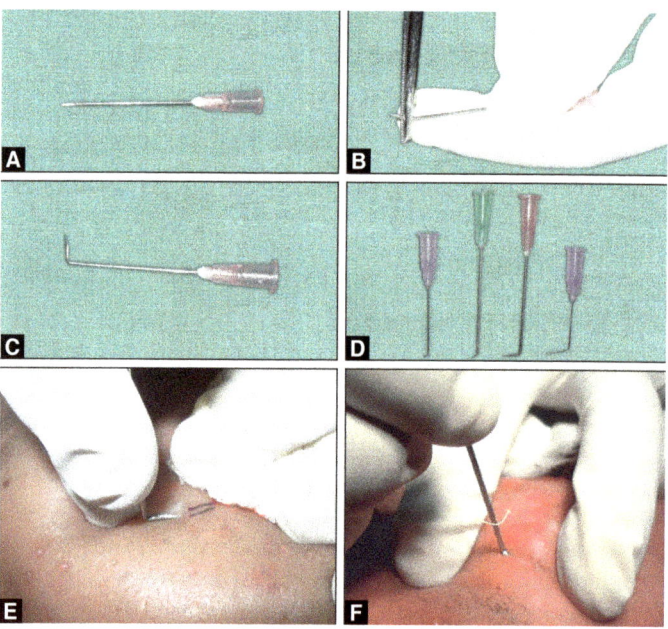

Figs. 4A to F: (A to D) Modification of the needle for subcision; (E and F) Modified subcision.

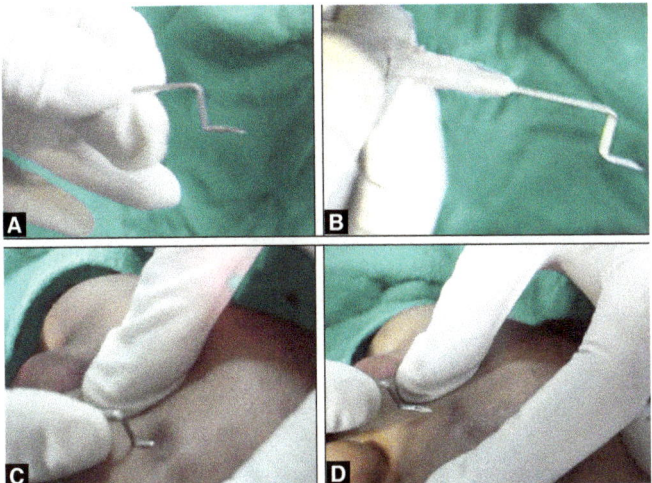

Figs. 5A to D: Further modification with mounting on a syringe for a better grip.

- If the scar is very large, multiple entry points may be used to cover the entire scar.
- Subcision can also be done as an aggressive procedure treating the entire cheek and not individual scars. Though this may be more effective in a single session, the risk of complications is also higher. Hematoma and fibrotic nodules may occur more commonly.
- The scars in the dependent area are subcised first as bleeding can obscure vision.
- All the scars are thus subcised individually, one by one. Firm pressure is given after the procedure for at least 5 minutes to stop bleeding and to prevent the formation of a large hematoma or bruise.
- The subcision should not be deep and great care should be taken to avoid injury to bigger vessels.

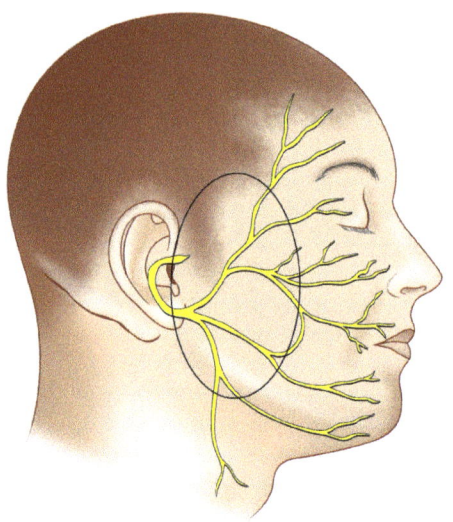

Fig. 6: Danger areas of subcision.

TABLE 1: Danger areas of subcision.		
Danger area	Nerve injured	Effect
Temporal	Temporal branch of facial nerve	• Brow ptosis—inability to frown • Reduced ability to close eyes tightly
Mandible	Marginal mandibular branch of facial nerve	Asymmetric smile

- The danger areas are the temporal and preauricular areas as the branches of the facial nerve are superficial and can be injured **(Fig. 6)**.
  Care should also be taken in the mandibular area because here the vessels are superficial **(Table 1)**. Any injury usually recovers spontaneously in 6 months.
- A topical antibiotic is applied after the procedure.

POSTPROCEDURE CARE

No special care is necessary. Topical antibiotics are advised. If there is excessive swelling, anti-inflammatory drugs may be given. If there is excessive bruising, Thrombophob® ointment may be applied. Sun exposure should be avoided in patients prone to postinflammatory hyperpigmentation (PIH).

EFFICACY

The efficacy varies between 15 and 80%.[4,6] Initial improvement is more because of edema. This is often followed by a reduction in improvement because of resorption of the edema. Hence, the procedure has to be repeated **(Figs. 7A and B)**. It can be repeated every 2–4 weeks till optimum response. Subcision has been combined with suction to make it more efficacious.[8] In a study, the protocol followed was that first subcision was done with a 23 gauge needle, followed by suctioning on the third day after subcision for flat and depressed subcised scars. Suction was performed with the handpiece of a microdermabrasion device and continued at least every other day for 2 weeks.

Better improvement was seen in patients who had suction done daily as compared to the group, who had suction done irregularly. The authors concluded that to have the best effect suction should be started on the third day of subcision,

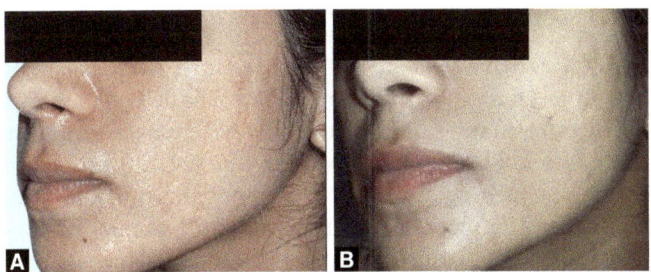

Figs. 7A and B: Subcision combined with suction and microneedling every 2 weeks.

continued daily for 1 week and then alternate day for 1 week. Subcision has also been performed with an 18 gauge spinal needle cannula with the authors reporting fewer sessions and side effects.[9] When compared with other methods, subcision was as effective or better than chemical reconstruction of skin scars (CROSS) technique for rolling scars with a lower incidence of complications. When compared to fillers, it was equally efficacious.[10]

COMPLICATIONS

Generally, subcision is a safe procedure and complications are rare. Bruising and swelling is common, if the subcision is done vigorously or a blood vessel is pierced. This can last for 1–2 weeks **(Fig. 8)**.

If it persists, it is drained by piercing with a no. 24 gauge needle. Pustules or cysts may occur if there is secondary infection. These should be drained with no. 24 gauge needle and systemic antibiotics should be given. Persistent nodules may rarely occur due to excessive fibrosis. If these do not reduce by 4 weeks, intralesional triamcinolone 2.5 mg/mL can be injected. If there is excessive inflammation, PIH can occur in darker skin patients.

Combination Treatment

Subcision can be combined with other treatments for acne scars to increase efficacy of the procedure, such as CROSS technique, punch excision, and fractional CO_2 laser. This can be done in the same session or at different sessions. The subcision is done first, followed by the second procedure when the bleeding subsides. A study comparing subcision combined with fractional CO_2 laser with the laser alone, found better efficacy with the combination treatment. However, side effects such as bruising and hyperpigmentation were seen in the combination treatment side.[11]

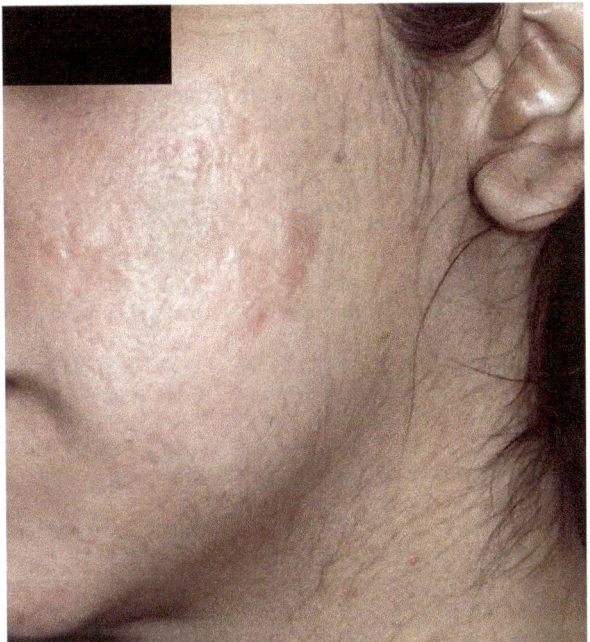

Fig. 8: Bruising and nodule formation 1 week after subcision.

CONCLUSION

Subcision is a safe and effective procedure for the treatment of depressed scars that can be carried out as a simple office procedure.

REFERENCES

1. Khunger N; IADVL Task Force. Standard guidelines of care for acne surgery. Indian J Dermatol Venereol Leprol. 2008;74(Suppl):S28-36.
2. Spangler AS. New treatment for pitted scar; preliminary report. AMA Arch Derm. 1957;76(6):708-11.
3. Orentreich DS, Orentreich N. Subcutaneous incisionless (subcision) surgery for the correction of depressed scars and wrinkles. Dermatol Surg. 1995;21(6):543-9.

4. Alam M, Omura N, Kaminer MS. Subcision for acne scarring: technique and outcomes in 40 patients. Dermatol Surg. 2005; 31(3):310-7.
5. Vaishnani JB. Subcision in rolling acne scars with 24G needle. Indian J Dermatol Venereol Leprol. 2008;74(6):677-9.
6. Chandrashekhar BS, Nandini AS. Acne scar subcision. J Cut Aesth Surg. 2010;3(2):125-6.
7. Khunger N, Khunger M. Subcision for depressed facial scars made easy using a simple modification. Dermatol Surg. 2011;37(4):514-7.
8. Harandi SA, Balighi K, Lajevardi V, Akbari E. Subcision-suction method: a new successful combination therapy in treatment of atrophic acne scars and other depressed scars. J Eur Acad Dermatol Venereol. 2011;25(1):92-9.
9. Nilforoushzadeh M, Lotfi E, Nickkholgh E, Salehi B, Shokrani M. Can subcision with the cannula be an acceptable alternative method in treatment of acne scars? Med Arch. 2015;69(6):384-6.
10. Ramadan SA, El-Komy MH, Bassiouny DA, El-Tobshy SA. Subcision versus 100% trichloroacetic acid in the treatment of rolling acne scars. Dermatol Surg. 2011;37(5):626-33.
11. Nilforoushzadeh MA, Faghihi G, Jaffary F, Haftbaradaran E, Hoseini SM, Mazaheri N. Fractional carbon dioxide laser and its combination with subcision in improving atrophic acne scars. Adv Biomed Res. 2017;6:20.

CHAPTER 9

Punch Excision Techniques

Niti Khunger

IN A NUTSHELL

- Punch excision techniques are utilized for deep punched out and boxcar scars.
- If the surface texture of the scar is relatively normal, punch elevation can be done.
- If the surface texture is abnormal, punch excision followed by punch grafting should be done.
- If the scar is wide >3.5 mm in diameter, punch excision followed by suturing is better.
- Punch excision technique should be followed by resurfacing for optimal result.

INTRODUCTION

Punch excision techniques are invaluable simple techniques for the treatment of deep depressed and large acne scars. The basic principle of excision techniques is to replace a prominent scar with a less obvious scar. There are various techniques of punch excision and the selection of technique depends on the type of scar. They can be combined with resurfacing techniques, either at the same session or at a later session to optimize results.

EQUIPMENT

- Disposable biopsy punches of various sizes—1.0, 1.5, 2.0, 2.5, 3.0, 3.5, 4.0, 4.5, and 5.0 mm

- Fine atraumatic or jewelers forceps
- Iris scissors
- Sterile Petri dish or stainless steel bowls for holding the grafts
- Needle holder
- Skin sutures 6-0 Prolene®
- Surgical glue or Steri-Strips®
- Local anesthesia lignocaine 1% with adrenaline
- Spirit and povidone-iodine for surgical cleansing
- Surgical marking pen.

INDICATIONS

Punch excision techniques are utilized for the treatment of deep depressed scars **(Table 1)**. They are particularly useful when the depth of the scars is more than what can be safely treated with resurfacing techniques, which is deep reticular dermis. They are most valuable for punched out scars with sharp walls that are adherent at the base and cannot be treated with resurfacing or fillers. When acne scarring involves large contiguous areas of the face or there are bridging scars with trapped sebum in the tunnels, or scars with persistent cysts, or the skin is lax and loose, elliptical excision followed by suturing in the direction of the relaxed skin tension lines (RSTL) is the best option. It may also be used cautiously in resistant hypertrophic or keloidal scars that are not responsive to intralesional steroids (ILS). In this case, excision should always be followed by ILS to prevent recurrence.

RELATIVE CONTRAINDICATIONS

- Patients with history of poor wound healing
- Patients with history of abnormal scarring
- Patients on isotretinoin in the last 6 months; should be done cautiously
- Patient with unrealistic expectations
- Patients with active nodulocystic acne.

TABLE 1: Excision techniques for acne scars.

Technique	Utility	Advantage	Complication
Punch elevation (flotation)	Depressed small scars <4 mm with normal surface texture, ice pick scars, and deep boxcar scars	Simple technique, no scarring, good color matching, and excellent quick procedure	• Ring scar, partial improvement due to sinking of the floating graft, and punch displacement • Cobblestoning
Punch excision and suturing	• Depressed scars >4 mm with abnormal surface texture • Deep boxcar scars	Round or irregular depressed scar replaced by a linear scar, simple procedure, and quick	Scar can widen; scars that are too close to each other cannot be treated at the same session
Punch excision and grafting	Depressed scars with abnormal surface texture <4 mm in diameter, ice pick scars, deep boxcar scars, hypertrophic and keloidal scars not responding to ILS	Atrophic scars can be treated adequately	• Color mismatch • Cobblestoning and scarring at donor site
Elliptical excision	• Large contiguous areas of atrophic scarring • Bridging scars • Skin laxity	Can be used for severe atrophic and bridging cars	Linear scars

(ILS: intralesional steroids)

PREPROCEDURE ASSESSMENT AND PREPARATION

Assess the patient for contraindications.

Counsel the patient about the degree of improvement expected, requirement of more than one procedure if scars are numerous and the necessity of a resurfacing technique to optimize results. If the scars are numerous and closely placed, all scars cannot be treated at the same time. Hence, more than one procedure may be required. The time interval is usually 4-6 weeks between the procedures. These excision techniques have to be complemented with a resurfacing procedure. This may be mechanical by dermabrasion or by a fractional resurfacing laser. The improvement expected is generally 60-70%, depending on the initial severity. It is usually not possible to eliminate all scars entirely.

Each scar should be assessed individually with attention to the surface, size, depth, and shape. Subcision can be done either by preceding the revision techniques or at the same session.

PROCEDURE[1,2]

Informed consent and photographs of the patient should be taken.

The size, shape, depth, and surface of each scar is assessed and the type of procedure to be undertaken is selected and noted. When there are multiple scars, it is advisable to first treat the scars that are most bothersome to the patient. These can be marked by asking the patient.

After surgical cleansing with spirit, povidone-iodine and again spirit, the scars are marked with marking ink with the patient in the sitting position. Some scars may get effaced or less noticeable with the patient lying down.

Local anesthesia, either with topical eutectic mixture of local anesthetics under occlusion for 2 hours prior, or infiltration with 1% lignocaine with adrenaline is used. Sedative can be given for an apprehensive patient. Nerve blocks can be given for multiple scars over extensive areas.

Subcision: Subcision is first done with a sterile no. 18 or 20 needle with the bevel pointing upwards and angulated as described. A Nokor needle may be used alternatively.

Punch elevation: If overlying skin is relatively normal, an appropriate size punch that exactly fits into the scar is selected and introduced up to the subcutaneous tissue. A sudden give will be felt once the subcutaneous tissue is reached. The excised punch is raised to the surface, without cutting at the base. It should be neither raised nor depressed. It can be manipulated upward with the tip of the needle **(Figs. 1A and B)**. The grafts are fixed with surgical glue or Steri-Strips.®

Punch closure: If there are few sharply punched out scars spaced apart from each other, or large scars 4 mm or more in diameter, they are excised and sutured along the RSTL with 5-0 or 6-0 Prolene® **(Figs. 2A to D)**.

Punch grafting: If scars are close to each other, surface and texture is atrophic and <4 mm in diameter, they are excised and replaced by punch grafts taken from either the postauricular area or gluteal area. Care should be taken that they are flush with the surface and snugly fitting. Too large a graft will pop up and cause cobblestoning and too small a graft will get depressed and heal with a ring-like scar.

Abraded punch grafting: In this technique, the epidermis at the donor site is first abraded with a motorized dermabrader. Then, punch grafts of the required size are harvested. In the recipient site, the entire affected area of acne scars is abraded.

The abraded donor grafts are then placed in recipient punched out sites. The advantage of this technique is that there is better color matching as the regenerating epidermis covers the grafted site and the area in between uniformly. There are reduced chances of cobblestoning and ring scar formation. In addition, duration of treatment is shortened as the procedure of grafting and resurfacing is carried out at one sitting **(Figs. 3A to F)**.

Dressing: A nonadherent dressing, either chlorhexidine gauze (Bactigras®) or paraffin gauze or semipermeable dressing such

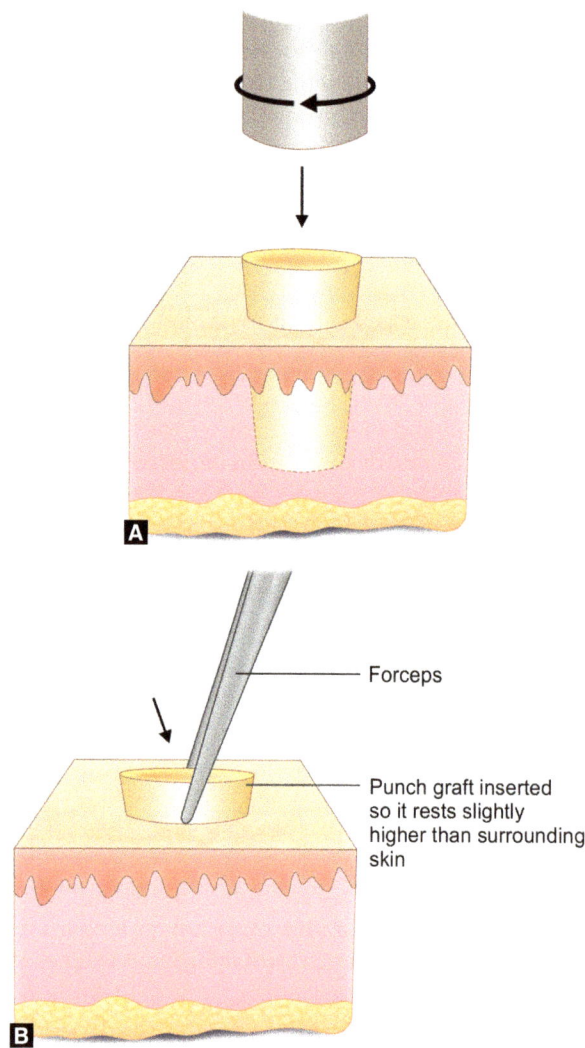

Figs. 1A and B: Principles of punch elevation.

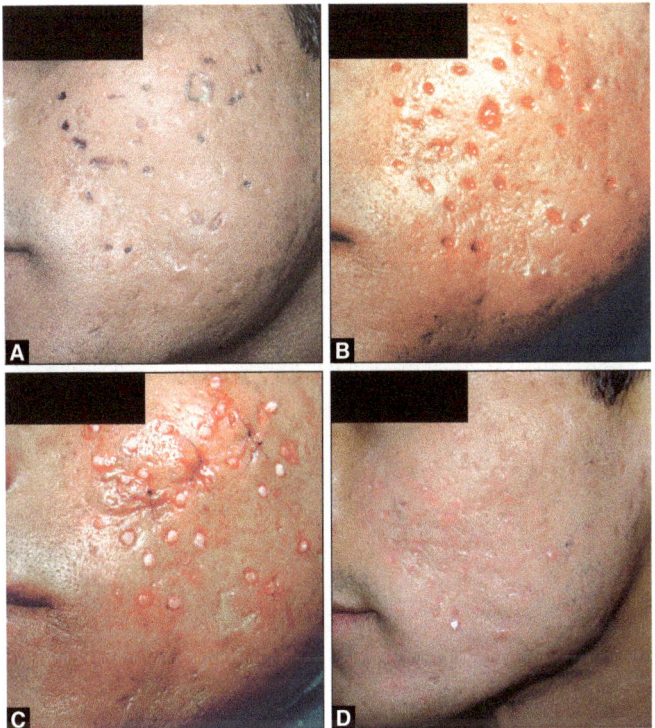

Figs. 2A to D: Punch grafting and punch excision followed by suturing.

as Vigilon or Tegaderm is used to cover the wound. Broad-spectrum antibiotics are given for 1 week.

POSTPROCEDURE CARE

The dressing is removed gently, after wetting with normal saline after 3–7 days. Care should be taken so that the grafts are not pulled out.

The priming regimen is restarted after re-epithelialization according to patient requirement.

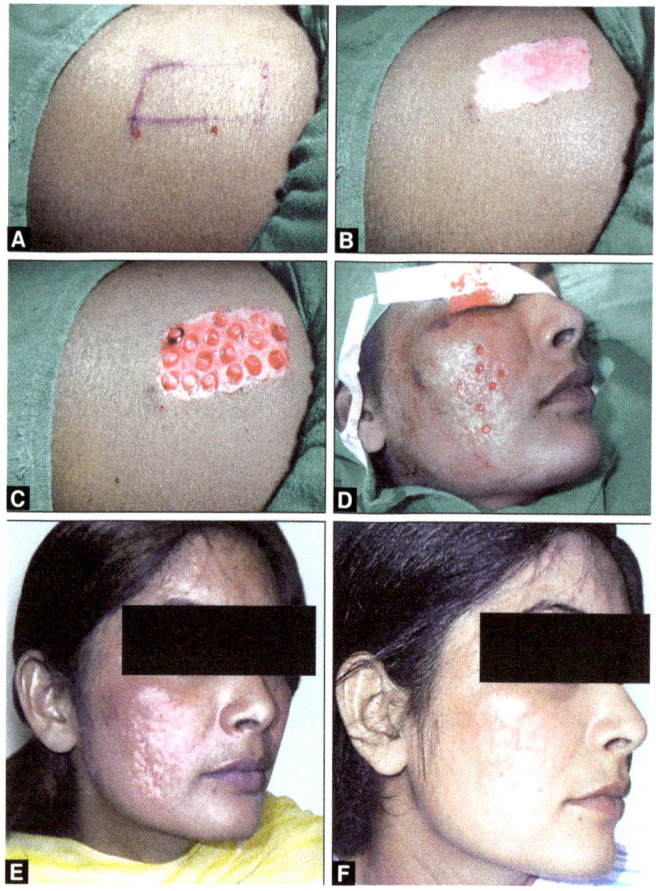

Figs. 3A to F: Abraded punch grafting. (A) Marking of donor site on the gluteal region; (B) Dermabrasion of the epidermis; (C) Punch excision of donor grafts; (D) Punch excision at recipient site; (E) One month after the procedure; (F) Three months after the procedure.

In severe scarring, the procedures of subcision and punch excision techniques may be repeated after 4-6 weeks, before resurfacing for better cosmetic results.

Resurfacing is done mechanically using a diamond fraise attached to a dermabrader or with a fractional CO_2 or fractional Er:YAG laser, according to the equipment available and expertise of the surgeon. It may be done in the same sitting or after 4–6 weeks.

COMPLICATIONS

- Poor graft uptake
- Graft extrusion
- Worsening of depression if elevated or grafted scar is extruded out
- Partial improvement with persisting depression
- Widening of the scar
- Ring-shaped scars (depressed grooves around the margins of the grafts) **(Fig. 4)**. Spot resurfacing is required for improvement.

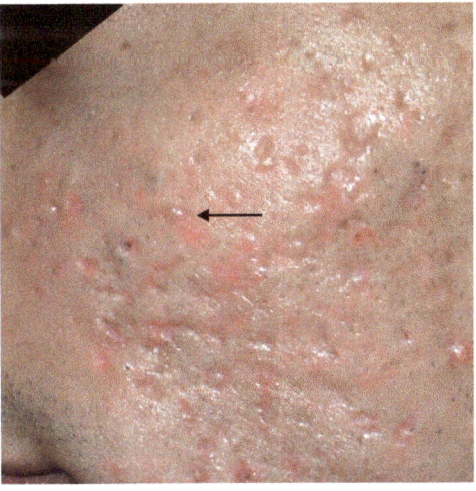

Fig. 4: Ring scars.

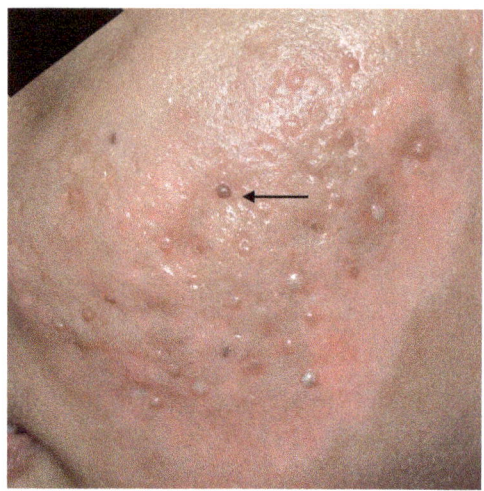

Fig. 5: Elevated scars following punch grafting.

- Elevated scars **(Fig. 5)**. Flattening the scars with radiofrequency ablation.
- Cobblestoning **(Fig. 6)**
- Color or texture mismatch in punch grafting **(Figs. 7A to D)**
- Persistent hyperpigmentation of the grafts **(Figs. 5 and 7C)**.

Complications of punch excision can be avoided by selecting the right technique according to the type of scar. The technique selected depends on the type of scars. Punch excision with elevation should be done only if the surface texture and color of the scar is normal. Underlying adhesions should be broken and it should be sufficiently elevated for a satisfactory response. While excising the scar, care should be taken to preserve as much subcutaneous tissue as possible to act as an anchoring foundation. Attention should be paid to meticulous technique and postoperative dressing and care. Precise suturing technique and use of Steri-Strips® (3M Corp., St. Paul, MN) or surgical glue for up to 7–10 days following the procedure can prevent scar spread. Where there are large

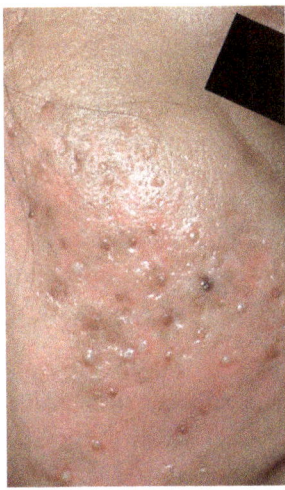

Fig. 6: Cobblestoning following punch grafting.

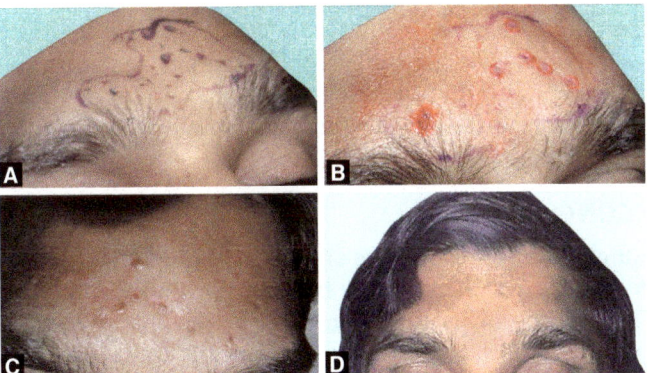

Figs. 7A to D: Color mismatch followed by improvement. (A) Marking of scars; (B) Punch grafts placed at recipient site; (C) Hyperpigmentation and elevation of grafts; (D) Spontaneous improvement at 3 months.

areas of scarring, it is better to avoid large excisions, which will give rise to longer linear scars. A series of small excisions will give better results performed at 4–6 weeks' intervals.

When removing the dressing, it is important to use very gentle traction. Wetting the site with saline for 10-15 minutes before change of dressing prevents detachment or extrusion of the graft. The risk of ring scars or depressed borders around the grafts or depression or elevation of the grafts themselves can be minimized by ensuring that the graft is slightly larger in diameter than the recipient site. Patients should be advised not to touch or press their graft sites and to minimize facial movements, talking, smiling, and chewing for the 3 days following the procedure.

PROS AND CONS

Punch excision and grafting is a simple office procedure as all dermatologists have an expertise in punch biopsy techniques. The advantage of these procedures is that it can lead to an instant "lift" of deep depressed scars. The surrounding normal skin is spared, hence healing is faster and there are fewer complications.

The disadvantage is that cobblestoning, ring scars, and hyperpigmentation in darker skins are common. Hence, fractional resurfacing following punch excision technique is usually required to optimize results.

CONCLUSION

Punch excision techniques are essential in the treatment of deep scars, which cannot be improved by resurfacing alone. They provide an instant "lift" to punched out boxcar scars and are also beneficial in larger ice pick scars. It is essential to select the correct size of the punch along with the right technique.

REFERENCES

1. Khunger N. Standard guidelines of care for acne surgery. Indian J Dermatol Venereol Leprol. 2008;74(Suppl):S28-36.
2. Savant SS. Acne and its scars. In: Savant SS (Ed). Textbook of Dermatosurgery and Cosmetology, 2nd edition. Mumbai, India: ASCAD; 2005. pp. 568-72.

CHAPTER 10

Microneedling

Jaishree Sharad

IN A NUTSHELL

- ❖ Microneedling is a minimally invasive treatment for acne scars.
- ❖ It is mainly useful for rolling, linear, and shallow boxcar scars.
- ❖ The instrument with needles attached on a drum is rolled over the skin.
- ❖ Microneedling causes dermal stimulation with increased dermal collagenization.
- ❖ Multiple sessions are done at intervals of 4–6 weeks.
- ❖ It is safe for all skin types.

INTRODUCTION

Microneedling is a relatively new and novel technique in the armamentarium of acne scar management. Skin needling has been used since 1995 to achieve percutaneous collagen induction (PCI). It is an effective method for treating acne scars (grades 2-3)[1] and other skin lesions. In 1995, Orentreich and Orentreich[2] described "subcision" with a needle to build connective tissue beneath retracted scars and wrinkles. Camirand and Doucet[3] treated scars with a tattoo gun to "needle abrade" them. Although this technique could be used on extensive areas, it was laboriously slow, and the holes in the epidermis were too close and too shallow. All these techniques worked because the needles disrupted old collagen strands in the upper dermis and induced new collagen formation.

PRINCIPLE OF MICRONEEDLING[4]

Microneedling involves the use of a handheld rolling instrument with tiny needles which create multiple superficial puncture wounds in the skin. Depending on the length of the needles, the needles penetrate into the dermis and initiate a complex chemical cascade including numerous growth factors, such as fibroblast growth factor, platelet-derived growth factor, and transforming growth factors alpha and beta, which result in an invasion of fibroblasts. This surge of activity inevitably leads to the production of more collagen and elastin by the fibroblasts. Keratinocytes migrate across the epidermal defect and proliferate, thickening the epidermis. Five days after the injury, a fibronectin matrix is laid down along the axis in which fibroblasts are aligned and collagen is deposited in the upper dermis just below the basal layer of the epidermis. Collagen type III is the dominant form in the early wound-healing phase. Tissue remodeling continues for months after the injury and is accomplished primarily by the fibroblast. Collagen type III is gradually replaced by collagen I over a period of a year or more.[4]

It has also been postulated that the body reacts to any epithelial injury with electrical signals that control a cascade of wound healing mechanisms. Under normal conditions, the interior of skin cells have a resting electrical potential of −70 mV. The extracellular space as well as the skin's surface is charged positively. If an epithelial injury occurs, the skin cells release potassium and proteins that in return changes the conductivity of the interstitium. At the same time, the inner cellular current increases dramatically to −120 mV and more. This potential difference forces fibroblast to migrate to the point of injury and finally forces them to proliferate and transform into collagen fibers.[5]

INSTRUMENTS

A standard microneedling device is made of plastic with a 12 cm handle that holds a drum-shaped cylinder at the end, similar to a small paint roller, 2 cm in diameter and 2 cm in width. The surface of the cylinder holds medical-grade stainless steel needles, the number of which ranges from 192 to 540 **(Fig. 1A)**. The needles come in varied lengths ranging from 0.5 to 2 mm, which control the depth of penetration. The one with a length of 1.5 mm serves best for acne scars. Needles have a radial arrangement of 15° in relation to the roller center in order to help in uniform depth of penetration. Depending on the applied pressure, the needles penetrated the scar tissue to a depth of 0.1–1.3 mm.

The other microneedling device which is gaining more popularity now is the electric-powered pen. This is available as the dermapen® **(Fig. 1B)** or dermapin. It can be either operated with an alternating current power cord or a battery pack. When used with corded power, the device speed can be adjusted ranging from 10,250 to 23,750 rpm. With battery power, the device speed is fixed at 13,500 rpm. Sterile disposable needle cartridges are made of 12 array count/32 gauge and 36 array count/30 gauge. Skin on the forehead is treated with needle depths ranging from 0.5 to 1.0 mm, whereas on the rest of the

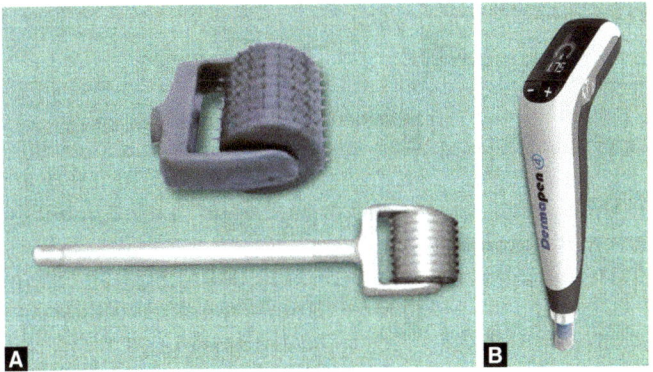

Figs. 1A and B: (A) Microneedling instrument—roller; (B) Dermapen®.

face, needle depths of 1.5–3.0 mm are preferred. Thicker or more fibrotic skin is usually treated with deeper needle depths.[6]

Variations in the Instrument[7]

- The needles in dermarollers are mostly made of medical-grade stainless steel, but some instruments have needles made of titanium or gold coating that are believed to be less traumatic and safer than the uncoated. High ratio of tip length versus diameter of 13:1 is an important property of good needles.
- *Automated rollers:* Instruments with disposable heads and hence can be used for many patients. They are battery driven.
- Instruments with a vibration mode to reduce pain.
- *Scalp rollers:* They have titanium needles unlike stainless steel rollers and are used to treat thinning hair.
- Instruments with a light-emitting diode (LED) photon light attached, mainly used for scarring and wrinkles. However, no published data is available regarding its efficacy. The various lights available are 405 nm blue, 633 nm red, 590 nm yellow, and 560 nm green.
- *Homecare dermarollers:* The needle size is <0.15 mm in length. They are used for treatment of open pores, fine lines, cellulite, and stretch marks, and to reduce sebum production. They are also used for transdermal delivery of substances such as lipopeptides and other antiaging products. They can be used twice a week for up to 100 times. After use, the rollers have to be cleaned in hot tap water and shaken dry.
- *Dermastamp:* They are the miniature versions of the Dermaroller® with diameter of 0.12 mm and needle length varying from 0.2 to 3 mm. They are used for localized scars (e.g. varicella scars) and wrinkles. The procedure with the dermastamp can be performed in 2 minutes.

- *Dermapen*: It is an automated microneedling device which looks like a pen. This ergonomic device makes use of disposable needles and guides to adjust needle length for fractional mechanical resurfacing. It has 9–12 needles arranged in rows. It makes use of a rechargeable battery to operate in two modes, namely, the high speed mode (700 cycles/min) and the low speed mode (412 cycles/min) in a vibrating stamp-like manner. The needles are disposable and hence it is reusable. It is safe as the needle tips are hidden inside the guide, and more convenient to treat narrow areas such as the nose, around the eyes and lips without damaging the adjoining skin.
- *DermaFrac*: It is a newer modification of microneedling combining microdermabrasion, microneedling, simultaneous deep tissue serum infusion, and LED. It can be used for acne, uneven skin tone, fine lines and wrinkles, open pores, and photodamaged skin. It is noninvasive and cost-effective with less down time with individualized selection of serums for infusion.
- *Microneedle (MN) delivery systems*: It is a painless method of transdermal drug administration, especially useful for vaccines.
- *Dermarollers with various types of MNs*:
    - Hollow MNs—for insertion into the skin and infusion of drug through the MN pore created.
    - Coated MNs—for deposition of active ingredient into the epidermis, followed by removal of the MN array.
    - Solid MNs—for skin pretreatment, followed by the application of an active-loaded reservoir.
    - Dissolving MNs—for delivery of active compound, incorporated into the matrix of the needles, into the skin.
    - Swellable MNs—for drug delivery through the hydrogel matrix from a drug-loaded reservoir.

Indications

Grades 2 and 3 boxcar and rolling scars and linear atrophic scars can be treated with microneedling. Microneedling can be an alternative to laser resurfacing in patients not suitable for laser treatment or wishing to have a less invasive procedure with fewer risks. It is a useful technique in patients prone to postinflammatory hyperpigmentation (PIH) as compared to lasers. In lasers, risk of PIH is higher because of the heat generated.

CONTRAINDICATIONS

Patients on anticoagulants or steroids should either be asked to stop the medication for a week or be treated with caution. Patients with verrucae, or skin infection, or any cancer should not be treated with microneedling to avoid spread of the existing disease. Microneedling should not be done in patients with history of keloids, uncontrolled diabetes, and collagen vascular disease. It is also better to avoid treating pregnant women purely for safety issues as no studies have been conducted on pregnant women. Patients with unrealistic expectations are also poor candidates.

LIMITATIONS

Minimal improvement has been seen when microneedling is performed in ice pick scars and grade 4 acne scars. Fresh scars or scars less than 1 year old respond best to this treatment. Old fibrosed scars may not show a good response.

The other limitation is the single usage of the instrument. Ideally, the instrument should be used only once as the needles have sharp and delicate tips which may become blunt after a single use. Blunt needles could lead to scarring. If you do not see any improvement in three sittings, it is advisable to switch to another treatment modality.

PRECAUTIONS

Any active infection and active acne should be treated well in advance before doing the microneedling procedure. Vitamin E, *Ginkgo biloba*, or aspirin should be stopped at least 3 days before microneedling in order to avoid bruising. Sun protection should be emphasized. Patients should be advised against picking at their skin, avoiding irritant cleansers such as chloroxylenol (Dettol® or Cetavlon) and avoiding scrubs, abrasive cleansers, and loofahs as all these habits may inadvertently lead to PIH during the healing period. If there is a past history of herpes simplex, it is important to give a course of oral acyclovir to the patient before microneedling is done. Never use the same instrument for more than one patient.

Priming a patient before any treatment is extremely important. It may be worthwhile to put the patient on topical clindamycin gel for about 2 weeks before doing the microneedling procedure, if there is a history of acne occurring occasionally. PIH could be a major concern in the Indian skin or skin types III–V. Hence, sun protection should be emphasized and topical skin lightening agents such as kojic acid, hydroquinone, and retinoic acid should be advocated for at least 2 weeks before the procedure.

Though it is said that isotretinoin should be stopped 6 months before any surgical procedure, it has been seen by experts that microneedling done when the patient is on a low dose, isotretinoin does not produce any side effects.

PREPROCEDURE PREPARATION

On the day of the treatment, written informed consent must be taken. Photographs should be taken both in front view and side profile with a standard camera and good light. Once this is done, cleanse the skin and apply topical anesthesia in the form of a eutectic mixture of 2.5% lidocaine and 2.5% prilocaine under occlusion. After an hour, remove the anesthetic cream with acetone. Cleanse the area with chlorhexidine, povidone-iodine, and isopropyl alcohol solutions. Normal saline is used as the final cleanser to prevent any irritation.

TECHNIQUE

With one hand, stretch the skin to be treated. With the other hand, grip the roller like a pen and roll it on the skin. By stretching the skin, the scars become flatter and this helps in reaching greater scar depth. Roll the instrument backward and forward 6-10 times in four directions horizontally, vertically, and diagonally right and left to cover an area of roughly 2 × 2 inches **(Fig. 2A)**. This ensures an even pricking pattern, resulting in about 250-300 pricks/cm^2. Roll until uniform pinpoint bleeding is seen which is taken as the clinical endpoint **(Fig. 2B)**. Keep the movements short in order to assure a more uniform depth of penetration.

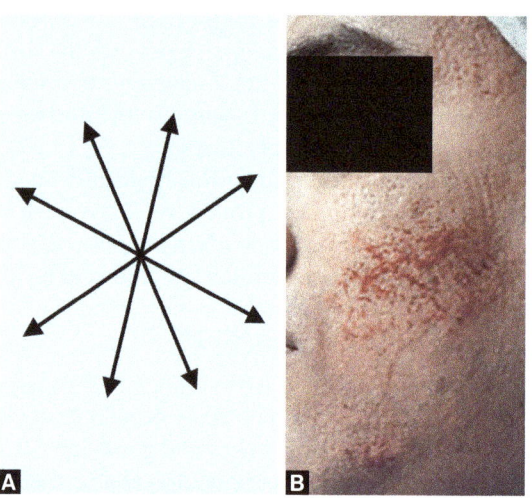

Figs. 2A and B: (A) Uniform direction of movement of roller; (B) Endpoint of microneedling is pinpoint bleeding.

The technique is operator dependent and therefore the depth of penetration depends on the pressure applied. Since the needles are sharp and penetrate the skin easily, only a moderate pressure is required. Aggressive rolling or lateral pressure can lead to scarring. Less pressure is required over bony areas such as the forehead and nose. It is advisable to use a roller with 0.5 mm length and apply mild pressure while treating the orbital region in order to minimize pain and prevent hematoma formation. Number of roller movements should be less in the orbital region. While treating the skin around the lips, ask the patient to clamp lips together so the vermillion borders touch. This ensures uniform treatment and leaves no skip areas.

Because the needles are set in a roller, every needle initially penetrates at an angle and then goes deeper as the roller turns. Finally, the needle is extracted at a converse angle, as it rolls into and then out of the skin for about 1.5-2 mm into the dermis.[8] The epidermis, particularly the stratum corneum, remains intact except for the miniscule holes or microchannels. These microchannels are closed within minutes after the treatment without any visible traces in the epidermis and stratum corneum. Hence, there is no profuse bleeding. The pinpoint bleeding stops immediately and there is a serous ooze which is wiped with a clean gauze soaked in normal saline.

POSTPROCEDURE CARE

A thin layer of antibacterial cream such as mupirocin may be applied to the treated areas. No dressing is required as there are no dermal injuries and the epidermal injury is minimal. There may be erythema and edema immediately after the treatment and may persist for up to 48 hours **(Fig. 3)**. Mild scabbing may occur in about 2-3 days. The scabs fall off without leaving any visible marks.

Patients should be advised to avoid sun exposure for a week to prevent PIH. A short course of systemic antibiotics may be

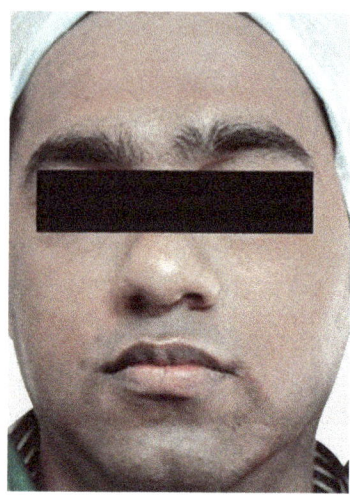

Fig. 3: Erythema postmicroneedling.

given to prevent secondary bacterial infection. The patients should be strictly advised to avoid the use of scrubs, loofahs, or any such abrasive cleansers for up to a week. There should be an interval of 6-8 weeks between two microneedling sessions to promote neocollagenesis.[9]

About 5-6 sessions are usually required to achieve cosmetically acceptable results.

Hyaluronic acid, vitamin C, tranexamic acid, and growth factors may also be applied immediately after microneedling as multiple microchannels in skin are said to increase transdermal drug penetration. However, there is no published evidence supporting their efficacy. Many patients complain that there is initially greater degree of improvement immediately after microneedling which slowly diminishes with time. This probably occurs because of postprocedure edema leading to a filling effect. When the edema gradually resolves, scars become more prominent.

In a comparative study between PCI and CROSS (chemical reconstruction of skin scars) technique for acne scars, it was reported that though there was no significant difference in efficacy between the two techniques, PCI was more efficacious in rolling acne scars, whereas CROSS was more effective in boxcar and ice pick scars.[10] PCI may also be more suitable for patients with darker skin types and those with a history of skin dyschromia because of a higher incidence of postinflammatory hyper- and hypopigmentation with 100% trichloroacetic acid (TCA) CROSS. CROSS technique also has a more prolonged downtime as compared to PCI.

In a study by Majid,[11] microneedling was performed in patients with acne scars. Good-to-excellent response was seen in rolling and boxcar scars, while pitted scars showed only moderate improvement. Deep tunnels and other complicated scars showed a poor response to treatment.

Microneedling can be combined with other treatment modalities such as peels, lasers, dermal fillers, and subcision to get better results in the treatment of acne scars.

In a study done by the author, microneedling was combined with 35% glycolic acid peel to treat acne scars in skin type III–IV. Microneedling was done once in 6 weeks. Thirty five percent glycolic acid peel was done 3 weeks after every session of microneedling. There was significant improvement in superficial and moderately deep scars. In addition, there was improvement in skin texture and reduction in postacne pigmentation[12] **(Figs. 4A to D)**. In a comparative study of three groups using GA 35% peel alone, microneedling with dermapen monotherapy and combined GA 35% peel and microneedling, significantly better results were obtained with the combination therapy.[13] Patients were treated at 2-weekly intervals for six sessions and rolling scars showed greater degree of improvement as compared to boxcar and ice pick scars.

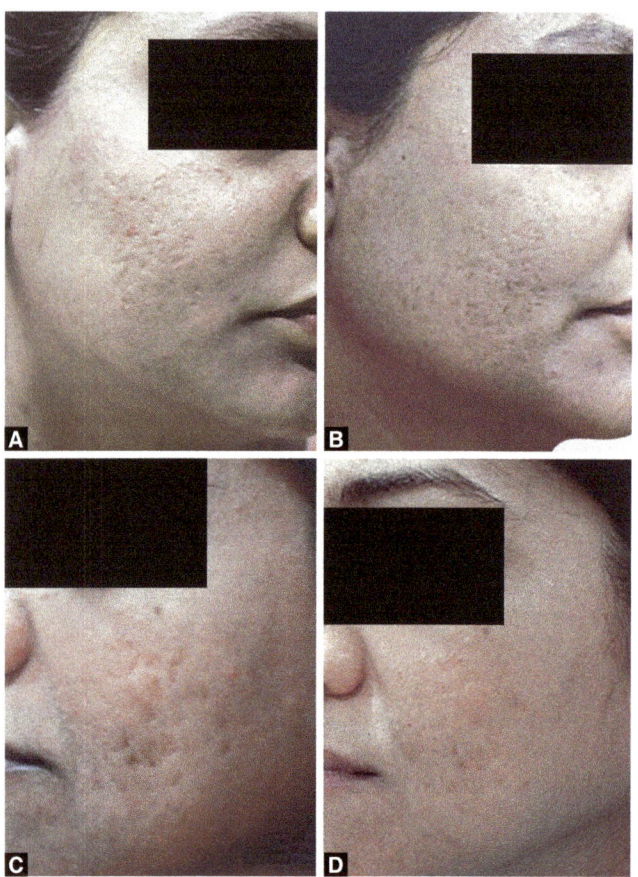

Figs. 4A to D: After three sessions of microneedling.

Fractional laser ablation with erbium or carbon dioxide laser can be combined in the same sitting with microneedling in the treatment of acne scars. However, this may lead to PIH increasing the need of postprocedure skin cooling, strict protection from sunlight, and postprocedure care. It is also advisable to avoid both the procedures at the same time in dark skinned individuals (skin types IV–VI) to avoid inadvertent PIH. There could be a 2-week interval between microneedling and fractional laser treatment in such individuals.

Advantages

- Simple office procedure
- Minimally invasive
- Safe and effective
- Minimal downtime
- Can be used in all skin types
- Can be combined with other techniques
- No expensive equipment required
- Affordable.

Disadvantages

- Slow improvement
- Requires repeated sessions
- Does not work for all scar types.

COMPLICATIONS

The procedure is well tolerated and patients usually resume their normal activities immediately after the treatment. Transient side effects such as milia, secondary bacterial infection, or PIH may be seen. The needled areas may show small bruising and mild redness for 1–2 days. Occasionally, a slight hematoma may occur on bony areas such as the dorsum of the nose or the forehead. Eventually all areas heal without a scar. There is no permanent injury to the dermis, hence the chances of severe infection and scarring are rare, unless the technique is incorrect.[14]

A tram-track appearance has been reported in one study[15] and the formation of granulomas in the other.[16]

CONCLUSION

Microneedling is a simple office procedure with minimal downtime. The recurring cost of the device is very affordable as it is a mechanical handheld device. It is safe in dark skin (skin types III–VI) as there is no thermal damage nor is the epidermis injured. The downside is that many treatment sessions are required. Secondly, all types of scars cannot be treated with microneedling.

REFERENCES

1. Goodman GJ, Baron JA. Postacne scarring: a qualitative global scarring grading system. Dermatol Surg. 2006;32(12):1458-66.
2. Orentreich DS, Orentreich N. Subcutaneous incisionless (subcision) surgery for the correction of depressed scars and wrinkles. Dermatol Surg. 1995;21(6):6543-9.
3. Camirand A, Doucet J. Needle dermabrasion. Aesthetic Plast Surg. 1997;21(1):48-51.
4. Cohen KI, Diegelmann RF, Lindbland WJ. Wound healing. Biochemical and clinical aspects. Philadelphia: WB Saunders Co; 1992. pp. 541-61.
5. Jaffe LF. Control of development by steady ionic currents. Fed Proc. 1981;40(2):125-7.
6. Alster TS, Graham PM. Microneedling: a review and practical guide. Dermatologic Surgery. 2018;44(3):397-404.
7. Sharad J. Microneedling. In: Venkataram M (Ed). ACS (I) Textbook on Cutaneous & Aesthetric Surgery. New Delhi: Jaypee Brothers Medical Publishers Pvt (Ltd); 2012. pp. 572-9.
8. Fabbrocini G, Fardella N, Monfrecola A, Proietti I, Innocenzi D. Acne scarring treatment using skin needling. Clin Exp Dermatol. 2009;34(8):874-9.
9. Doddaballapur SJ. Microneedling with dermaroller. Cutan Aesthet Surg. 2009;2(2):110-1.
10. Leheta T, El Tawdy A, Abdel Hay R, Farid S. Percutaneous collagen induction versus full-concentration trichloroacetic acid in the treatment of atrophic acne scars. Dermatol Surg. 2011;37(2):207-16.
11. Majid I. Microneedling therapy in atrophic facial scars: an objective assessment. J Cutan Aesthetic Surg. 2009;2(1):26-30.

12. Sharad J. Combination of microneedling and glycolic acid peels for the treatment of acne scars in dark skin. J Cosmet Dermatol. 2011;10(4):317-23.
13. Saadawi AN, Esawy AM, Kandeel AH, El-Sayed W. Microneedling by dermapen and glycolic acid peel for the treatment of acne scars: Comparative study. J Cosmet Dermatol. 2019;18(1):107-14.
14. Fernandes D, Signorini M. Combating photoaging with percutaneous collagen induction. Clin Dermatol. 2008;26(2):192-9.
15. Pahwa M, Pahwa P, Zaheer A. "Tram track effect" after treatment of acne scars using a microneedling device. Dermatol Surg. 2012;38 (7 Pt 1):1107-8.
16. Soltani-Arabshahi R, Wong JW, Duffy KL, Powell DL. Facial allergic granulomatous reaction and systemic hypersensitivity associated with microneedle therapy for skin rejuvenation. JAMA Dermatol. 2014;150(1):68-72.

CHAPTER 11

Microdermabrasion

Apratim Goel

IN A NUTSHELL

- ❖ Microdermabrasion is an effective modality for the treatment of superficial acne scars, but not for deep scars.
- ❖ It can be combined with superficial peels and lasers for facial rejuvenation and improvement of surface texture.
- ❖ It can be done using either crystal or diamond tips.
- ❖ It is a safe, noninvasive office procedure with minimal or no downtime.

INTRODUCTION

Microdermabrasion is a type of mechanical exfoliation or microresurfacing technique that uses a mechanical medium for exfoliation along with adjustable suction to remove the outermost layer of dead skin cells from the epidermis. It is a noninvasive procedure, which is performed in-office by a trained skin care professional.

Since its development in Italy in 1985, the procedure has gained popularity over the years as other skin resurfacing techniques are efficacious, but have the potential for significant complications. Microdermabrasion can be an effective treatment with minimal risk and rapid recovery for a variety of cosmetic conditions including mild acne scars, fine lines, hyperpigmentation and stretch marks.

PRINCIPLE

Microdermabrasion causes partial skin ablation to the level of the stratum corneum. More aggressive treatments can reach the superficial papillary dermis. The body interprets this as an injury and rushes to replace the lost skin with new and healthy cells. Thus, microdermabrasion produces clinical improvement by a mechanism resembling a reparative process at the dermal and epidermal levels. According to histopathological studies, significant epidermal and papillary dermal thickening is seen.[1,2] There is flattening of the rete ridges and thinning of the stratum corneum with homogenization. All treated areas show an increase in the basal cell activity. Collagen fibers in treated areas show hyalinization with thicker, more tightly packed, horizontally oriented collagen bundles. Improved appearance of elastic fibers and changes in microcirculation are also noted.[3]

This process has a few beneficial effects. The surface of the skin is smoother and improved. The healing process brings newer skin cells that look and feel smoother. Also, without the stratum corneum acting as a barrier, medicinal creams and lotions are more effective because of more or better absorption of active ingredients.[4,5]

INSTRUMENTS

All professional microdermabrasion machines work in basically the same way using four main components:
1. Vacuum/air pump
2. Tube
3. Wand or handpiece
4. Crystals or diamond tips.

The vacuum is the engine of the microdermabrasion machine and performs two functions. It is responsible for pumping the crystals through the tube onto the skin. Once the microdermabrasion crystals have been used, it then sucks them away from the skin and deposits them in a container which is later disposed off. The tube is the passage through which the crystals travel from the microdermabrasion machine to the handpiece. The handpiece is attached to the end of the tube and is the part of the machine that the professional holds while performing the microdermabrasion treatment. Microdermabrasion wands are usually made of steel or glass. The top of the wand is what touches the patient's skin. The microdermabrasion crystals are pumped to the skin at high speed to exfoliate the skin before being sucked away and disposed off.

How do Microdermabrasion Machines Work?

The mechanical technique of microdermabrasion uses a flow of inert microcrystals through a controlled graduated vacuum to gently ablate the skin. Particles of microcrystals are drawn, under suction, from a container and passed over the skin through a small hole at the end of the handpiece. At the same time, the skin is sucked into the handpiece under the vacuum pressure while the crystals pass over that area. Most machines use a 4-6 mm opening at the tip of the handpiece. The crystals along with dead skin cells are then collected in a reservoir and discarded. The particle flow rate and vacuum pressure determine the amount of skin contact with the particles.

Some microdermabrasion machines allow an increase in the rate and speed at which microdermabrasion crystals are delivered giving a more thorough treatment, which may be necessary in some cases. Usually, the most powerful microdermabrasion machines are only needed for severe cases of scarring and are only used by dermatologists. At beauty spas, less powerful microdermabrasion machines are seen that are suitable for the majority of cases. These are known as esthetician grade microdermabrasion machines.

Types of Microdermabrasion Machines

There are two main types of microdermabrasion machines:
1. Crystal microdermabrasion machines
2. Diamond microdermabrasion machines or crystal-free microdermabrasion.

Crystal Microdermabrasion Machines

Microdermabrasion crystals are the key ingredients in the crystal microdermabrasion process that are responsible for exfoliating facial or body skin. Crystals are loaded into cartridges or crystal jars that fit onto the microdermabrasion equipment. When the machine is turned on, the microdermabrasion crystals are fed from the cartridge into the microdermabrasion tubing, handpiece and tip until they make contact with the skin. Microdermabrasion crystals are then sucked back into the machine and deposited in another cartridge or residual crystal jar before being disposed of.

There are four types of crystals that can be used in microdermabrasion machines:
1. Aluminum oxide
2. Sodium bicarbonate
3. Sodium chloride
4. Magnesium oxide.

Aluminum oxide microdermabrasion crystals

Aluminum oxide is the most popular crystal used in microdermabrasion machines. Although aluminum oxide can come in a variety of different colors, including red and green, the crystals used in microdermabrasion are almost always white **(Figs. 1A to C)** Aluminum oxide crystals or corundum crystals as they are sometimes known to possess several special qualities which make them particularly good for microdermabrasion.

Hard: Aluminum oxide is one of the hardest known materials, second only to diamonds.

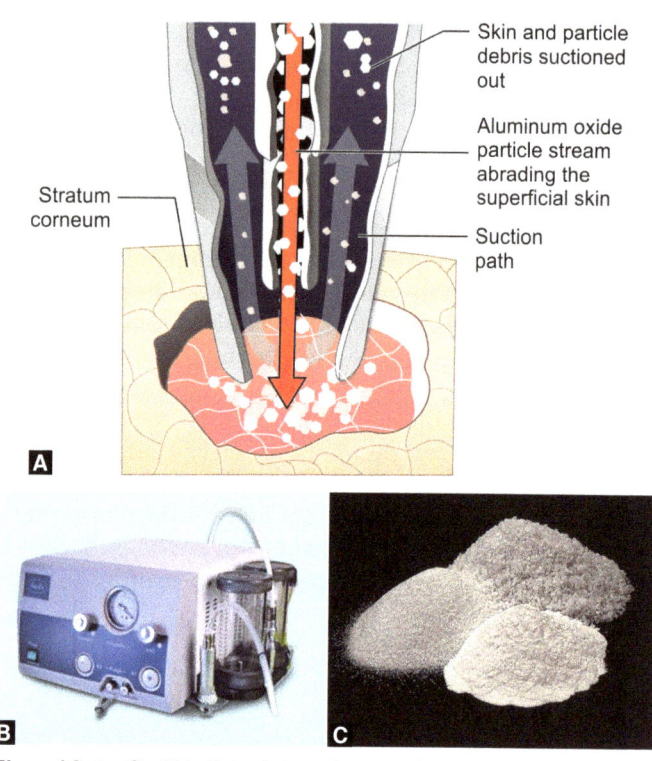

Figs. 1A to C: (A) Principle of crystal microdermabrasion; (B) Crystal microdermabrasion machine; and (C) Aluminum oxide crystals.

This hardness makes them well suited for microdermabrasion as they are strong enough to be blasted onto the skin without fragmenting.

Rough: Aluminum oxide crystals used in microdermabrasion have rough, jagged surfaces. This makes them excellent for abrading against and exfoliating the top layer of skin.

Cheap: Aluminum oxide microdermabrasion crystals are cheap which makes it easy to buy them in large quantities.

Light: Microdermabrasion crystals made from aluminum oxide are much lighter than other metallic crystals. This means they can be blasted through microdermabrasion machines easily without applying too much air pressure.

Although there has been some recent controversy in the microdermabrasion industry regarding the safety of aluminum oxide, the traditional belief has been that these microdermabrasion crystals are safe because they are nontoxic and there is no possibility of a chemical reaction with the skin. The main risk associated with aluminum oxide microdermabrasion crystals is the possibility of accidental inhalation which may cause some temporary respiratory problems. It is important to remember that only people who come into regular prolonged contact with these microdermabrasion crystals have these complaints. They can be avoided by proper precautions taken by the skincare professional such as wearing masks, gloves, etc. Patients undergoing a few sessions of microdermabrasion treatments need not worry about these risks. Patients with chronic respiratory problems may be given crystal-free microdermabrasion treatments.

Sodium bicarbonate microdermabrasion crystals
Sodium bicarbonate microdermabrasion crystals point to a number of benefits:

Organic: Sodium bicarbonate microdermabrasion crystals are organic which means it decomposes naturally once it is disposed off. This is helpful for the environment.

Water soluble: Microdermabrasion crystals made from sodium bicarbonate are water soluble. Therefore, any crystals stuck on the face after the microdermabrasion treatment can simply be washed off.

Neutral pH balance: The neutral pH balance of these microdermabrasion crystals means they will not irritate the skin. In fact, sodium bicarbonate has soothing qualities which can make the skin feel better.

No definitive comparative studies have been carried out between the different types of microdermabrasion crystals making it impossible to say which one is better.

However, the other metallic crystals are not as abrasive as aluminum oxide crystals. Being harder, aluminum oxide microdermabrasion crystals are more suitable for heavy microdermabrasion treatment such as acne scars.

Choosing the size of microdermabrasion crystals

Size is the other important factor in using microdermabrasion crystals. Crystals between 100 and 120 µm are considered good for microdermabrasion. The larger the size of microdermabrasion crystal, the more harsh the process will be. Thus, to achieve a deeper depth of exfoliation in case of acne scars, larger size of crystals may be used.

Diamond Microdermabrasion

Diamond microdermabrasion relies on micro-dermabrasion tips covered with tiny diamonds to perform skin exfoliation. When the diamond microdermabrasion tip makes contact with the skin, it abrades against the top layer pulling it off. The microdermabrasion machine then sucks the loose dead skin cells away from the face. Otherwise, diamond and crystal microdermabrasion peel procedures are exactly the same in that the treatment provider passes the wand over each area of the skin three times. One advantage of diamond crystal-free microdermabrasion is that the dead skin cells are accumulated onto a cotton filter and the operator can see exactly what was removed from the skin after the treatment is finished.

Diamond microdermabrasion tips

Microdermabrasion tips are actually thousands of tiny diamond particles which are uniformly sized. Diamond microdermabrasion machines come with an assortment of

tips of varying sizes (**Figs. 2A to D**). The appropriate diamond tip to use depends on the patient's individual skin condition:
- 100 for coarse skin
- 200 for normal skin
- 300 for sensitive skin.

Diamond microdermabrasion machines can come with anywhere between 2 and 9 different microdermabrasion tips. These tips are not disposable which means great care has to be taken in cleaning them between treatments. Diamond microdermabrasion tips are sterilized in steam, alcohol or ultraviolet light.

Compared to crystal microdermabrasion machines, diamond microdermabrasion machines are smaller in size and have a lower maintenance cost. The disadvantage is that

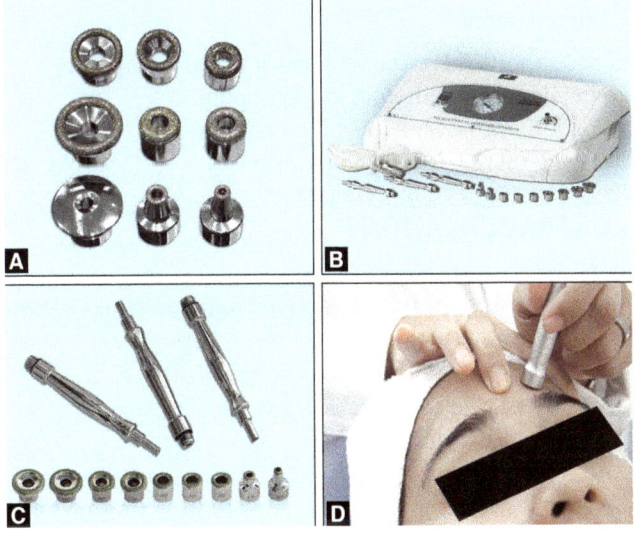

Figs. 2A to D: (A) Diamond tips suitable for microdermabrasion; (B) Microdermabrasion machine; (C) Microdermabrasion tips; and (D) Diamond peel.

since the tips are not disposable, theoretically, there is a risk of transmission of infection, if the tips are not cleaned thoroughly and sterilized.

INDICATIONS

As with all cosmetic procedures, proper patient selection is imperative. Microdermabrasion is most effective with superficial skin conditions because it produces a superficial depth of injury.[6] It is well suited for patients with busy lifestyles because the only real downtime is that of the treatment itself. Even patients with Fitzpatrick skin types IV-VI, who may be at more risk of complications with other resurfacing techniques, may be treated with relative safety.

- Superficial acne scars
- Comedones
- Dilated pores

Besides superficial postacne scars, it can also improve:
- Fine lines, mild photoaging, age spots
- Postinflammatory hyperpigmentation
- Stretch marks.

CONTRAINDICATIONS

The contraindications for microdermabrasion are similar to those for other resurfacing procedures. These relative contraindications include:
- Active herpes infection
- Malignant skin tumors
- Keloids
- Active acne
- Active rosacea
- Warts
- Erosions or ulcers
- Open cuts or wounds

- Eczema
- Psoriasis
- Lupus erythematosus
- Uncontrolled diabetes mellitus
- Evolving dermatoses, and certain keratoses
- Vascular lesions
- Recent surgery (<6 weeks) on the area to be treated
- Recent chemical peels or other resurfacing treatments.

Active herpes simplex, warts, and other lesions should be treated prior to microdermabrasion.

LIMITATIONS

Microdermabrasion produces a superficial ablation, primarily in the epidermis; therefore, this procedure is ineffective for deeper acne scars. However, for fine lines and more superficial scars, microdermabrasion can be an effective treatment with minimal risk and rapid recovery.

Patients also must be prepared for the number and frequency of treatments. If patients are unwilling to commit to a series of treatments, then they are unlikely to see significant results and will not be satisfied with the outcome. While some tightening of the skin may occur using microdermabrasion, facial contour is not significantly affected (i.e., jowling, midface ptosis, neck laxity).

PRECAUTIONS

Consultation for any resurfacing procedure should address the patient's concerns and expectations. Carefully evaluate the quality of the patient's skin for active acne, or other skin infections. Deep scars and rhytides must be distinguished from those that are superficial because greater depth of injury is required for effective treatment of the deeper lesions. If the patient has any significant upcoming event, consider this information in order to allow adequate recovery time from any resurfacing treatment. The limitations of the procedure and results expected should be clearly explained.

PREPROCEDURE PREPARATION

No premedication is necessary, unless desired. Prior to the procedure, the skin is cleaned of all makeup and oil. No topical or local anesthetic is necessary. Contact lenses are removed, and eye protection is placed to prevent injury from stray particles. Eye protection is very important to prevent stray particles from entering the eye.

TECHNIQUE

The technical key to microdermabrasion is placing the skin under tension so that an effective vacuum is achieved. Typically, stretching the treatment area with the nondominant hand and using the dominant hand to guide the handpiece is the method used to achieve this effect. When treating the neck, the neck is placed in extension to assist in skin tension.

The pressure of the crystal stream and suction pressure is adjusted as desired. The handpiece is moved over the treatment area in a single, smooth stroke. A second treatment perpendicular to the first treatment is generally performed. Thicker skin, such as that on the forehead, chin, and nose, can be treated more aggressively (i.e., adjust the speed of handpiece movement or number of passes). Decrease the pressure when treating the thinner skin, e.g., upper cheek and neck. Vertically orient all strokes when treating the neck. Between treatments, the face is cleaned of any residual crystals. The desired endpoint of treatment is erythema (**Fig. 3**). Specific areas, such as acne scars or age spots, can be focally treated more aggressively with additional passes. Treatment sessions generally last approximately 30–40 minutes for the face and neck.

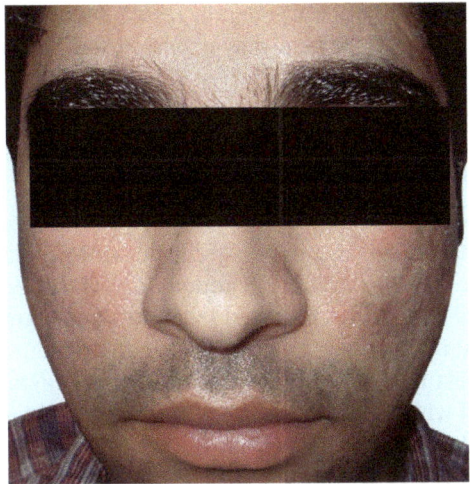

Fig. 3: Erythema after desired endpoint of microdermabrasion.

Partial skin ablation to the level of the stratum corneum is desirable. More aggressive treatments that can reach the superficial papillary dermis are required while treating acne scars. The degree of exfoliation is determined by the vacuum pressure, particle flow, the speed and movement of each pass, as well as the number of passes over a given area of skin. Repeated passes over one area, or excessive contact time on one area, may result in pinpoint bleeding, petechiae and bruising. Vacuum pressure (negative pressure) varies inversely with particle flow, and the pressure varies depending on the manufacturer.

As the vacuum pressure increases, so does the risk of bleeding and bruising.

POSTPROCEDURE CARE

The treated area is cleaned thoroughly to remove any residual crystals. A cold compress is applied to calm and soothe the skin post treatment. Erythema generally resolves within hours after treatment, but the patient may experience a mild sunburn-like sensation for a couple of days. Sunscreen should be used liberally because photosensitivity may be increased.

Follow Up

Effective microdermabrasion usually requires a series of 5-12 treatments. The series can be significantly longer, particularly with acne scarring. Initially, treatments are weekly or biweekly for several treatments, followed by monthly to biannually for maintenance treatments, depending on the patient.

The results achieved with microdermabrasion can be enhanced with medical therapies in the form of topical skin treatments. Common adjuncts to microdermabrasion include tretinoin, alpha-hydroxy acids, retinoic acid, and topical vitamin C. In patients with a tendency to hyperpigmentation, the application of hydroquinone between treatments can be useful. Liberal use of sunscreen and moisturizers is also beneficial. Postoperatively, these products serve to address exfoliation and photosensitization. Long-term benefits include reduction of sun damage and photoaging and improved skin moisture.

COMPLICATIONS

The great advantage of microdermabrasion is its relative lack of complications.

In early years of use, reports cited redness of the eyes, photophobia, and epiphora after examination by an ophthalmologist. The examination revealed conjunctival congestion, crystals adherent to the cornea, and superficial punctate keratopathy. Using eye protection virtually eliminates ocular complications, but corneal abrasion from stray crystals remains a theoretic risk. The erythema generally resolves within hours after treatment, allowing patients a rapid return to their usual activities. Scarring has not been documented from microdermabrasion, although scarring is theoretically possible when producing any injury to the skin. However, microdermabrasion barely extends through the epidermis, so the depth of injury is very superficial. This fact is both its advantage and its limitation. Superficial injury means rapid healing and recovery with little risk; however, only superficial skin conditions, such as fine lines, and shallow scars, can be treated.

CONCLUSION

In conclusion, the success rate of microdermabrasion acne scar treatment is influenced by four important factors: size, location, number and depth of the acne scars. As microdermabrasion works by exfoliating the superficial surface of the skin, it is effective in treating superficial acne scars. To eliminate deeper ice pick and other atrophic scars, other acne scarring treatments in conjunction with microdermabrasion are required.

REFERENCES

1. Spencer JM. Microdermabrasion. Am J Clin Dermatol. 2005;6(2): 89-92.
2. Freedman BM, Rueda-Pedraza E, Waddell SP. The epidermal and dermal changes associated with microdermabrasion. Dermatol Surg. 2001;27(12):1031-3.
3. Karimpour DJ, Kang S, Johnson TM, Orringer JS, Hamilton T, Hammerberg C, et al. Microdermabrasion: a molecular analysis following a single treatment. J Am Acad Dermatol. 2005;52(2): 215-23.
4. Lee WR, Shen SC, Kuo-Hsien W, Hu CH, Fang JY. Lasers and microdermabrasion enhance and control topical delivery of vitamin C. J Invest Dermatol. 2003;121(5):1118-25.
5. Rajan P, Grimes PE. Skin barrier changes induced by aluminium oxide and sodium chloride microdermabrasion. Dermatol Surg. 2002;28(5):390-3.
6. Tsai RY, Wang CN, Chan HL. Aluminum oxide crystal microdermabrasion: a new technique for treating facial scarring. Dermatol Surg. 1995;21(6):539-42.

CHAPTER 12

Lasers and Light Devices

Sanjeev Aurangabadkar

IN A NUTSHELL

- Fractional CO_2 and fractional Er:YAG lasers are most effective for atrophic acne scars.
- Fractional nonablative lasers are also effective for mild atrophic scars. They have lower downtime but require more sessions to give a significant response.
- Ideally lasers should be combined with other modalities such as subcision and chemical reconstruction of skin scars technique to give optimum results.

INTRODUCTION

Acne scarring is a commonly encountered problem in clinical practice. Though a plethora of treatment options are available, no single modality seems to be uniformly effective in all patients. The type and severity of acne scars is important as it allows one to choose the best modality or combination that will yield the best outcome in a given patient.

Rapid technological advancement has taken place in the field of lasers and light devices over the past decade, allowing better and safer treatments. Laser and light devices used in acne scarring are given in **Table 1**. Laser resurfacing includes devices employing ablative, nonablative, and fractional ablative technologies. The three approaches largely differ in their method of thermal damage, varying degrees of efficacy, downtime, and side-effect profiles.

TABLE 1: Laser and light devices used to treat acne scars.

Laser, light device and wavelength	Chromophore and mode of action	Clinical application
CO_2 laser 10,600 nm ablative and fractional CO_2	Water, nonselective tissue ablation, thermal damage and collagen shrinkage	Grade 4 atrophic and hypertrophic scars
Er:YAG 2,940 nm ablative and fractional Er:YAG	Water, nonselective ablation, minimal thermal damage	Grade 2–3 atrophic and hypertrophic scars
Er:Glass 1,540/1,550 nm nonablative fractional	Water, nonablative, columns of thermal damage in dermis	Grade 1–2 atrophic and hypertrophic acne scars
1,320/1,440-nm nonablative fractional	Water, nonablative, columns of thermal damage in dermis	Grade 1–2 atrophic and hypertrophic acne scars
Pulsed dye laser 585 nm	Selective photothermolysis; oxyhemoglobin	Hypertrophic scars and keloids, persistent erythematous macules
Intense pulsed light	Selective photothermolysis; hemoglobin, melanin	Hypertrophic scars, erythematous and hyperpigmented macular scars
Nd:YAG 1,064 nm	Hemoglobin, water	Grade 1 atrophic scars
Diode 1,450 nm	Water	Grade 1 atrophic scars

(CO_2: carbon dioxide; Er:YAG: erbium:yttrium-aluminum-garnet)

Fractional laser technology, introduced by Manstein et al. in 2004,[1] represents a major advantage over the previous conventional ablative methods [carbon dioxide (CO_2) and erbium:yttrium-aluminum-garnet (Er:YAG) lasers].

Though ablative lasers had the advantages of predictability in the depth of tissue ablation and thermal denaturation, traditional ablative laser resurfacing suffered from several disadvantages. The need for effective anesthesia, prolonged downtime, the risk of dyspigmentation and scarring particularly in darker skin types were the major downsides. The need for intensive postoperative care, the longlasting erythema and need for prolonged avoidance of sun exposure after treatment were the further disadvantages. Fractional lasers were developed to overcome these shortcomings.[2]

PRINCIPLE

The principle of selective photothermolysis postulated by Anderson and Parrish forms the basis for most of the lasers and light devices used for the treatment of acne scars.[3] According to this theory, when a wavelength that is selectively absorbed by the target chromophore is used with sufficient energy, in a pulse duration that is equal to or shorter than the thermal relaxation time of the target, thermal injury is selectively confined to the target without producing collateral thermal damage.

The fractional device delivers light in microscopic columns sparing normal skin in between, producing an array of microthermal zones (MTZs). This creates small columns of thermal injury. Fractional producing microscopic columns of thermal damage in the epidermis and dermis up to a depth of 300–400 μm in regularly space arrays over a fraction of the skin surface. This is in contrast to ablative resurfacing where the entire epidermis and part of the dermis is removed.[4]

Fractional photothermolysis, therefore, denotes induction of thermal alteration of a fraction or a column of skin, leaving intervening areas of normal skin untouched, which rapidly repopulate the ablated columns of tissue. The number, size and depth of the vertical columns can be varied depending on the type of machine used, the wavelength, fluence and the number of stacks or applications of the laser. An average of 15–25% of the skin surface is treated in a single treatment session. The resulting dermal–epidermal debris is eliminated by the phenomenon of transepidermal elimination through the MTZs of injury. Further, the degenerated dermal material is incorporated into the columns of microscopic epidermal necrotic debris (MENDs) and is shuttled up the epidermis and, ultimately, exfoliated through the stratum corneum **(Fig. 1)**.

Similar to ablative laser resurfacing, the areas of thermally ablated tissue are repopulated by fibroblast derived neocollagenesis and epidermal stem cell reproduction.

Since a major portion of intervening skin is left unaffected, healing occurs quickly, thereby reducing the downtime. At each subsequent session, such fractions are treated and in over 3–6 sittings with an interval of 4 weeks between sessions, treatment is completed.

Fractional technology is available for both ablative and nonablative lasers and both technologies have found several applications including treatment of acne scars.[5]

Though ablative laser resurfacing still remains the gold standard, fractional lasers and nonablative lasers have become more popular due to the added safety and lower downtime

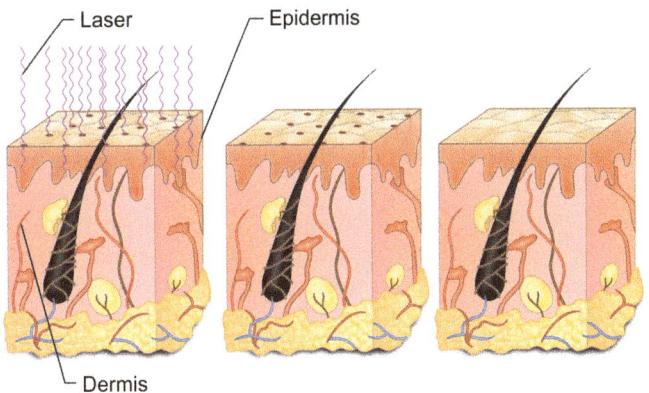

Fig. 1: Principle of fractional CO_2 laser.

with acceptable clinical results. The downside is that multiple sessions may be necessary for getting a satisfactory result as compared to a single full face laser resurfacing.

ABLATIVE CO_2 LASER RESURFACING

The carbon dioxide laser has a wavelength of 10,600 nm and its target chromophore is extracellular and intracellular water. This treatment is aggressive but remains at a specific depth of 20–30 μm with thermal damage of 50–150 μm. Treatment is usually bloodless but still achieves total ablation of the epidermis and a portion of the dermis. In addition to the ablation, there may also be stimulation of collagen by the procedure. The usefulness is primarily for hypertrophic scars, boxcar scars (preferably shallow), and, less effectively, keloids. Improvement may be seen as early as 2 weeks but may continue over a period of 18 months due to wound-healing phase. A single treatment is usually sufficient. Recovery time postprocedure is usually 1–3 months. Side effects include protracted visible healing, prolonged erythema, eczema, hyperpigmentation or hypopigmentation, milia, acne, cysts, infection, telangiectases or additional scarring. It is now rarely used because of the prolonged downtime and pigmentary alterations in dark skins and should be avoided.

ERBIUM:YAG LASER RESURFACING

At a wavelength of 2,940 nm, the Er:YAG has 16 times greater absorption in water than the CO_2 laser. The treatment with the Er:YAG laser is more gentler than the CO_2 laser but penetration is more superficial leading to less collateral thermal damage and faster healing. The downside is that it is less efficacious than the CO_2 laser with regard to dermal remodeling and collagen stimulation. Er:YAG laser is available in a short pulse, variable pulse and dual-pulsed modes. It is useful for hypertrophic scars, superficial boxcar scars and mild rolling scars. Side effects include edema, erythema, delayed healing, acne, hyperpigmentation or hypopigmentation, milia, infection, or scarring.[6]

ABLATIVE FRACTIONAL LASER RESURFACING

Fractional CO_2 Lasers

Fractional CO_2 laser treats columnar microscopic areas of the skin leaving uninvolved islands of normal skin between the treated zones. The intervening normal skin allows rapid re-epithelialization, thereby minimizing the downtime and the risk of side effects. The CO_2 lasers are available with either a computerized scanner that allows modulation in the number of dots, the spacing between the dots and the energy delivered per dot as well as the pattern of the scan or with a stamping handpiece that produces a 7 × 7 grid of pixels or dots that offers 49 pixels per 1 cm square **(Fig. 2)**. With the stamping handpiece, multiple stacks can be performed over the same

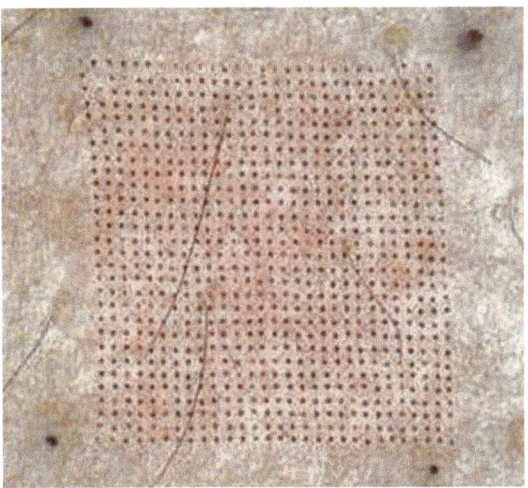

Fig. 2: Impression after stamping handpiece.

site or multiple passes can be done to cover the entire area. Treatments are usually done once a month for 2–5 sessions. The fractional CO_2 laser is useful for the treatment of mild-to-moderate acne scars, including rolling and boxcar scars[7] **(Figs. 3A and B)**. A newer modified approach using the CO_2 laser focally on the scars has been reported.[8]

The fractional lasers can be combined with other techniques such as subcision, microneedling, trichloroacetic acid (TCA) CROSS (Chemical reconstruction of skin scars, dot peels), tissue augmentation, chemical peels and microdermabrasion to enhance the efficacy and results.

Fractional Er:YAG Laser

The nonablative fractional lasers are safe in darker skin types but the clinical improvement noted in patients is often quiet subtle. The fractional ablative lasers have proven to be a safe and effective option for the treatment of acne scarring even in patients of skin of color[8] **(Figs. 4A and B)**.

The Er:YAG has a wavelength of 2,940 nm and is highly absorbed by tissue water. Fractional Er:YAG lasers have been developed that split the laser beam into micro beams that allow fractional treatment in a grid of 7×7 and/or 9×9 dots/cm^2. The 7×7 tip is used for scars whereas the 9×9 tip is used for rejuvenation.

Treatments can be delivered either by performing multiple passes or by stacking pulses, thereby increasing the depth of penetration and inducing collagen remodeling. The number of stacks used depends on the structure, topography (acne scars vs. hypertrophic scar vs. wrinkles) and the desired level of penetration, i.e., the greater the number of stacks, the higher the penetration. The laser can be used in the short (1 ms), medium (1.5 ms) or long pulse mode (2 ms). For fractional treatment of acne scars, the long pulse mode is selected during treatment. Generally, multiple sittings are performed (average of 5) at intervals of 4 weeks between sessions **(Figs. 5A and B)**.

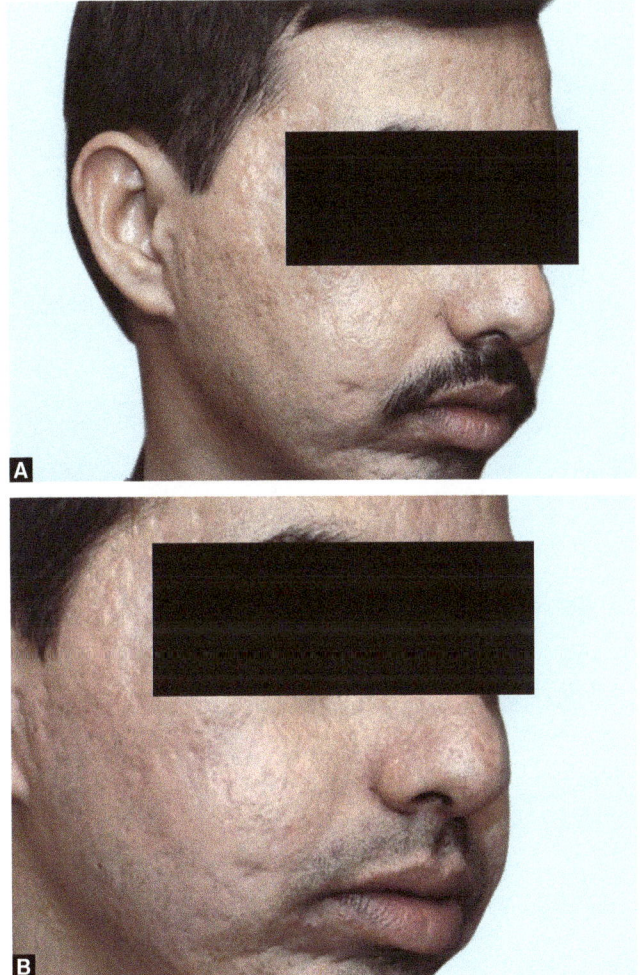

Figs. 3A and B: (A) Severe acne scarring in a skin type 4 male patient; (B) Good improvement in scarring after five fractional CO_2 laser treatments.

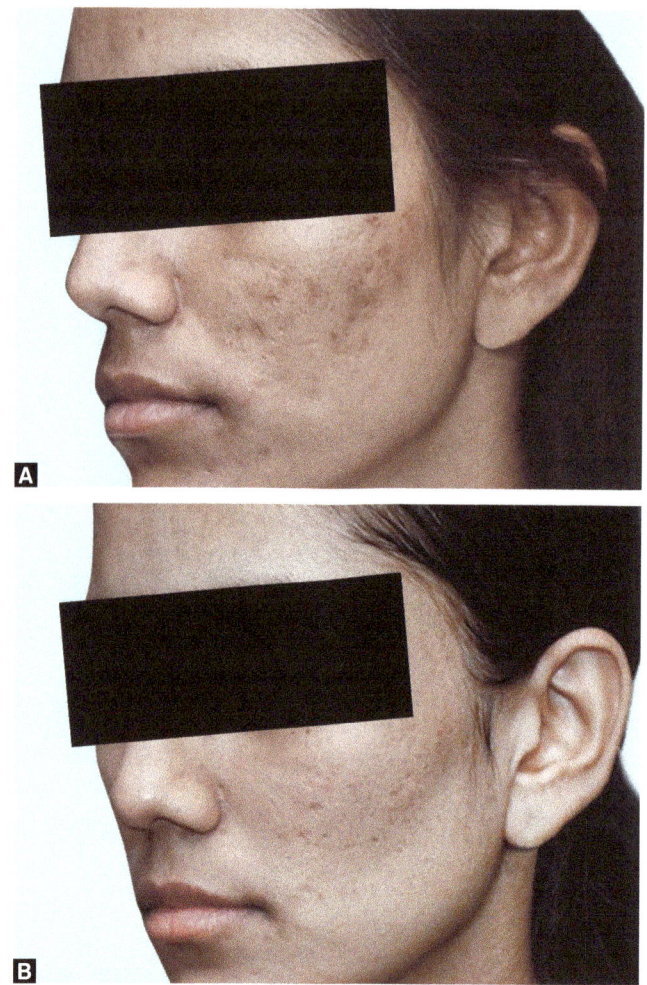

Figs. 4A and B: (A) Macular acne scars and shallow boxcar scars before treatment; (B) Marked improvement in scarring after five erbium fractional laser sessions.

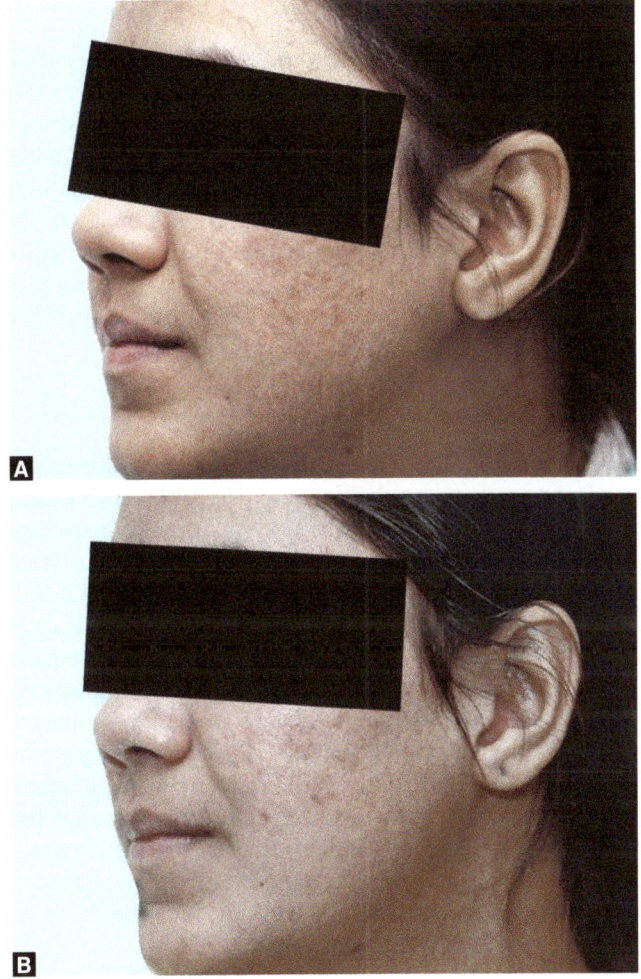

Figs. 5A and B: (A) Acne scars in type 4 skin; (B) Acne scars after four fractional Er:YAG (erbium:yttrium-aluminum-garnet) laser sessions.

NONABLATIVE LASERS

Ablative lasers carry certain amount of risk in treating patients with darker skin types. To overcome these limitations, nonablative devices of varying wavelengths were developed that allow safer treatment in the skin of color. These devices produce selective thermal stimulation of dermal collagen while sparing the epidermis. These lasers also employ cooling techniques to protect the epidermis from thermal injury. Because these modalities are less aggressive, they are more suitable for mild rolling scars, superficial atrophic scars than ice pick scars, boxcar scars and keloids.

Nonablative Fractional Er:Glass Laser

The fractional erbium glass laser is a 1,540 or 1,550 nm glass fiber laser producing subablative pulses of laser that range from 1 to 30 mJ.[9] The Er:Glass laser wavelength penetrates up to the papillary dermis inducing neocollagenesis and skin tightening. The chromophore here is tissue water and is minimally absorbed by melanin. Fixed pattern of pulses per pass can be deposited with the help of the scanner-enabled computerized handpiece. A metal-armored fiberoptic cable delivers the laser light to the handpiece. A sapphire window on the disposable tip is usually in skin contact and is programmed to allow 100 minutes of use. This helps to prevent degradation of the optical characteristics of the tip from repeated laser exposure or mechanical damage during cutaneous contact. Treatments are repeated once a month for 4-5 sessions with resultant improvement of 20-30% in acne scarring.[10]

Pulsed Dye Lasers

The 585-nm pulsed dye laser (PDL) is best suited for the treatment of hypertrophic scars and keloids. The laser targets the vascularity and erythema of the scars due to its excellent absorption in oxyhemoglobin and is best done when scars are less than 1 year old.[11] This laser is more suited for patients with Fitzpatrick skin type's I–III due to the less competition by melanin. The beneficial effect is due to decreased vascularity and stimulation of collagen production. Dierickz treated 15 patients with erythematous hyperpigmented scars with PDL and reported 77% improvement with an average of 1.8 treatments.[11]

1,064-nm Nd:YAG Laser

The 1,064-nm wavelength is poorly absorbed by melanin with a higher absorption in hemoglobin allowing treatment of vascular lesions, hypertrophic scars and keloids. The mechanism of action and effects are similar to PDL treatment. The laser can be used for the treatment of erythematous acne scars, hypertrophic scars and keloids. Studies have shown the laser to be useful for mild-to-moderate atrophic acne scars. Treatments are performed once in 4–6 weeks for a total of 5 sessions. Histologically, increase in dermal collagen is observed after Nd:YAG laser treatments. Keller et al.[12] reported that acne scarring improved in 100% of nine patients with the nonablative 1,064-nm Nd:YAG laser. The mean improvement was 29.36% with 89% of patients having greater than 10% improvement.

1,320-nm Nd:YAG Laser

Poor melanin absorption, and deep papillary and midreticular effects are seen with this laser. The 1,320-nm Nd:YAG has deeper penetration and has good affinity for tissue water. Dermal remodeling and neocollagenesis is seen histologically after multiple treatments.[13]

Patient satisfaction with treatment was rated as 62% of 32 patients studied and textural improvement was reported at 31% at the end of six treatments[13] **(Figs. 6A and B)**.

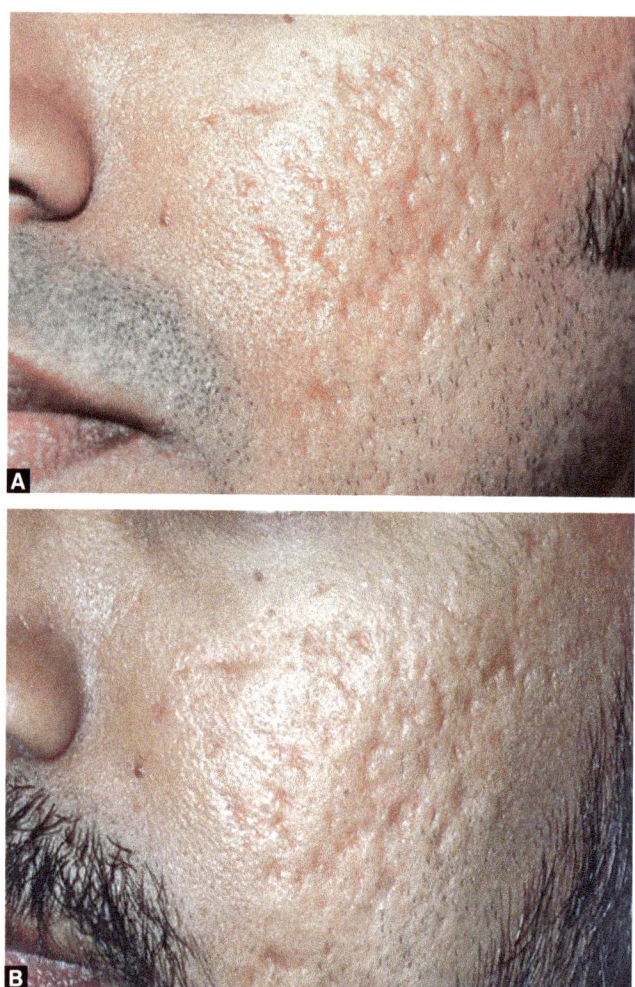

Figs. 6A and B: (A) Moderate acne scars before treatment; (B) After four sessions of 1,320-nm fractional nonablative laser.

1,450-nm Diode Laser

Similar to the 1,320 and 1,064-nm Nd:YAG laser, the 1,450-nm diode laser also targets tissue water and produces nonablative effects with dermal heating and collagen remodeling. Due to these effects, the laser can be used for the treatment of atrophic and hypertrophic acne scarring. Eleven subjects were treated with a 1,450-nm diode laser in a split-face study. One-half of the face received a single pass consisting of stacked double pulses. The other side received a double-pass treatment of single pulse. Settings were 11 J/cm^2 or lower as tolerated. Overall acne scar improvement was seen in 83% of patients.[14]

INTENSE PULSED LIGHT DEVICES

Intense pulsed light devices (IPLs) are polychromatic, noncoherent intense pulsed light devices that use cut-off filters to narrow the wavelength to target specific structures in the skin. The pulse duration, interval between pulses and the energy (joules) can be varied to fine tune the system to selectively treat vascular and pigmented lesions, hair reduction, acne, etc. After a series of 4–5 treatments, histopathology studies show an increase in papillary dermal fibrosis with increase in the number of fibroblasts.[15] IPLs can be used to treat atrophic or depressed acne scars as well as hypertrophic scarring. IPLs may be a good substitute to PDL for the treatment of hypertrophic scars. They produce less purpura compared to PDL but may cause greater discomfort during treatments **(Figs. 7A and B)**.

PATIENT SELECTION AND PREOPERATIVE CARE

- Evaluate and counsel the patient thoroughly
- Obtain a detailed informed consent
- Ask about history of herpes simplex
- Rule out contraindications **(Box 1)**

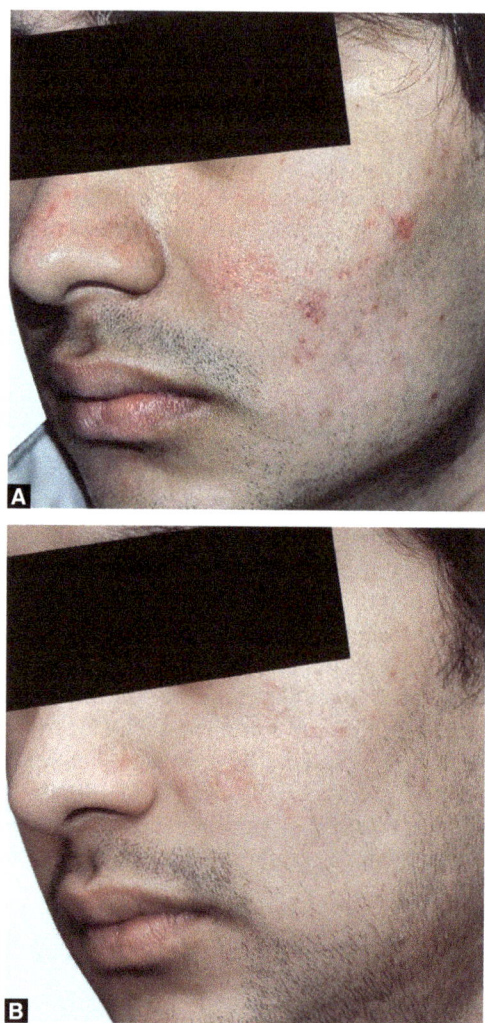

Figs. 7A and B: (A) Erythematous macular scars and boxcar scars; (B) Marked improvement in scarring after four intense pulsed light and five fractional Er:YAG (erbium:yttrium-aluminum-garnet) laser sessions.

> **Box 1:** Contraindications for laser therapy.
>
> - History of immunocompromised status
> - Active systemic disease that might interfere with wound healing
> - Active local or systemic infection
> - Connective tissue disorders
> - Pregnancy and lactation
> - History of allergy to any medication necessary for treatment
> - Active psoriasis or vitiligo
> - Unrealistic expectations
> - Body dismorphophobic disorder

- Patient should be instructed about the nature and procedure of treatment, the expected outcomes and the need for multiple sittings.
- Patient should have realistic expectations that the treatment may only improve acne scars and not completely eliminate them.
- Number of sessions depends on the type and depth of acne scars and the machine used. On an average, 4-6 sessions are needed to get a satisfactory outcome.
- Take minimum three photographs front and two side views
- Choose the laser according to the type of acne scar and patients' skin type **(Table 2)**.
- Test patches are recommended in darker skin patients. Treatment is safe and well tolerated even in darker individuals but it is better to be cautious in patients with a risk of dyschromias and test spots are recommended.
- Patients undergoing laser skin resurfacing with a history of herpes labialis should receive prophylactic oral antiviral therapy. Acyclovir, famciclovir or valacyclovir should be started 1 day before and continued for 5 days, postoperatively.
- Oral antibiotics, such as dicloxacillin or azithromycin, may be prescribed to patients with a history of bacterial infections of the facial skin to reduce the chance of secondary bacterial infection.

TABLE 2: The recommended choice of treatment for the different types of acne scars.

Type of scars	Lasers and light device used	Combination and other options
Erythematous macular scars	IPL and PDL	Microdermabrasion and peels may help
Acne hypermelanotic macules	IPL, ablative fractional lasers	Can be combined with peels as an adjuvant
Atrophic rolling and superficial boxcar scars	Ablative and nonablative fractional lasers, nonablative mid-infrared lasers	Can be combined with peels, dermaroller
Significant rolling and deep boxcar scars and ice pick scars	Ablative and nonablative fractional lasers, laser skin resurfacing	Subcision, TCA CROSS, microneedling may be added to treatment program
Hypertrophic and keloidal scars	PDL, IPL	Intralesional steroids, 5 FU

(CROSS: chemical reconstruction of skin scars; FU: fluorouracil; IPL: intense pulsed light; PDL: pulsed dye laser; TCA: trichloroacetic acid)

- *Priming:* While treating patients with darker skin, adequate priming with sunscreens and skin lightening agents should be done at least 4 weeks prior to initiating therapy.
- *Isotretinoin:* It was earlier believed that patients should stop isotretinoin at least 6 months before undergoing laser treatment. This recommendation was based on previous reports of keloid formation and atypical scar formation after use of dermabrasion and argon lasers, which are more invasive and ablative procedures. This belief is now changing, particularly with regard to functional lasers. Patients may continue isotretinoin under supervision.
- *Pregnancy:* Pregnancy is a contraindication for laser skin resurfacing.

ANESTHESIA

Most ablative and nonablative laser procedures are performed under topical anesthesia with mixture of lidocaine and prilocaine applied under occlusion for 60 minutes prior to the procedure. As an alternative, cold air may be used to minimize discomfort.[16]

POSTOPERATIVE CARE

Minimal care is needed post procedure. Ice packs immediately postprocedure and emollients or moisturizers may be needed till re-epithelialization is complete. Sunscreens and photoprotection should be started soon after the procedure and diligently used daily. Mild topical steroid may be prescribed if erythema and edema persist. Postoperative antibiotics are usually not necessary.

COMPLICATIONS (BOX 2)

In general, the side effects of lasers are minimal and transient. Mild erythema, edema, and peeling are common and can be managed by use of sunscreens, and moisturizers. However,

---

Box 2: Complications of laser or intense pulsed light treatment.

Mild:
- Erythema and edema
- Acneiform eruptions
- Milia
- Delayed purpura
- Superficial erosions

Moderate:
- Persistent erythema
- Bacterial infections
- Activation of herpes simplex
- Postinflammatory hyper- and hypopigmentation

Severe:
- Hypertrophic scarring
- Ectropion formation

side effects do occur, commonly when aggressive doses/higher stacking is used, particularly in patients with darker skins **(Box 2)**. Fractional ablative lasers are more likely to produce side effects than fractional nonablative lasers.[16]

Erythema: Postoperative erythema is usually mild and lasts for 2–3 days, but can persist up to a week. However, more prolonged erythema and linear abrasions, often persisting up to 3–4 weeks have been observed when fractional laser treatments with higher fluences and when multiple stackings are used[17] **(Fig. 8)**.

Edema: Post-treatment edema is machine- and patient-dependent. The average patient experiences edema for 1–3 days, though in some patients, it may last up to 1 week. The risk of edema also increases with higher fluences. It can be treated easily by applying ice at 10 minutes intervals for the first 24 hours after treatment. Some physicians advocate the use of

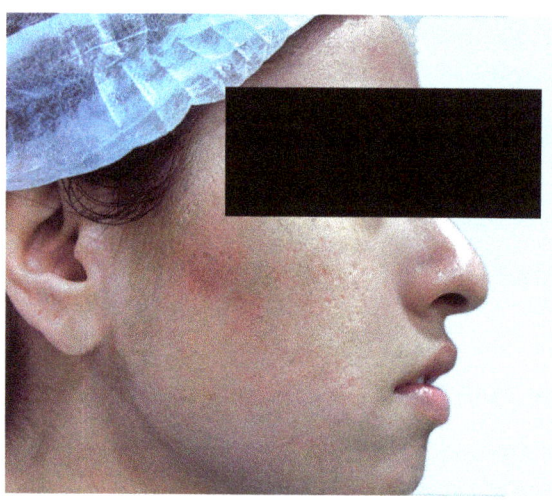

Fig. 8: Persistent erythema after fractional Er:YAG (erbium:yttrium-aluminum-garnet) laser. (*Courtesy:* Dr Shehnaz Arsiwala, Mumbai)

topical or short course systemic corticosteroids following treatment.

Petechiae: Occasional petechiae can be seen especially in periorbital area following use of higher fluences.[18] Often such petichiae are delayed occurring after 3 days. Avoidance of nonsteroidal anti-inflammatory drugs, aspirin, and other blood thinners in the immediate postoperative period are recommended to decrease the risk of purpura in such patients. Patients should also be advised to avoid rubbing or scratching of treated skin, because of increased skin fragility during the immediate post-treatment period.

Postinflammatory hypo- and hyperpigmentation: Though incidence of hyperpigmentation is considerably less than that with ablative lasers, it may be seen in darker skin patients, particularly in those patients with history of postinflammatory hyperpigmentation (PIH) or melasma[19] **(Fig. 9)**. Caution should

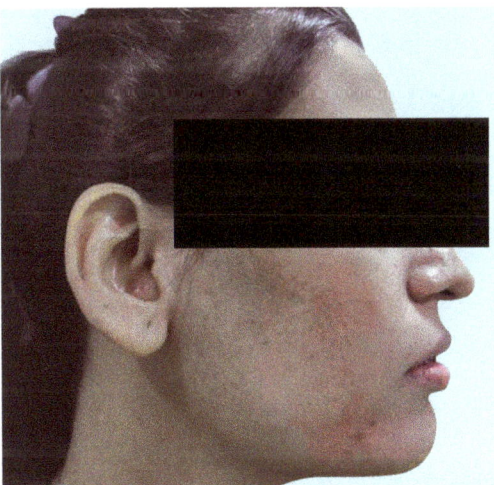

Fig. 9: Postinflammatory hyperpigmentation after fractional Er:YAG (erbium:yttrium-aluminum-garnet) laser. (*Courtesy:* Dr Shehnaz Arsiwala, Mumbai)

be exercised while using higher fluences or multiple stackings in such patients. Precautionary 2–4 weeks pretreatment with skin lightening agents and strict sun protection is advisable. Hypopigmentation is rare and when it occurs is difficult to treat.

Bacterial infection is rare, but has been reported in 0.1% of cases.[20]

Transient acneiform eruptions and milia may occur.[21] Antibiotics can be used to prevent flare-ups of acneiform eruptions **(Fig. 10)**.

Hypertrophic scarring, though rare, has been reported after fractional CO_2 laser use for neck rejuvenation.[22] Focal areas of erythema and induration 2–4 weeks after treatment are the first signs of potential scar formation. Neck is an area prone for such scarring. Postoperative wound infection, contact dermatitis, and tendency for keloidal scarring are other potential risk factors.

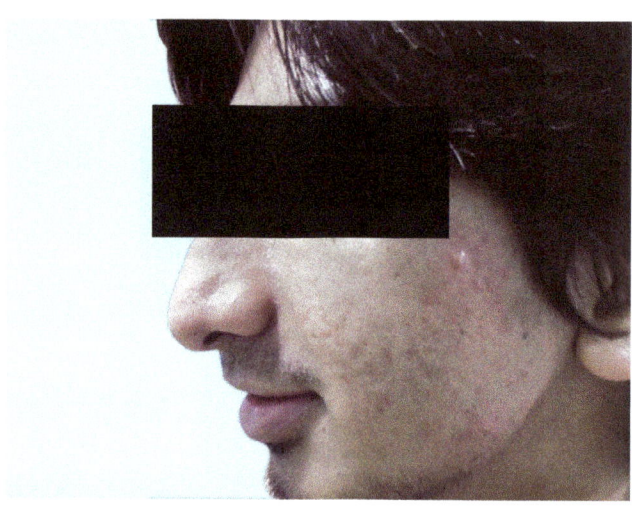

Fig. 10: Acneiform eruption folliculitis after Er:YAG (erbium:yttrium-aluminum-garnet) laser. (*Courtesy:* Dr Shehnaz Arsiwala, Mumbai)

Cicatricial ectropion is a rare, but potentially serious complication and has been reported after fractional CO_2 laser treatment.[23]

NEWER LASER TECHNOLOGIES FOR ACNE SCARS

Picosecond alexandrite and picosecond Nd:YAG lasers have been evaluated in the management of acne scars. These extremely short-pulsed lasers have a pulse duration in the picosecond (10^{-12}) range. Both the 755-nm alexandrite and the 532/1,064-nm Nd:YAG lasers have been tried in acne scars. Histologic examination after treatment showed evidence of laser-induced optical breakdown consistent with a localized plasma formation in the epidermis. This breakdown is initiated by absorption of the picosecond light by melanin. These changes led to dermal wound healing with formation of new collagen, elastic tissue, and mucin.[24]

In a retrospective study of 42 patients with atrophic acne scars, treated with the 755-nm picosecond laser, all patients showed improvement in scars and skin texture after 2–6 sessions, with a mean session count of 4.28 sessions. The laser was safe in darker skins and PIH was seen in 2 out of 42 patients (4.7%).[25] The advantage of this technology is that it is very safe up to skin phototype V and has minimal adverse effects. No vesiculation, crusting, scarring or PIH was noted in a study conducted by Tanghetti et al.[24] However, these lasers are expensive at the present moment.

CONCLUSION

An array of treatment options are available for the treatment of acne scars, but none is singly or wholly effective. Treatments have to be individualized to cater to the type and severity of scars and the goal of the physician and patient should be to improve the scarring rather than eliminate it. Ablative lasers have a higher incidence of side effects especially in darker skin types, whereas results are mild and slow with nonablative technologies. Fractional laser technology represents a major advantage over the previous conventional ablative methods and these fractional lasers are gaining popularity because of their favorable side-effect profile, reduced recovery time, and good clinical outcome. The picosecond lasers are promising and safe in darker skin types. Often, multiple modalities may have to be used to deliver the best results. Proper patient selection, counseling and priming of the patients is essential to obtain a good result.

REFERENCES

1. Manstein D, Herron GS, Sink RK, Tanner H, Anderson RR. Fractional photothermolysis: A new concept for cutaneous remodeling using microscopic patterns of thermal injury. Lasers Surg Med. 2004;34:426-38.
2. Hu S, Chen MC, Lee MC, Yang LC, Keoprasom N. Fractional resurfacing for the treatment of atrophic facial acne scars in Asian skin. Dermatol Surg. 2009;35(5):826-32.
3. Anderson RR, Parrish JA. Selective photothermolysis: precise microsurgery by selective absorption of pulsed radiation. Science. 1983;220:524-7.
4. Hantash BM, Bedi VP, Sudireddy V, Struck SK, Herron GS, Chan KF. Laser-induced transepidermal elimination of dermal content by fractional photothermolysis. J Biomed Opt. 2006;11:041115.
5. Goel A, Krupashankar DS, Aurangabadkar S, Nischal KC, Omprakash HM, Mysore V. Fractional lasers in dermatology—Current status and recommendations. Indian J Dermatol Venereol Leprol. 2011;77:369-79.
6. Woo SH, Park JH, Kye YC. Resurfacing of different types of facial acne scar with short-pulsed, variable-pulsed, and dual-mode Er:YAG laser. Dermatol Surg. 2004;30:488-93.
7. Chapas AM, Brightman L, Sukal S, Hale E, Daniel D, Bernstein LJ, et al. Successful treatment of acneiform scarring with CO_2 ablative fractional resurfacing. Lasers Surg Med. 2008;40:381-6.
8. Schweiger ES, Sundick L. Focal acne scar treatment (FAST), a new approach to atrophic acne scars: A case series. J Drugs Dermatol. 2013;12:1163-7.

9. Chiu RJ, Kridel RW. Fractionated photothermolysis: The Fraxel 1550 nm glass fiber laser treatment. Facial Plast Surg Clin North Am. 2007;15:229-37.
10. Kim HJ, Kim TG, Kwon YS, Park JM, Lee JH. Comparison of a 1,550 nm Erbium: Glass fractional laser and a chemical reconstruction of skin scars (CROSS) method in the treatment of acne scars: a simultaneous split-face trial. Lasers Surg Med. 2009;41:545-9.
11. Dierickx C, Goldman MP, Fitzpatrick RE. Laser treatment of erythematous/hypertrophic and pigmented scars in 26 patients. Plast Reconstr Surg. 1995;95:84-90.
12. Keller R, Belda Júnior W, Valente NY, Rodrigues CJ. Nonablative 1,064 nm Nd:YAG laser for treating atrophic facial acne scars: histologic and clinical analysis. Dermatol Surg. 2007;33:1470-6.
13. Rogachefsky AS, Hussain M, Goldberg DJ. Atrophic and a mixed pattern of acne scars improved with a 1320 nm Nd:YAG laser. Dermatol Surg. 2003;29:904-8.
14. Uebelhoer NS, Bogle MA, Dover JS, Arndt KA, Rohrer TE. Comparison of stacked pulses versus double-pass treatments of facial acne with a 1,450 nm laser. Dermatol Surg. 2007;33:552-9.
15. Goldberg DJ. New collagen formation after dermal remodeling with an intense pulsed light source. J Cutan Laser Ther. 2000;2:59-61.
16. Fisher GH, Kim KH, Bernstein LJ, Geronemus RG. Concurent use of a hand-held forced cold air device minimizes patient discomfort during fractional photothermolysis. Dermatol Surg. 2005;31:1242-3.
17. Ross RB, Spencer J. Scarring and persistent erythema after fractionated ablative CO_2 laser resurfacing. J Drugs Dermatol. 2008;7:1072-3.
18. Fife DJ, Zachary CB. Delayed pinpoint purpura after fractionated carbon dioxide treatment in a patient taking ibuprofen in the postoperative period. Dermatol Surg. 2009;35:553.
19. Chan HH, Manstein D, Yu CS. The prevalence and risk factors of post-inflammatory hyperpigmentation after fractional resurfacing in Asians. Lasers Surg Med. 2007;39:381-5.
20. Setyadi HG, Jacobs AA, Markus RF. Infectious complications after nonablative fractional resurfacing treatment. Dermatol Surg. 2008;34:1595-8.
21. Graber EM, Tanzi EL, Alster TS. Side effects and complications of fractional laser photothermolysis: Experience with 961 treatments. Dermatol Surg. 2008;34:301-5.

22. Avram MM, Tope WD, Yu T, Szachowicz E, Nelson JS. Hypertrophic scarring of the neck following ablative fractional carbon dioxide laser resurfacing. Lasers Surg Med. 2009;41:185-8.
23. Fife DJ, Fitzpatrick RE, Zachary CB. Complications of fractional CO2 laser resurfacing: Four cases. Lasers Surg Med. 2009;41:179-84.
24. Tanghetti EA. The histology of skin treated with a picosecond alexandrite laser and a fractional lens array. Lasers Surg Med. 2016;48:646-52.
25. Huang CH, Chern E, Peng JH, Hsien-Li Peng P. Noninvasive atrophic acne scar treatment in Asians with a 755-nm picosecond laser using a diffractive optic lens-a retrospective photographic review. Dermatol Surg. 2019;45:195-202.

CHAPTER 13

Fillers

Amit Luthra

IN A NUTSHELL

- Fillers are best used for shallow distensible acne scars.
- They give instant results but its use is limited by the need for repeated injection.
- Hyaluronic acid is most widely used.
- Complications can occur if proper aseptic techniques are not followed.

INTRODUCTION

Since 95% of acne patients will develop scarring to some degree, the earlier the treatment appropriate for the severity of acne is initiated, the lesser will be the scarring. Differences in location, depth, size and number of scars all affect treatment decisions. Each procedure has its own risks and benefits, and several procedures are normally combined to create the smoothest appearing skin.

Injections for acne scars utilize dermal fillers to raise the depressed acne scars to the same level as the surrounding skin. To create a pocket and achieve better results, subcision should be performed prior to injection or filling. There are many types of dermal fillers that can be injected into acne scars to raise the surface of the skin and give a smoother look. Examples of dermal fillers are fat, bovine collagen, human collagen, hyaluronic acid derivatives, and polymethyl-methacrylate microspheres with collagen. The correction with fillers is not permanent, so further injections are necessary.

Fat has gained popularity in recent times mainly because of the longevity and the comparative low cost. The transplantation utilizes a patient's own fat removed by a small liposuction cannula, prepared and reinjected into the dermal defect. While none of these methods are permanent, fat can last for a long time (see Chapter 14).

PRINCIPLE[1]

The basic principle of scar correction by fillers is to raise the depressed scar to the same level as the surrounding skin. In order to achieve an optimum result, an adequate space should be created before the filling substance is introduced, otherwise it can result in an uneven appearance due to the fibrosis that occurs. Hence, subcision should always be done prior to introducing a filler or fat for acne scars.

INSTRUMENTS AND MATERIALS[2-4]

An ideal filler material should be physiologic, i.e., be easily incorporated into the body's tissues, simple to place, permanent, undergoes minimal degradation, and be risk free, with no complications or side effects. Superficial skin products include collagen or hyaluronic acid and deep skin products include fat, silicone implants, and permanent fillers. Although close, none available meets all of these criteria completely.

Hyaluronic Acid

The most common filler material to be used is hyaluronic acid. Commercial preparations that are available are the Merz range (Belotero®), Galderma range (Restylane® and Perlane®) and the Allergan range (Juvéderm Ultra® and Juvederm Ultra

Plus®). Other brands like Yvoire, Princess, Perfectha, etc. are now available, giving varied options.

Hyaluronic acid is a highly hydrophilic, natural, linear polysaccharide (alternating residues of D-glucuronic acid and N-acetyl-D-glucosamine) component of connective tissue in all mammals so is not tissue- or species specific. It displays isovolemic degradation in which molecules of HA degrade allowing those remaining to absorb more water. Thus, the total volume of gel remains stable. The injectable concentration steadily decreases through reabsorption while the relative volume is essentially unchanged. The duration of effect for acne scars is roughly a year or more. In a study of 12 patients with acne scars, treated with 2 mL of nonstabilized hyaluronic acid as a filler showed improvement, with minimal side effects.[5]

Collagen

This is not available in India and is sparingly used in Europe and USA. The most popular collagen products employed to refill natural collagen and create raised acne scars include, Zyplast®, Zyderm®, CosmoDerm®, and CosmoPlast.® Zyplast® and Zyderm® are not recommended for patients with autoimmune diseases as they are derived from bovine collagen. Skin testing is required before injecting. Patients with possible allergic reactions can use CosmoDerm® or CosmoPlast.® These products are human derived and no skin testing is required to be injected with these substances. Most collagen injections for acne scars can last for 3-6 months.

Newer Acne Scars Fillers

The polylactic acids are a more recent addition to the treatment options available for injection to scars. Previously, these materials were used in suture materials and other treatments. New-Fill®, the primary brand for Europe, was available in 1999, as freeze-dried polylactic acid available for reconstitution with water. Poly-L-lactic acid was rebranded in the United States in 2000 as Sculptra.® A frequent use, other than scars, is in lipoatrophy because of human immunodeficiency virus (HIV). It is thought to stimulate neocollagenesis over 3-6 months and is for long-term augmentation. Side effects are possibly worsened by excess injection material, inadequate duration between injections, or multiple single-session injections. No skin tests are necessary with the use of polylactic acids.

Radiesse® contains 25-45 µm diameter calcium hydroxyapatite microspheres in polysaccharide (carboxymethylcellulose) aqueous gel. It is categorized as "semipermanent" with earlier claimed durations of 2-5 years, but more recent estimates of 12-16 months. There is little inflammation, a low side-effect profile and no allergy testing is required.

Reviderm Intra® consists of 40-60 µm Sephadex® (dextran) beads suspended in bacterial-derived hyaluronic acid. It stimulates inflammation and neocollagenesis.

ProFill® is a polyoxyethylene and polyoxypropylene polymer forming an injectable gel that must be refrigerated as a liquid until used. Skin testing is not necessary.

Fibrel is patient plasma that is mixed with porcine gelatin plus epsilon-aminocaproic acid and lidocaine. It serves as a physical filler and a media for neocollagenesis. This product requires a patient blood draw and may be more painful on injection or lead to a local inflammatory response.

Others

More substances are now available and many new ones continue to be introduced. Polyacrylamides (PA) comprise yet another form of injectable augmentation products and, once again, several products exist. Outline® is composed of absorbable hydrophilic PA gel particles that are positively charged, thus attracting negatively charged glycosaminoglycans already in the skin such as hyaluronic acid. Similarly, Evolution®, where positively charged polyvinyl microspheres in hydrophilic gel, also attracts the negatively charged molecules. *Bio-Alcamid*® is a polyalkylimide gel that is 96% water and 4% synthetic polymer that stimulates a fibrous response after injection. *Agriform* is a 5% water and 95% hydrophilic PA gel combination, in contrast to Aquamid, a 97.5% water and 2.5% hydrophilic polyacrylamide gel mixture. Extra precautions are necessary when doing the permanent fillers because of the increased likelihood of granulomas.

INDICATIONS

Filler substances are best used for shallow, saucer-shaped acne scars[6] **(Fig. 1)**. Most of these are applicable to depressed scars such as the atrophic rolling variety. Postsurgical and traumatic scars can also be treated with fillers. Fat transplantation,

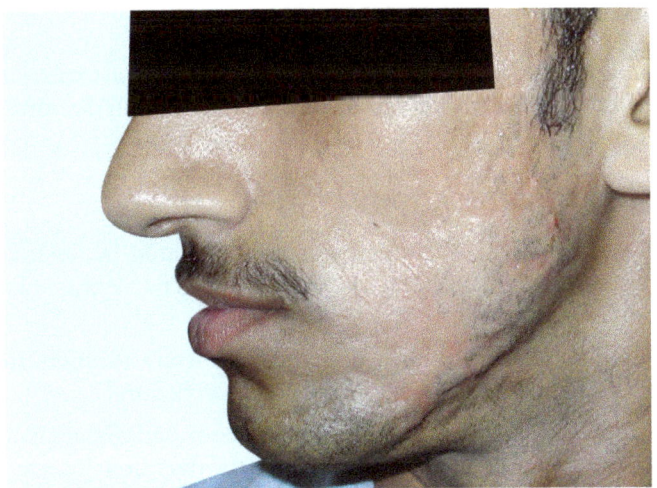

Fig. 1: Shallow depressed scars.
(*Courtesy:* Dr Niti Khunger)

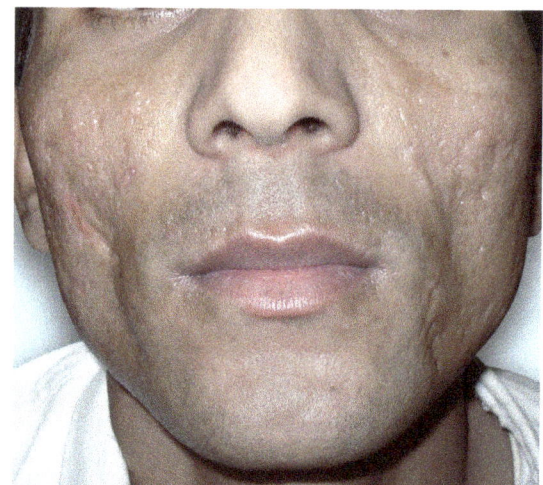

Fig. 2: Lipoatrophic acne scars.
(*Courtesy:* Dr Niti Khunger)

collagen, and filler injection is recommended in the treatment of depressed scars and scars with resulting contour deformity **(Fig. 2)**.

CONTRAINDICATIONS

Hypersensitivity to products as demonstrated by positive skin testing for collagen products. Testing is not required for products like hyaluronic acid and PAs.

Unrealistic expectations: It is very important to align the patients on the results before the actual procedure.

Inflammation: Injection site should be free of any inflammation and any acne should be treated before the treatment for scars.

Pregnancy and lactation: As with other esthetic procedures, fillers should be avoided during pregnancy and lactation.

Herpes simplex infection: Patients need to start antivirals before the procedure, if there is a history of herpes simplex.

Bleeding diathesis and anticoagulant therapy: Possible bruising is likely.

LIMITATIONS

Using temporary fillers gives only modest results which last for 6-9 months. Most people are left desiring more improvement. The introduction of new technologies of cross linkage of hyaluronic acid has given us increased longevity. Other ways to lift the scar include subcision technique, where a needle is used to lift the scar up so that it sits level with the plane of the rest of the skin. This can be done in conjunction with fillers and should precede the fillers by a week. Fillers are not useful for ice pick scars.

PRECAUTIONS

Aseptic precautions during the procedure are very important to prevent any post filler infections and infectious granulomas.

Laser treatment should follow temporary fillers like hyaluronic acid after a month at least and PAs after 6 months.

PREPROCEDURE PREPARATION

Informed Consent

- Photographs before the procedure are the most important as there is a tendency to forget what one looked like before the procedure
- Careful cleaning with spirit, povidone-iodine (Betadine®) and then spirit
- Filler should be chosen carefully.

TECHNIQUE[3,4,7-9]

Of the various techniques for injecting fillers, linear threading, serial puncture and the fan technique are useful for acne scars. The technique is chosen according to the type and size of the scars **(Figs. 3A to D)**.

Bigger scars: The linear threading technique is preferred wherein the length of the needle is inserted in the scar and the substance is injected while pulling the needle slowly backwards so that the threads of the gel are placed along the scar **(Fig. 3A)**.

Smaller scars size: The serial puncture technique is utilized. Multiple injections are placed serially along the scar. It is made

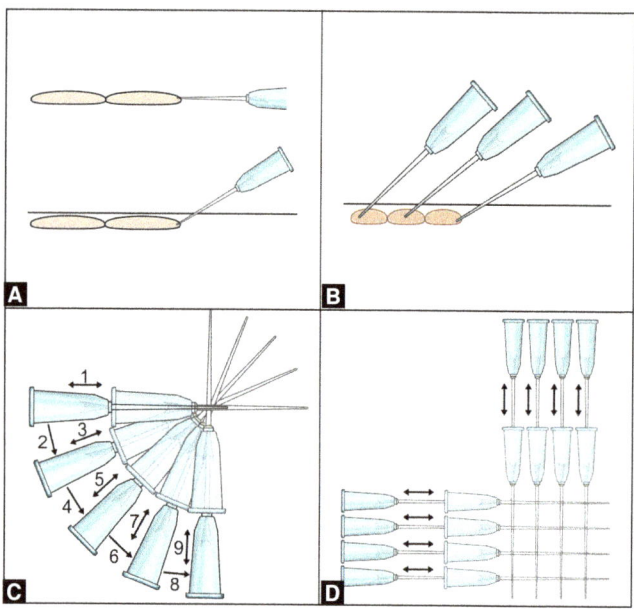

Figs. 3A to D: Injection techniques of fillers: (A) Linear threading technique; (B) Serial puncture technique; (C) Fan technique; and (D) Cross-hatching technique.

closely together so that it merges into a smooth continuous contour, which lifts the scar **(Fig. 3B)**.

Wide scars: The *fan technique* can be used to treat the scar from one entry point. The needle is inserted at the periphery of the scar as and when using the linear threading technique. After injecting one line, the direction of the needle is changed and injected as before along a new line, till the entire scar is treated **(Fig. 3C)**. The cross-hatch technique may be used for very wide, large scars **(Fig. 3D)**. It is important to do adequate subcision before injecting fillers or fat to create a pocket and avoid lumpiness of the surface.

The treated area will appear swollen immediately after and bruises may occur after the procedure. The patient should be warned about these. The area should be gently massaged to get an even contour **(Figs. 4A to C)**.

Treatment of scars dispersed over the cheeks and temples present a practical challenge. Using a 25G cannula, one can do subcision and global filling of the cheeks and temples at the same time. This gives a stretching effect to the scars and they appear less visible **(Figs. 5A and B)**. A tower technique has been described, where the filler is injected directly below the depressed acne scar to provide support to the depressed tissues.[9] Another technique is the combination of microfocused ultrasound followed by the filler, calcium hydroxylapatite dermal filler microsound immediately followed by the filler.[10]

POSTPROCEDURE CARE

Strict instructions to the patient should be given to ensure optimum results. Oral and topical antibiotics should be used in case of permanent fillers. Too much manipulation of the treated site should be avoided for 7 days. Exposure to extreme hot or cold conditions should also be avoided.

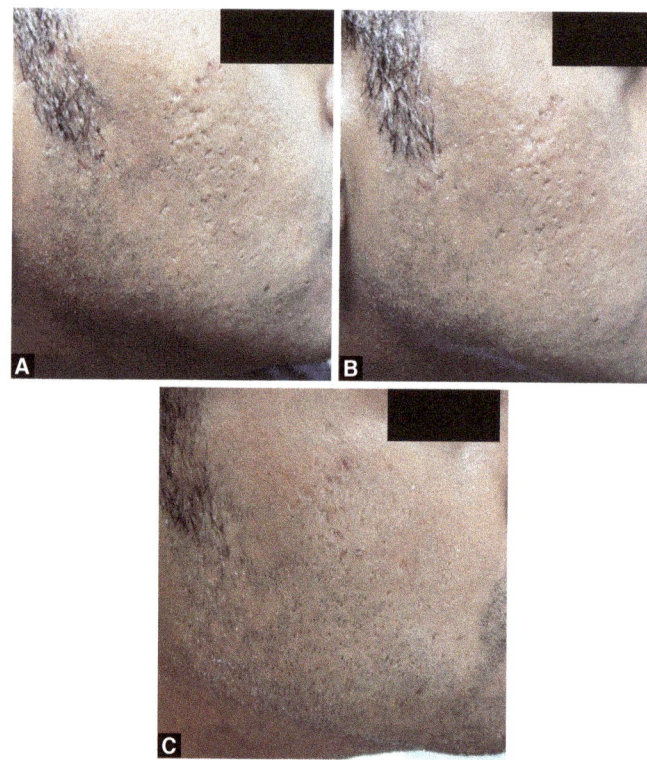

Figs. 4A to C: (A) Before the filler; (B) Immediately after hyaluronic acid filler; and (C) Three months after the filler.

Parlor procedures which involve massage should be deferred for at least 2 weeks. The touch up treatment can be given after 2–4 weeks, if necessary.

COMPLICATIONS

Side effects potentially include erythema, edema, bruising, inflammation, lumping, delayed reactions, infection, pain, milia and acne.

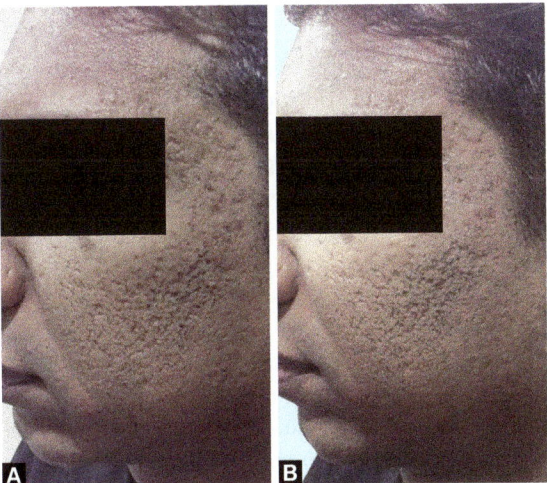

Figs. 5A and B: (A) Before the filler; (B) After the filler.

Potential rare side effects include pigmentary changes, allergic reaction, hypertrophic scarring or keloids, possible granulomas, migration of product, ulceration, tissue death, significant distortion, or technical error on placement.

There is very low true allergic potential so skin testing is not required although some physicians prefer to do so.

If a permanent filler is chosen and is placed too deep, too shallow, or overcorrected, or if there is a persistent defect, minor surgical removal, excision, electrodessication, or steroid treatment could be required.

Hyaluronic acid lumps can be resolved using hyaluronidase injections.

ADVANTAGES

Fillers are a practical and instant solution relatively free of side effects for patients who wish to get quick results.

DISADVANTAGES

However, the effects of fillers like hyaluronic acid are temporary and injections need to be repeated once in 6–10 months. Fillers may not be the treatment of first choice for somebody looking for permanent results. They are expensive; hence, price-conscious patients can be suggested cheaper alternatives like chemical peels and microneedling.

The final results depend a lot on physician expertise and proper placement.

CONCLUSION

While fillers are generally safe, effectiveness is related to areas of injection and physician expertise. Each has its own specific properties and longevity that makes it more suitable for certain uses than for others. Semipermanent fillers must be repeated at regular intervals, although with certain products, the filler is replaced by the patients' own collagen over the course of several treatments. Permanent fillers require minimal touch-ups and have long-lasting effects of 5 years and longer. Overall fillers are a good choice for acne scars but with lots of limitations.

REFERENCES

1. Sclafani AP, Romo T IIIrd, Jacono AA, McCormick SA, Cocker R, Parker A. Evaluation of acellular dermal graft (Alloderm) sheet for soft-tissue augmentation: a 1-year follow-up of clinical observations and histological findings. Arch Facial Plast Surg. 2001;3:101-3.
2. Multimodal Treatment of Acne, Acne Scars and Pigmentation. Dermatol Clin. 2009;27(4):459-71.
3. Wollina U, Goldman A. Fillers for the improvement in acne scars. Clin Cosmet Investig Dermatol. 2015;8:493-9.
4. Forbat E, Ali FR, Al-Niaimi F. The role of fillers in the management of acne scars. Clin Exp Dermatol. 2017;42:374-80.

5. Dierickx C, Larsson MK, Blomster S. Effectiveness and safety of acne scar treatment with nonanimal stabilized hyaluronic acid gel. Dermatol Surg. 2018;44(Suppl 1):S10-8.
6. Rivera AE. Acne scarring: A review and current treatment modalities. J Am Acad Dermatol. 2008;59(4):659-76.
7. Cooper JS. Treatment of facial scarring: lasers, filler, and nonoperative techniques. Facial Plast Surg. 2009;25:311-5.
8. Vedamurthy M. Soft tissue augmentation—Use of hyaluronic acid as dermal filler. Indian J Dermatol Venereol Leprol. 2004;70:383-7.
9. Goodman GJ, Van Den Broek A. The modified tower vertical filler technique for the treatment of post-acne scarring. Australas J Dermatol. 2016;57:19-23.
10. Casabona G. Combined use of microfocused ultrasound and a calcium hydroxylapatite dermal filler for treating atrophic acne scars: A pilot study. J Cosmet Laser Ther. 2018;20:301-6.

CHAPTER 14

Autologous Fat Transfer for Acne Scars

Vivek Kumar, Niti Khunger, Ridhima Lakhani

IN A NUTSHELL

- The focus on fat grafting has been shifting from mere lipofilling to its regenerative properties and overall improvement of skin texture, which is a major advantage.
- Autologous fat grafting is an effective treatment for atrophic acne scars that have volume loss such as lipoatrophic scars and scars that improve on stretching the skin such as rolling acne scars.
- It can be injected in the form of macrofat, microfat or nanofat, depending on particle size.
- Nanofat is prepared using a standard emulsification and filtration protocol and is injected intradermally or subcutaneously.
- It is a minimally invasive technique with few complications and is safe in all skin types.
- Efficacy and survival of the fat is still variable, which is the only disadvantage of this technique.

INTRODUCTION

In the 1980s, when the liposuction procedure became more widely available, plastic surgeons started offering their patients autologous fat transfer for cosmetic reasons. Neuber was the first to report autologous fat transfer on the face for scars in 1893 and the technique was later refined by Coleman, when it became more popular and widely used.[1] Essentially, fat is harvested from one region and transferred to another where it is required. Fat transfer, also known as fat grafting,

Autologous Fat Transfer for Acne Scars

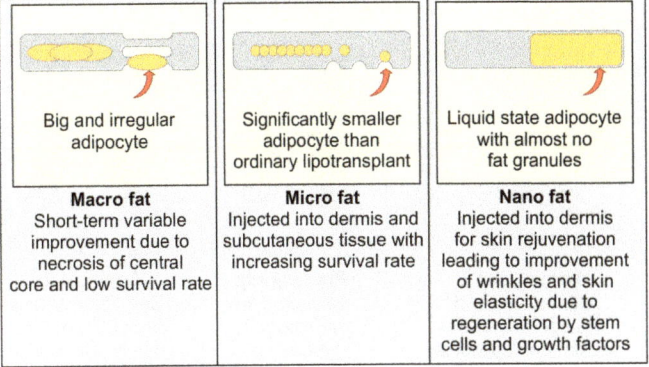

Fig. 1: Various types of fat grafts.

fat autografts, autologous fat transplantation, fat injection or lipofilling, is being increasingly used in cosmetic surgery to restore volume loss and for atrophic acne scars. The technique has undergone several changes over time to improve survival of the transplanted fat. Previously, large boluses of fat obtained from a 3-mm cannula (macrofat) or smaller boluses from a 1-mm cannula (microfat) were injected, but results were unpredictable as chances of fat necrosis of the central core of fat tissue were higher.[2] The recent technique to process the fat by emulsification to finer components (nanofat) as described by Tonnard et al.[3] gives more predictable results. The microfat or nanofat grafts contain predominantly adipose-derived stem cells (ADSC), which have an important role in regeneration of collagen[4,5] **(Fig. 1)**.

PRINCIPLE

The main principle is that fat is harvested from a donor site by an atraumatic technique, it is processed and made suitable for injection at the recipient site **(Fig. 2)**. The aim is to raise the depressed scar to the same level as surrounding skin.

Lipo-structure technique

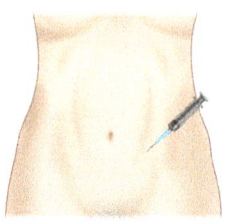

Harvest: 3-mm cannula moved through adipose to loosen and collect fat

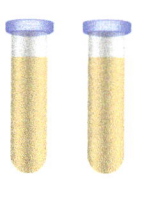

Processing: Collected fat transferred to tubes for centrifugation

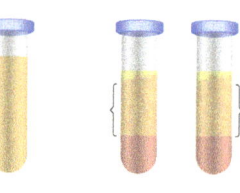

Separation: Centrifuge setting at 3000 rpm for 3 min is standard to separate fractions

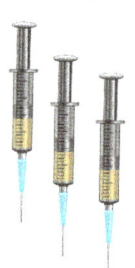

Isolation: Middle layer of viable adipocytes is transferred to 1 cc syringes

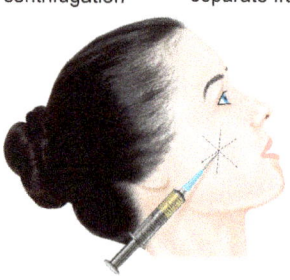

Implantation: Small aliquots of fat injected at different depths of defect

Fig. 2: Technique of lipografting.

The variations in technique are chiefly based on different methods of processing the fat and injecting in the recipient sites. However, all techniques still lack standardization and predictable results.

INSTRUMENTS

- Fat harvesting (**Figs. 3A and B**)
  - 1 cc syringe with LA (2% lignocaine with premixed adrenaline)

Autologous Fat Transfer for Acne Scars

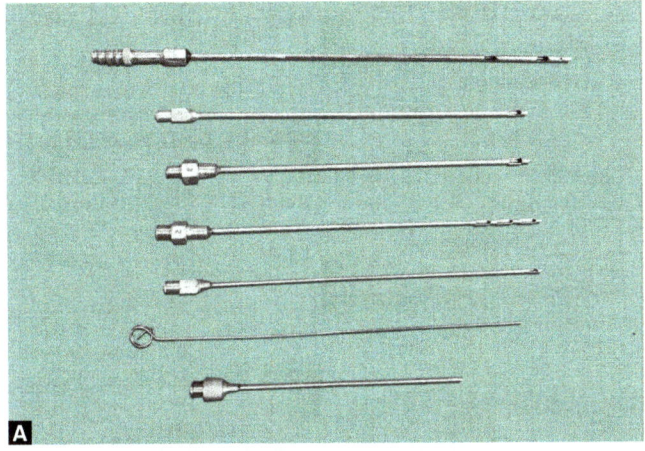

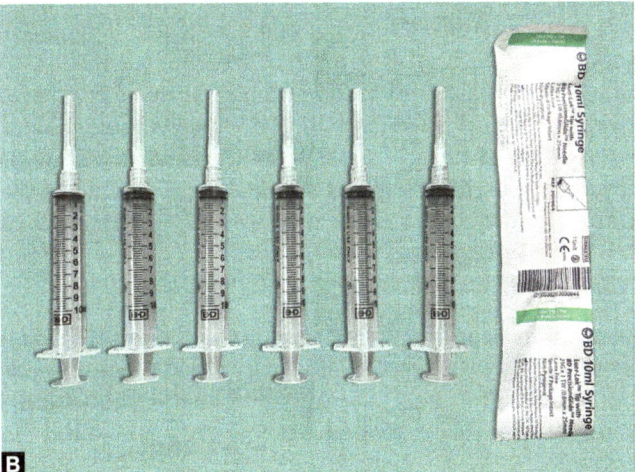

Figs. 3A and B: Instruments for fat grafting.
(A) Liposuction cannula; (B) Syringe.

- Blade 11 no. for incision at the donor site
- Cannula (2 mm or 3 mm) mercedes port/multihole
- Tumescent solution

- Luer-lock disposable syringes (10 cc)
- Syringe stand.
- Fat processing or nanofat preparation
  - Centrifuge (optional)
  - Luer to luer connector (1.2 and 1.4 mm)
  - Filter
  - Petridish
  - 1 cc syringes.
- Fat reinjection
  - Injection cannulas – 22G (0.8 mm) –19G (1 mm)
  - Needles –26G –18G

INDICATIONS

Fat transfer is indicated for volume loss that occurs due to cystic acne and atrophic depressed acne scars. Rolling scars that improve on stretching the skin give the best results. It is the preferred treatment for lipoatrophic scars where there is large volume loss. Such scars require large volume of fillers, making it very expensive. For ice pick scars and boxcar scars, it may not give desired results as a standalone technique, but can improve the texture of the skin after lasers or punch techniques.

CONTRAINDICATIONS

Contraindications to fat grafting include the presence of any disease processes that adversely affect wound healing and poor overall health status of the individual such as immunosuppression, diabetes, hepatic or renal failure and pregnancy.

PRECAUTIONS

As fat grafting involves use of large amounts of tumescent anesthesia, the patient must be thoroughly assessed before the procedure. Routine clinical examination for general status of the patient and preoperative investigations such as hemogram, liver and kidney function tests, blood sugar, ECG, etc., must be carried out. Patients who have undergone previous radiotherapy or chemotherapy or are on immunosuppressive drugs should be treated cautiously. Any active infection should first be treated before undergoing the procedure. Recent treatment of the recipient site by steroid injections in the last 1 month may not give optimum results. In such patients, it is better to wait for at least 3 months before fat transfer. Patients with history of easy bleeding or bruising should have coagulation parameters and platelets checked.

ADVANTAGES

Autologous fat for transfer to atrophic areas is readily available, inexpensive, longlasting, gives a natural feel and does not cause adverse immunologic reactions. The complication rate is also low as compared to fillers.[2] Large volumes can be injected as required.

DISADVANTAGES

The main disadvantage of fat transfer is that retention of fat is very variable and resorption can occur. The resorption rates vary from 20-60%.[6] It is believed that mature adipocytes are sensitive to ischemia, while preadipocytes and ADSCs are less sensitive and might be the only tissues that survive transplantation. The variability of these cells between individuals may be one of the reasons for variable survival of fat grafts.[1]

PREPROCEDURE PREPARATION

Proper counseling of the patient is the most important step to success. The patient should be counseled regarding results expected and variability of long-term results. Patient consent and photographs are taken. Carefully look for any active infection in the donor or recipient site.

TECHNIQUE

First, carefully mark the recipient sites in the upright position. Surgically prepare and drape both the harvest site and the recipient site with strict aseptic precautions.

Fat Grafting Technique

The basic fat grafting procedure is divided into four parts:[7-9]
1. Donor site selection and anesthesia
2. Fat harvesting
3. Fat processing
4. Fat placement

Donor Site Selection and Anesthesia[7-9]

The lower abdomen, thigh or flank are preferred donor sites **(Fig. 4)**. Lower abdomen and inner thigh yield higher concentrations of processed lipoaspirate cells. The amount of connective tissue is less in these regions so less bleeding will occur after syringe aspiration. High levels of lipoprotein lipase within adipocytes harvested from the above regions indicate that these fat grafts may be more resistant to anoxia.

After selection of the donor site, the port through which the cannula will be inserted is marked and 1 mL of 2% lignocaine is injected. A small stab incision is made with a no. 11 or no. 15 blade and the cannula is inserted. The donor site is anesthetized by tumescent anesthesia (900 mL NaCl 0.9%, 0.25 mL adrenaline 1 mg/mL, 20 mL of lignocaine 20 mg/mL). Tumescent fluid is injected till the area becomes turgid. The advantage of tumescent anesthesia is that larger volume of diluted lignocaine provides adequate anesthesia without reaching the toxic dose. Lignocaine also acts as a bacteriostatic agent.

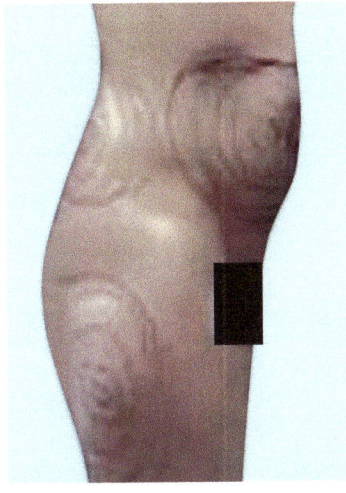

Fig. 4: Preferred donor sites for fat grafting.

Adrenaline provides a bloodless surgical field and also reduces the chances of post-liposuction hematoma. Modification of Klein's solution: 100 mL normal saline + 10 mL lignocaine + 1 mL adrenaline.

Fat Harvesting

Superiority of atraumatic technique for harvest of fat graft over conventional liposuction has been well established. The Coleman technique using a syringe yields a greater number of viable adipocytes and sustains a more optimal level of cellular function within the fat graft.[4] The viability of fat graft is significantly better when fat graft is harvested by 2 mm diameter cannula with a blunt tip and several side holes. Syringe aspiration is a relatively atraumatic technique, and a better procedure for harvesting of fat graft **(Fig. 5)**. Vacuum by syringe aspiration is around 0.2 atm as compared to by suction machine (1 atm). After waiting for 10–15 minutes following

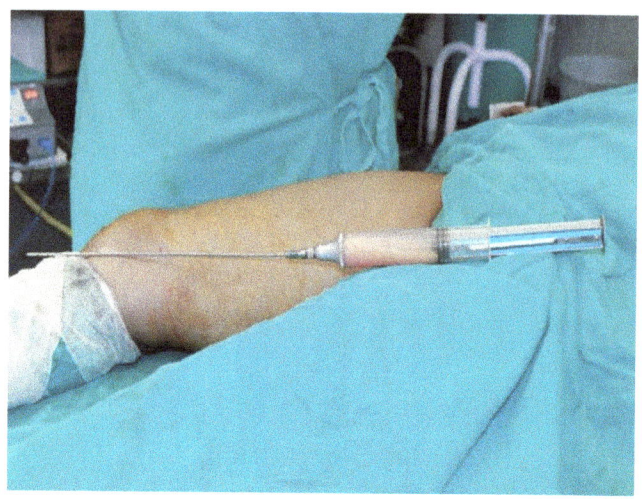

Fig. 5: Aspiration of fat with a cannula and syringe.

tumescent anesthesia, till the action of adrenaline has started, a 2-mm blunt cannula attached to a 10 mL Luer-lock syringe is inserted. It is gently manipulated. The plunger is pulled back for up to 3–5 cc to create a vacuum. Then the fat is aspirated using a back and forth motion, with the plunger steady. When the syringe is full, it is slowly detached from the cannula and another syringe is attached and then fat withdrawn. The nondominant hand is used as a guide to the tip of the cannula. The process is repeated till the required amount of fat is withdrawn, changing the direction of the cannula. Around 10–20 mL fat is usually considered adequate for acne scars, depending on the severity.

Fat Processing

It is important to process the fat because the lipoaspirate contains not only adipocyte and stem cells, but also blood cells, tumescent fluid and oil released from lysed adipocytes. The syringes containing aspirated fat are closed with a needle or syringe cap and put on a syringe stand to allow for decantation, with the hub facing down and the plunger on top. Alternatively, the aspirated fat can be centrifuged. Centrifugation at 50 g for 2 minutes separates fat, lipids, and blood cells with more viable adipocytes being found at the middle portion while oil is in the upper portion and blood cells in the lower. Centrifugation with 3,000 rpm for 3 minutes is optimal and should be recommended for processing fat grafts.[5] Significantly distorted and fractured adipocytes are seen when the centrifugal speed reaches 4,000 rpm.

Fat preparation
Centrifugation separates the harvested fat into three layers **(Fig. 6)**:
1. A top-level oily fluid which contains chylomicrons and triglycerides resulting from cell lysis

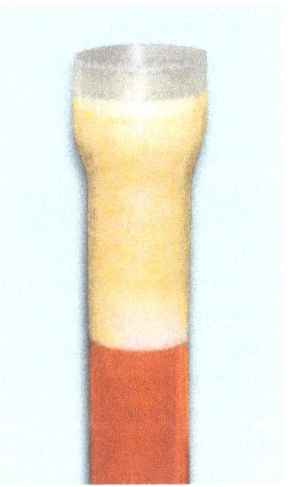

Fig. 6: Aspirated fat.

2. A lower level of blood residues and serum
3. A middle layer of purified fat

The lower liquid layer containing blood, serum and residues is discarded and the pure fat is transferred to another syringe using a connector. It may be washed with saline if it is bloody. This is macrofat which is used for filling large lipoatrophic acne scars. For preparation of nanofat, the syringe containing pure aspirated fat is connected to a 1.4-mm connector and moved back and forth around 30 times. The color changes from yellow to whitish or cream. For further preparation of nanofat, a filter is added and it is made to pass through 1.4 mm and then 1.2 mm cannula, progressively. The filter removes the connective tissue threads and strands that may be present. The final fat obtained is smooth and can pass through a 26-27 gauge cannula, for injecting fat safely. It is transferred to 1 mL syringes and made ready for injection.

Fat Injection and Placement

The donor site can be anesthetized by local anesthesia or regional block if required, depending on patient tolerance and area to be injected. The access incisions or needle piercing should be as less as possible and away from danger areas. Fat is placed intradermally or subcutaneously in the desired plane using linear threading and fan technique. Small aliquots of fat are placed. Ability of fat grafts to obtain nutrition through plasmatic imbibition occurs approximately 1.5 ± 0.5 mm from the edge of the vascularized tissue. The percentage of fat graft viability depends on the thickness and geometric shape of the grafts in the recipient bed. The goal with any grafting procedure is to gently apply the graft to a well-vascularized bed to maximize graft take. Every part of the graft should be within 1.5 mm of living, vascularized tissue. *Multipoint*, *multitunnel*, and *multilayer* injections are the basic techniques for prolonged fat survival **(Figs. 7 and 8)**. The fat grafts are placed

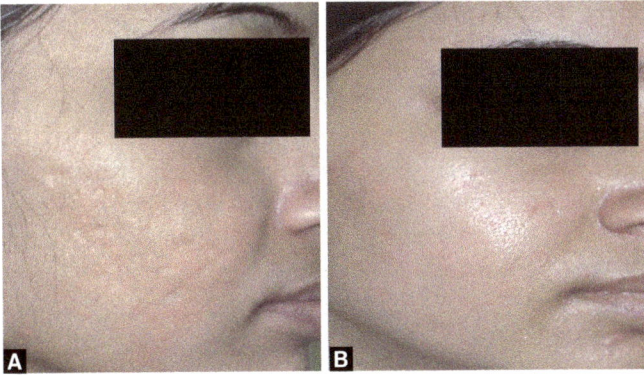

Figs. 7A and B: Acne scars after treatment with autologous fat grafting: (A) Preoperative; and (B) Postoperative.

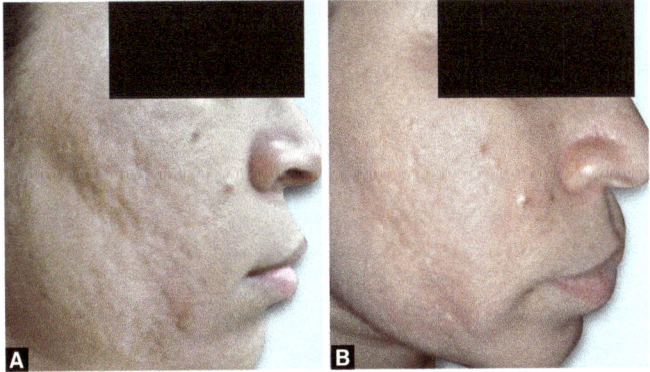

Figs. 8A and B: Acne scars treated with subcision followed by autologous fat grafting: (A) Preoperative; and (B) Postoperative.

in a small amount with each pass as the cannula is withdrawn. It is gently moulded to give an even surface. Fat grafts become vascularized around day 7 after transplantation. Significant overcorrection may increase the incidence of fat necrosis and subsequent calcification or even infection.

POSTOPERATIVE CARE

Discourage massage and excessive exercise immediately following fat grafting. These restrictions are to prevent migration of fat away from the desired areas of treatment. The patient should be counseled regarding sequelae of bruising and edema which may occur. Ice pack applications can be advised for first 72 hours. Analgesic and antibiotics may be given for 5 days. Recovery takes 2–6 weeks.

FOLLOW-UP[8]

Patients should be seen in the first week postoperatively to check the donor and recipient sites. Some edema and a minimal amount of bruising may be apparent. Reassurance is sufficient. An additional follow-up appointment should be made for approximately 6–8 weeks. At this point, most of the edema has subsided, and early results can be assessed. If a repeat procedure is to be performed, a waiting period of 6 months is prudent to allow the first graft to revascularize and to allow any edema to resolve.

Azzam et al.[10] compared the results of fractional CO_2 laser versus fat transfer in 10 patients each. Fat grafting showed better results as compared to CO_2 laser, with improvement in skin texture as well as scars.

Uyulmaz et al.[11] treated 52 patients with nanofat transfer for scars, wrinkles and dyspigmentation. The nanofat was injected to the entire face intradermally using a 24-, 25-, or 27-gauge sharp needles into the scar tissue or the dermis. The endpoint of injection was the appearance of yellowish discoloration of the skin during the injection process. In four cases, nanofat treatment was performed twice. Of the patient with scars, 74% had good improvement, 8% were satisfactory and only 8% of all treated scars were rated as unchanged post-treatment.

EFFICACY AND SURVIVAL OF FAT

Though fat grafting has been practiced for a long time, efficacy and survival of the transplanted fat still shows wide variation. Basically, there are three zones of the transplanted fat[12,13] **(Fig. 9)**. The outermost layer is the surviving zone which is in contact with the surrounding tissue and gets its nutrition by imbibition in the first 24–48 hours before vascular supply develops. Usually both adipocytes and ADSC survive in this zone as adipocytes are sensitive to hypoxia and ischemia. The middle layer is the regenerating zone, where the adipocytes undergo apoptosis (programmed cell death) due to hypoxia, whereas ADSCs survive because they are relatively resistant to hypoxia. Death of adipocytes stimulates macrophages and cytokine release, which signals the ADSCs to initiate differentiation and proliferation into adipocytes and also stimulates neoangiogenesis. The innermost layer is the necrotic zone where both adipocytes and ADSCs die and are replaced by oily cysts or scar tissue. The efficacy and survival of the fat mainly depends on the regenerating zone. Hence, small pearls of fat should be deposited to reduce the size of the innermost necrotic zone. Enrichment of the transferred fat with stromal vascular fraction (SVF) cells[14] or by platelet-rich plasma (PRP) increases fat survival.[15]

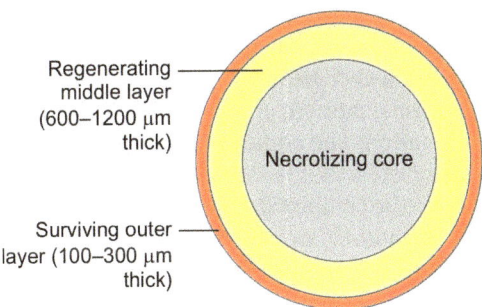

Fig. 9: Zones of transplanted fat.

COMPLICATIONS

As compared to traditional liposuction, autologous fat transfer involves small volumes and is a minimally invasive procedure; hence, there are few complications. The most common complication is minimal graft retention, which leads to patient dissatisfaction and poor results. Hematoma, oil cysts, infection and calcification are other adverse effects that can occur, which are related to fat necrosis. Irregularity and dimpling of the fat can occur in the scarred area, if lipofilling is not preceded by adequate subcision.

The most serious complication of fat grafting is embolization that can occur after inadvertent intravascular injection. Hence, aspiration is important before injection. Fat should always be injected while withdrawing the needle. Embolization can result in blindness, tissue necrosis or stroke, if large volumes or boluses are injected in an artery or forcefully injected. These complications are rare with microfat and nanofat and can be avoided by using blunt needles or cannulas.[16] Complications at the donor site include irregularities, bruising, hematoma or seroma. Rarely pain can persist for few months.

COMBINATION TREATMENTS

In the treatment of acne scars, it is advisable to combine subcision with fat grafting to give smoother results **(Fig. 10)**. Two to three sessions of subcision must be done prior to the procedure. Sezgin and Ozmen[17] combined microneedling with fat grafting in the treatment of scars and reported better results in the combination. The addition of PRP to the fat is reported to give better results as it is said to improve fat survival.[18] Fat grafting can also be combined with laser ablative or nonablative resurfacing to optimize treatment.[18] The lasers should ideally be done prior to fat grafting. Tenna et al.[18] treated 20 patients with acne scars with fat grafting in combination with PRP. Ten patients additionally received fractional CO_2 laser treatment.

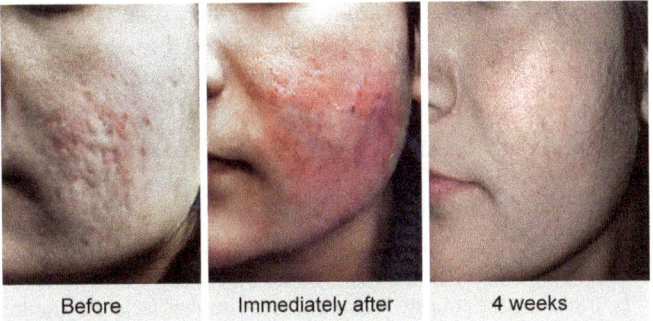

Fig. 10: Combination of two procedures—subcision and fat grafting.

They reported improvement in both the groups with no significant difference between the two groups.

FUTURE OF FAT

Enriching adipose grafts with stromal vascular fraction, ex vivo cultured adipose stem cells and platelet-derived growth factor among others is one method under active investigation which may assist graft survival through a range of mechanisms including increased angiogenesis.[2] The application of low-volume injections using autoclavable microguns represents a significant shift in thinking away from mere volume expansion.

CONCLUSION

Autologous fat grafting is an effective treatment for atrophic acne scars that have volume loss such as lipoatrophic scars and scars that improve on stretching the skin such as rolling acne scars. There are many variations in the technique of processing the fat. Fat can be injected in the form of macrofat, which has adipocytes; microfat, which has few adipocytes, but mainly ADSCs; and nanofat, which has no viable adipocytes, but mainly ADSCs. The success of fat grafting is dependent on the survival and regeneration of fat cells, which is variable. Fat grafting not only improves volume loss, but also leads to improvement in skin texture through the action of ADSCs. This is a major advantage of fat grafting. There are very few complications and it can be safely done on all skin types.

REFERENCES

1. Bellini E, Grieco MP, Raposio E. The science behind autologous fat grafting. Ann Med Surg (Lond). 2017;24:65-73.
2. Brooker JE, Rubin JP, Marra KG. The future of facial fat grafting. Craniofac Surg. 2019;30:644-51.
3. Tonnard P, Verpaele A, Peeters G, et al. Nanofat grafting: basic research and clinical applications. Plast Reconstr Surg. 2013;132:1017-26.
4. Kim WS, Park BS, Sung JH, Yang JM, Park SB, Kwak SJ, et al. Wound healing effect of adipose-derived stem cells: a critical role of secretory factors on human dermal fibroblasts. J Dermatol Sci. 2007;48:15-24.
5. Frese L, Dijkman PE, Hoerstrup SP. Adipose tissue-derived stem cells in regenerative medicine. Transfus Med Hemother. 2016;43:268-74.
6. Arcuri F, Brucoli M, Baragiotta N, Stellin L, Giarda M, Benech A, et al. The role of fat grafting in the treatment of posttraumatic maxillofacial deformities. Craniomaxillofac Trauma Reconstr. 2013;6:121-6.
7. Coleman SR. Structural fat grafts: the ideal filler? Clin Plast Surg. 2011;28:111-9.
8. Bhooshan LS, Devi MG, Aniraj R, Binod P, Lekshmi M. Autologous emulsified fat injection for rejuvenation of scars: A prospective observational study. Indian J Plast Surg. 2018;51:77-83.
9. Simonacci F, Bertozzi N, Grieco MP, Grignaffini E, Raposio E. Procedure, applications, and outcomes of autologous fat grafting. Ann Med Surg (Lond). 2017;20:49-60.
10. Azzam OA, Atta AT, Sobhi RM, Mostafa PI. Fractional CO_2 laser treatment vs autologous fat transfer in the treatment of acne scars: A comparative study. J Drugs Dermatol. 2013;12:e7-13.
11. Uyulmaz S, Macedo NS, Rezaeian F, Giovanoli P, Lindenblatt N. Nanofat grafting for scar treatment and skin quality improvement. Aesthet Surg J. 2018;38:421-8.

12. Eto H, Kato H, Suga H, Aoi N, Doi K, Kuno S, et al. The fate of adipocytes after nonvascularized fat grafting: evidence of early death and replacement of adipocytes. Plast Reconstr Surg. 2012;129: 1081-92.
13. Kato H, Mineda K, Eto H, Doi K, Kuno S, Kinoshita K, et al. Degeneration, regeneration, and cicatrization after fat grafting: dynamic total tissue remodeling during the first 3 months. Plast Reconstr Surg. 2014;133:303e-13e.
14. Tanikawa DY, Aguena M, Bueno DF, Passos-Bueno MR, Alonso N. Fat grafts supplemented with adipose-derived stromal cells in the rehabilitation of patients with craniofacial microsomia. Plast Reconstr Surg. 2013;132(1):141-52.
15. Serra-Mestre JM, Serra-Renom JM, Martinez L, Almadori A, D'Andrea F. Platelet-rich plasma mixed-fat grafting: a reasonable prosurvival strategy for fat grafts? Aesthetic Plast Surg. 2014;38(5):1041-9.
16. Yoshimura K, Coleman SR. Complications of fat grafting: how they occur and how to find, avoid, and treat them. Clin Plast Surg. 2015;42(3):383-8.
17. Sezgin B, Ozmen S. Fat grafting to the face with adjunctive microneedling: a simple technique with high patient satisfaction. Turk J Med Sci. 2018;48:592-601.
18. Tenna S, Cogliandro A, Barone M, Panasiti V, Tirindelli M, Nobile C, et al. Comparative study using autologous fat grafts plus platelet-rich plasma with or without fractional CO_2 laser resurfacing in treatment of acne scars: analysis of outcomes and satisfaction with FACE-Q. Aesth Plast Surg. 2017;4:661-6.

CHAPTER 15

Ice Pick Scars

Niti Khunger

IN A NUTSHELL

- ❖ Ice pick scars are common atrophic scars following acne.
- ❖ They are difficult to treat.
- ❖ Chemical reconstruction of skin scars (CROSS) technique or pinpoint CO_2 laser irradiation are methods of choice.
- ❖ Minipunch elevation can be done for very deep scars.
- ❖ Priming with skin lightening agents is essential before CROSS technique.
- ❖ There is a downtime of 3–7 days following CROSS.
- ❖ Subcision, minipunch elevation and laser resurfacing are supplementary procedures to enhance results.
- ❖ Camouflage by makeup fills the pits and gives satisfactory temporary relief.

INTRODUCTION

Ice pick scars are one of the most common type of atrophic scars seen following acne and also the most difficult to treat. They are so called because it appears as if the skin has been pricked with an ice pick. They are deep, narrow, sharply defined epithelial tracts extending vertically to the deep dermis or subcutaneous tissue fixed with bands of collagen.

The surface opening is wider than the deeper portion as it tapers into a "V" **(Figs. 1A and B)**. When they are mild and not very deep, they give the appearance of open pores and tend

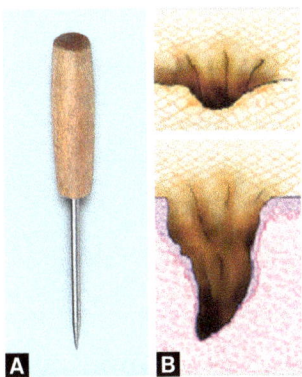

Figs. 1A and B: (A) Ice pick; (B) V-shape epithelial tract of the ice pick scar extending deep, wide at the surface.

to worsen with age as the skin becomes lax. They are more commonly seen on the cheeks, glabellar region and nose. They may be mild, moderate or deep **(Figs. 2A to C)**.

METHODS OF TREATMENT[1]

The depth of ice pick scars is often well below that can be reached with conventional skin resurfacing options like dermabrasion or ablative lasers, hence they are difficult to eliminate entirely by resurfacing **(Fig. 3)**. The successful treatment of ice pick scars requires destruction of the deep epithelial tract and collagenization of the underlying atrophic dermis. As they are not distensible, fillers are also not successful. On the contrary ice pick scars tend to become more prominent following fillers due to the filling of the surrounding more elastic tissue.

Ice pick scars are commonly treated by the following methods:
- Chemical reconstruction of skin scars (CROSS)
- Subcision

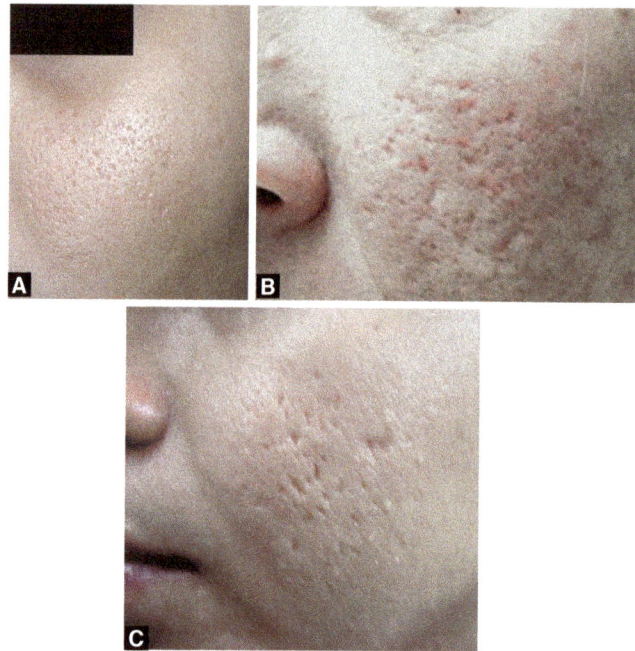

Figs. 2A to C: (A) Mild superficial ice pick scars; (B) Moderate ice pick scars; (C) Deep ice pick scars.

- Minipunch elevation or minipunch grafting
- Microneedling
- Fractional laser resurfacing (ablative or nonablative)

The best treatment is by combination of CROSS technique and subcision followed by microneedling or fractional laser resurfacing.

LIMITATIONS

It may not be possible to entirely eliminate deep ice pick scars, though they can be reduced.

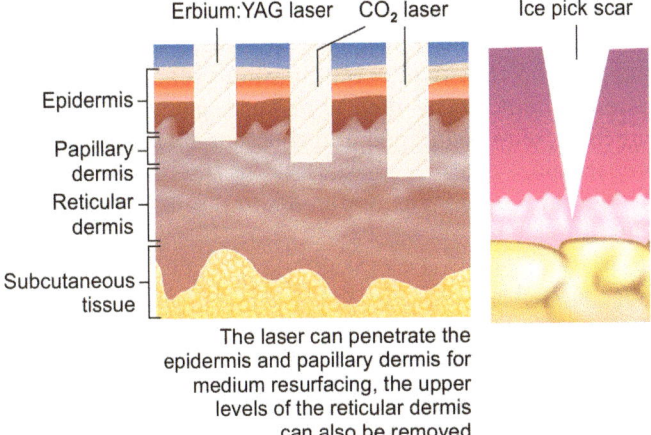

Fig. 3: Depth of ice pick scar is deeper than the depth of the laser beam.

PRECAUTIONS

Fillers should not be used initially, if the patient has predominantly ice pick scars as they tend to become more noticeable. It is better to treat the ice pick scars first before soft tissue augmentation by fillers or fat. Most of the techniques used for the treatment of ice pick scars require some downtime. Hence, this should be discussed first with the patient before beginning treatment.

PREPROCEDURE PREPARATION

Acne should be well controlled. Antiviral therapy with acyclovir or famciclovir beginning 2 days prior to the procedure and continued for 5 days or until complete healing may be required in patients with a history of facial herpes simplex. Priming is very important before the CROSS technique, particularly in darker skins prone to postinflammatory hyperpigmentation. Education about proper sunscreen use and topical tretinoin or adapalene cream along with a skin-lightening agent such as hydroquinone or kojic acid or low-strength glycolic acid are important prerequisites before CROSS treatment. It is emphasized that triple combination creams containing steroids should be avoided to prevent aggravation of acne. Punch excision techniques and subcision do not require any preparation.

Plan the procedures required and discuss the roadmap with the patient.

TECHNIQUE[2]

- Informed consent and pretreatment photographs with indirect lighting are important. Three views should be taken, front, side and oblique views
- Assess the sites, number, size and depth of the ice pick scars
- Scrub the sites with spirit, povidone-iodine and again spirit
- Degrease with acetone
- No anesthesia is required for CROSS
- Topical anesthesia may be given for subcision
- Infiltration anesthesia is required for punch excision techniques if combined with CROSS
- Do subcision first and wait for the bleeding to subside
- Pinpoint narrow (<2 mm), deeper ice pick scars should be treated with the CROSS technique, using a fine sharpened wooden toothpick (For details see Chapter 8) **(Fig. 4)**. Beginners may use 35–50% trichloroacetic acid (TCA). However, 90–100% TCA gives optimal results
- The CROSS technique should be carried out with the patient in the sitting patient, under oblique lighting
- It should not be used for large wide scars as it can cause further atrophy and worsening of the scars
- Wider (>2 mm) deep scars are treated with minipunch excision techniques (see Chapter 8)
- Care is taken to reach down to the subcutaneous tissue, or else there will not be significant improvement.

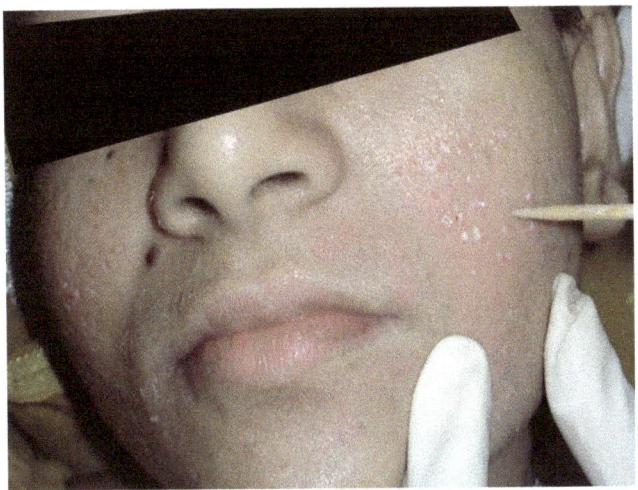

Fig. 4: Pinpoint frosting with 100% TCA following CROSS technique. (CROSS: chemical reconstruction of skin scars; TCA: trichloroacetic acid)

- Procedures can be repeated every 2–4 weeks till a satisfactory response is obtained. About 2–3 procedures are usually required, depending on the initial severity of the scars **(Figs. 5A and B)**.
- Fractional resurfacing with lasers can be done as a final procedure after CROSS treatment to enhance the results.

In a study of 30 dark-skinned patients (Type 4 and 5) with ice pick scars, excellent results (>70% improvement) were seen in 22 (73.3%) patients, while 8 patients had fair-to-good results.[3] Transient hyperpigmentation was seen in two patients. Phenol 88% has also been used instead of TCA for the CROSS technique. In a study comparing the two reagents, it was observed that though results were comparable, discomfort was less with TCA 90% but hyperpigmentation and widening of the scar was seen with TCA as compared to phenol.[4] Recently, the pinpoint irradiation technique using the CO_2 laser has

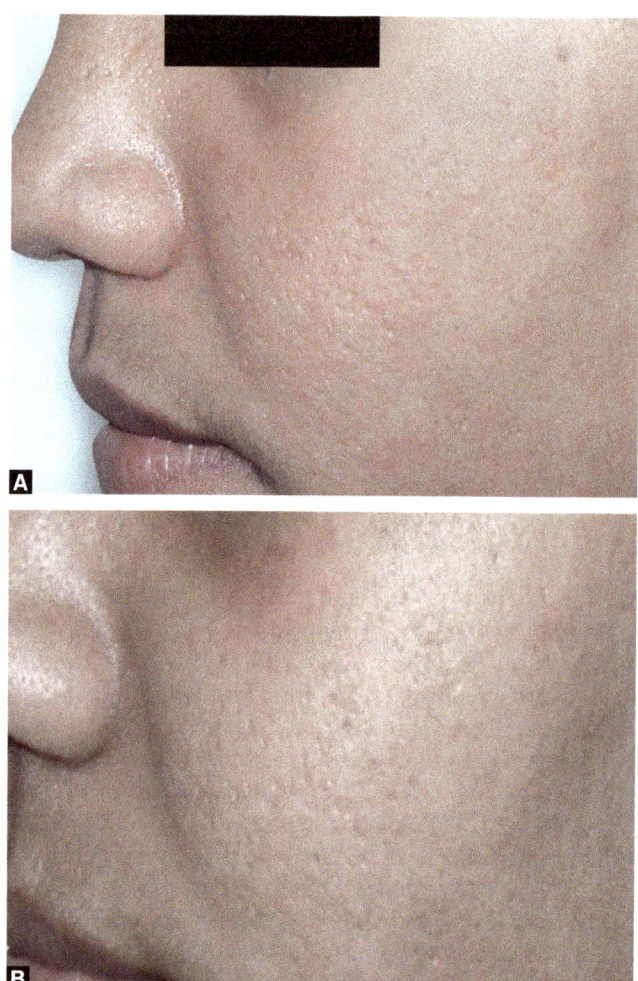

Figs. 5A and B: (A) Ice pick acne scars in type IV skin; and (B) Moderate improvement after three sessions of chemical reconstruction of skin scars (CROSS) at interval of 2 weeks.

been used for the treatment of ice pick acne scars.[4-6] In this technique, a conventional CO_2 laser with pinpoint irradiation is used, instead of the standard fractional laser. In a study by Mohammed G[6] in 60 patients with ice pick scars, the technique was compared with and without needling. Significant improvement in the scars was seen in all patients. However, there was no significant difference between the two groups, with or without needling.

Another report used low viscosity hyaluronic acid (HA) (Restylane® vital) for the treatment of ice pick acne scars after laser resurfacing.[7] In this study 12 subjects underwent microinjections of 20 mg/mL HA gel into discrete depressed acne scars on the face. Immediate improvement was seen in all patients. However, it is to be remembered that results are temporary lasting for an average of 3-6 months with temporary fillers. Adequate subcision is an important prerequisite for treatment with fillers.

Camouflaging the scars with makeup gives good satisfaction to the patient and should be advised before important events to relieve stress (for details see Chapter 25).

POSTPROCEDURE CARE

Immediate postprocedure erythema can be intense in fair skin patients **(Fig. 6)**. This reduces spontaneously in 2-3 hours or ice gel packs can be applied immediately after the procedure. Sun exposure should be minimized following the CROSS technique. The downtime for CROSS technique is 3-5 days till the crusts fall off **(Fig. 7)**. The priming regimen should be restarted. Following punch elevation or grafting, the graft should be immobilized with a dressing to prevent dislodging the graft or cobblestoning. The dressing should be kept for at least 5-7 days.

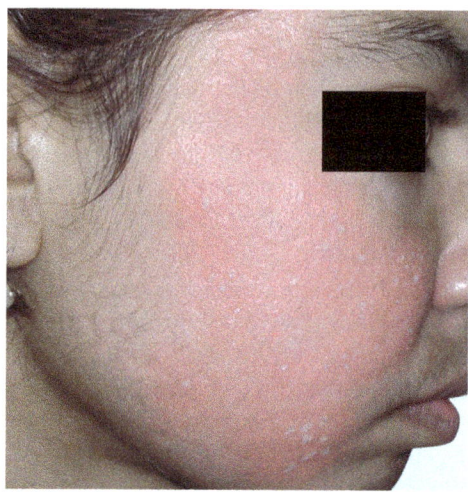

Fig. 6: Intense erythema immediately following chemical reconstruction of skin scars (CROSS) technique.

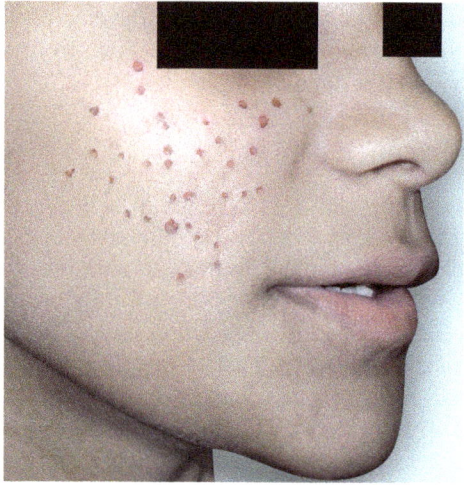

Fig. 7: Crusting following chemical reconstruction of skin scars (CROSS) technique.

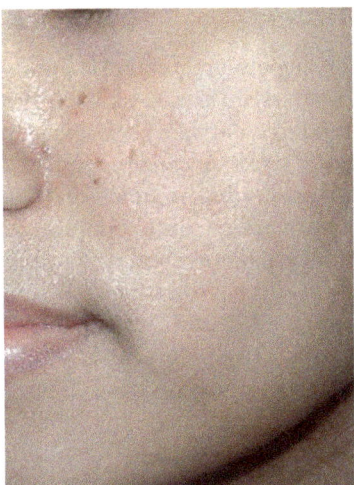

Fig. 8: Postinflammatory hyperpigmentation following chemical reconstruction of skin scars (CROSS) technique.

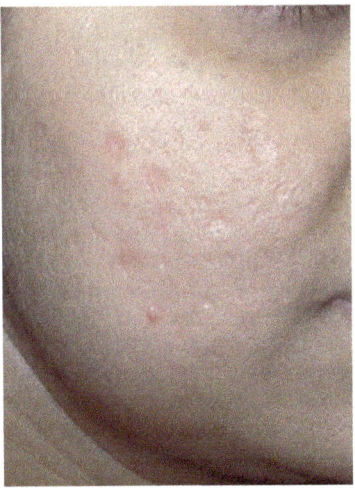

Fig. 9: Worsening of ice pick scars following incorrect chemical reconstruction of skin scars (CROSS) technique.

COMPLICATIONS

Postinflammatory hyperpigmentation is common after CROSS technique, particularly in darker skins, if the patient is not adequately primed or is careless about sun exposure **(Fig. 8)**. Worsening of the ice pick scar can occur following CROSS if the TCA spills to the surrounding normal skin **(Fig. 9)**. Premature removal of the crust can also cause suboptimal collagenization or worsening. Hence, patients should be warned not to pick at the crusts. Following punch elevation, a sunken pit or elevated popped up graft (cobblestone appearance) are common complications, which can be avoided by proper technique. To minimize complications, priming the patient with skin lightening agents, using a very fine toothpick which has been sharpened and a carefully practiced technique to avoid spillage of the reagent to the surrounding skin are essential.

CONCLUSION

Ice pick scars are one of the most difficult scars to treat. Subcision, CROSS technique and punch excision techniques in combination, followed by resurfacing give optimal results.

REFERENCES

1. Fabbrocini G, Annunziata MC, D'Arco V, De Vita V, Lodi G, Mauriello MC, et al. Acne scars: pathogenesis, classification and treatment. Dermatol Res Pract. 2010;2010:893080.
2. Bhardwaj D, Khunger N. An assessment of the efficacy and safety of CROSS technique with 100% TCA in the management of ice pick acne scars. J Cutan Aesthet Surg. 2010;3:93-6.
3. Khunger N, Bhardwaj D, Khunger M. Evaluation of CROSS technique with 100% TCA in the management of ice pick acne scars in darker skin types. J Cosmet Dermatol. 2011;10:51-7.
4. Dalpizzol M, Weber MB, Mattiazzi AP, Manzoni AP. Comparative Study of the use of trichloroacetic acid and phenolic acid in the treatment of atrophic-type acne scars. Dermatol Surg. 2016;42:377-83.

5. Kim S. Clinical trial of a pinpoint irradiation technique with the CO_2 laser for the treatment of atrophic acne scars. J Cosmet Laser Ther. 2008;10:177-80.
6. Mohammed G. Randomized clinical trial of CO_2 laser pinpoint irradiation technique with/without needling for ice pick acne scars. J Cosmet Laser Ther. 2013;15:177-82.
7. Halachmi S, Amitai DB, Lapidoth M. Treatment of acne scars with hyaluronic acid: an improved approach. J Drugs Dermatol. 2013;12:e121-e3.

CHAPTER 16

Boxcar Scars

Niti Khunger, Shikha Bansal

IN A NUTSHELL

- ❖ Boxcar scars are punched-out scars with vertical sharp edges that are not effaced while stretching the skin. They may be shallow or deep.
- ❖ Shallow scars are treated with subcision followed by laser resurfacing or microneedling.
- ❖ Deep scars are treated with punch excision techniques followed by resurfacing.

INTRODUCTION

Boxcar scars are round, oval, or irregular depressed scars with sharp vertical edges. They appear punched out and may be shallow (0.1–0.5 mm) or deep (0.5–4 mm), similar to varicella scars (**Figs. 1A and B**). Most often, they are 1.5–4.0 mm in diameter. These scars tend to be wider at the surface than an ice pick scar and do not have the tapering V shape. They occur due to inflammation occurring deep down into the dermis and extending even up to the subcutaneous tissue.

The principles of treatment include bringing the bottom of the scar to the surface level, making them less apparent or ablating the surrounding raised edges to the level of the floor of the scar. Shallow boxcar scars are within the dermal reach of skin resurfacing treatments such as laser resurfacing but deeper boxcar scars are resistant to improvement by resurfacing

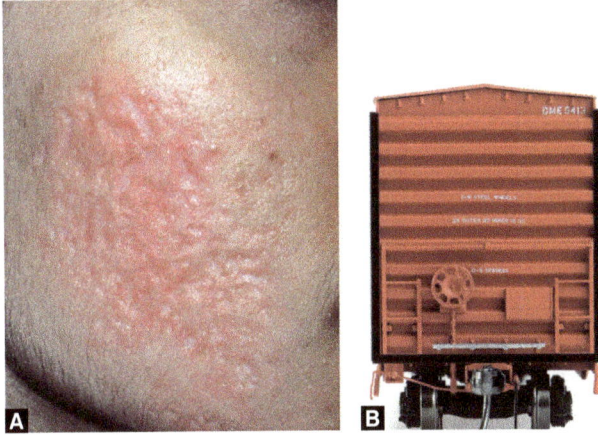

Figs. 1A and B: (A) Multiple punched-out boxcar scars; and (B) A boxcar with sharp vertical contours.

alone and require treatment of the full thickness of the scar in addition.

SITES

They are most common on the cheeks, forehead, and nose (**Fig. 2**).

METHODS OF TREATMENT

For Shallow Scars

- Subcision
- Fillers or autologous fat after subcision
- Microneedling
- Followed by resurfacing either by spot dermabrasion, spot microdermabrasion, or ablative fractional laser or fractional radiofrequency
- Subcision combined with microneedling (dermaroller) or dermastamping is a useful minimally invasive technique, particularly if lasers are not available or are not affordable.

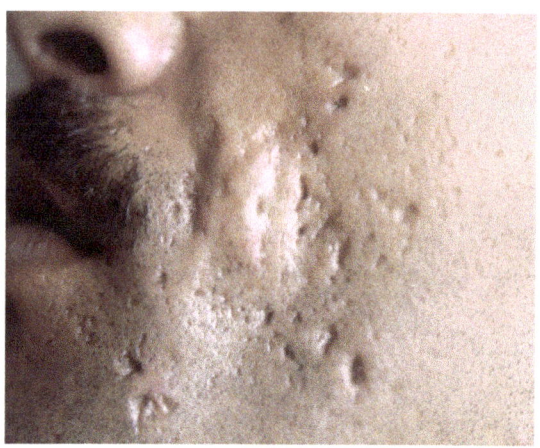

Fig. 2: Deep boxcar scars on the cheeks.

For Deep Scars

- Subcision
- Punch elevation
- Punch excision and suturing or grafting
- Followed by resurfacing.

These scars should not be treated with chemical reconstruction of skin scars (CROSS) technique as they usually worsen and become more prominent after CROSS.

INDICATIONS

Boxcar scars are generally very noticeable and psychologically disturbing. Hence, patients usually demand treatment.

CONTRAINDICATIONS

Active inflammation, active infection—bacterial, viral, or fungal, active acne, and bleeding tendencies.

LIMITATIONS

Not all scars can be effaced. Depending on scar severity, the improvement expected can be 60-80% after these techniques. Proper counseling with the patient regarding expectations, downtime, and outcomes is important. There is a downtime of 5-7 days following punch excision techniques.

PRECAUTIONS

Detailed history including important points like keloidal tendency, immunocompromised conditions, smoking, and degree of sun exposure are essential. Control of any active infection is important. Antiviral therapy with acyclovir or famciclovir beginning 2 days prior to the procedure and continued for 7-10 days until complete healing will be required in patients with a history of herpes simplex.

PREPROCEDURE PREPARATION

Preprocedure treatment with sunscreens, topical retinoid, hydroquinone, and glycolic acid is mandatory in patients with a tendency for pigmentation and in all patients with skin types IV-VI.

TECHNIQUE[1-4]

A proper informed consent and adequate photographs in frontal and oblique views with standardized uniform lighting are essential. Photographs with indirect lighting should also be taken.

Subcision

This is the first procedure that should be performed (for details, see Chapter 8). This technique involves undermining of the depressed acne scars and releasing the scar from the underlying fibrous tissue. The procedure produces a collection of blood under the defect. The blood acts as a spacer keeping the scar base from immediately reattaching to the surface layers. The subsequent organization of this blood clot is thought to induce longer-term correction by the formation of collagen. A single treatment will produce partial correction and successive treatments are usually required to produce further improvement. This technique may be readily combined with resurfacing. A bent sharp hypodermic needle or Nokor needle is inserted under the skin immediately adjacent to the scar and aimed at the level appropriate for that scar until it abuts resistance in the scar **(Fig. 3)**. An initial backward and forward motion much like the tunneling of a liposuction procedure is used, but after resistance to tunneling starts to decline and the scar is almost freed from the surface, the direction is changed. The instrument is now passed sideways in a sweeping action

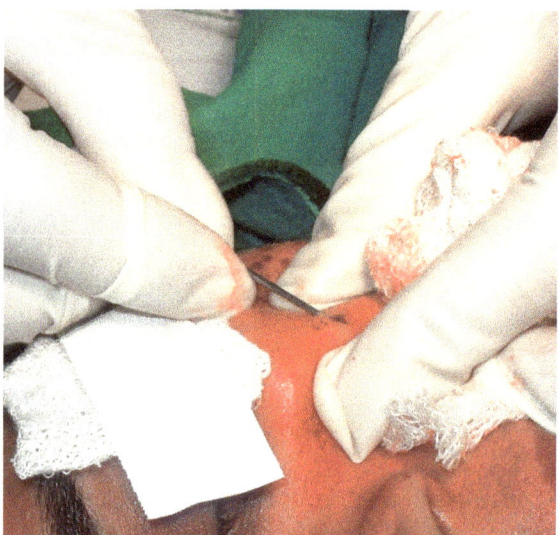

Fig. 3: Subcision to elevate the scars.

to complete the freeing up of the skin from its base. The depression should be seen to visibly lift at the completion of the procedure. Subcision can be repeated every 2-4 weeks till adequate response is achieved. Additional improvement may be achieved when it is combined with resurfacing procedures. For deeper boxcar scars, punch excision techniques are essential to give a good cosmetic result (the details are described in Chapter 9) **(Fig. 4)**.

If the surface texture of the scar is relatively normal, punch elevation (punch flotation) is adequate. In this technique, a biopsy punch corresponding to the size of the scar is selected and driven deep into the scar right up to the subcutaneous tissue, till a "give" is felt. It is then raised to the surface so that it is flush with the surrounding skin. If the surface texture of the scar is atrophic and abnormal, the scar is excised and discarded. It is replaced by a punch graft from the donor skin if

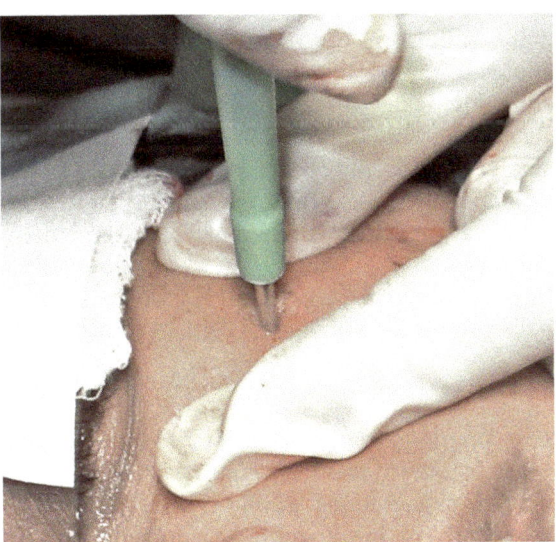

Fig. 4: Punch excision to elevate deep scars.

it is less than 3.5 mm and excised and sutured along the relaxed skin tension line (RSTL) if it is more than 3.5 mm.

If there are multiple deep boxcar scars, the uplifting procedures can be repeated till all scars and their depth have been treated. This is then followed by resurfacing by fractional carbon dioxide (CO_2) or erbium-doped yttrium aluminum garnet (Er:YAG) laser. The advantage of the fractional CO_2 laser is that it also causes skin tightening though it has a downtime of 3-5 days. If lasers are not available, subcision combined with microneedling or dermastamping is a good alternative. The subcision is done first followed by microneedling. The advantage of this combination technique is that it has a minimal downtime of 4-6 hours till erythema and edema subside. The disadvantage is that the improvement is slow and the sessions have to be repeated every 2-4 weeks.

POSTPROCEDURE CARE

Following subcision, light pressure should be given for 10 minutes to reduce bleeding. Following punch excision, care should be taken to prevent dislodgement of the punch graft. Excessive facial movements should be avoided and an adhesive dressing should be in place for at least 3-5 days. After resurfacing, adequate sun protection and skin lightening agents are essential to prevent postinflammatory hyperpigmentation (PIH).

The procedures can be repeated at monthly intervals till a satisfactory response is obtained **(Figs. 5A to D)**.

COMPLICATIONS

The most common complication of boxcar scars is inadequate correction, leading to dissatisfaction after the procedure and inadequate improvement. Complications of subcision include hematoma and nodule formation, if it is done vigorously. These usually subside spontaneously in 1-2 weeks. Complications

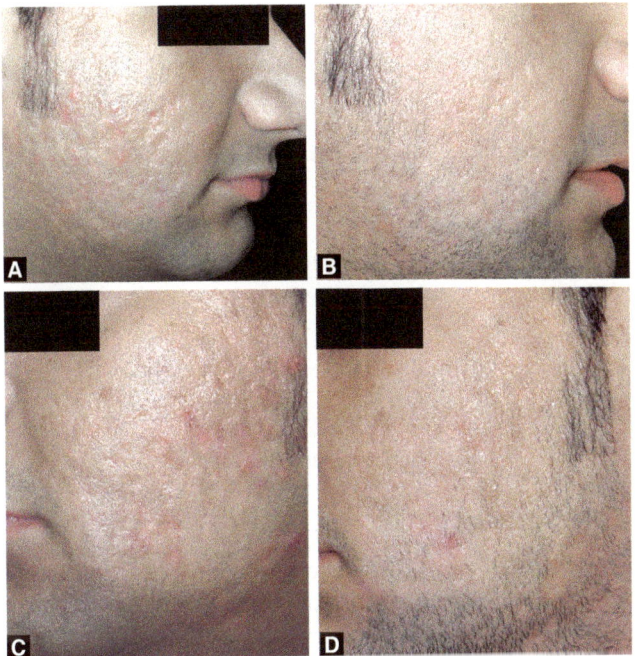

Figs. 5A to D: (A and B) Multiple boxcar scars; and (C and D) Significant improvement after subcision punch elevation and resurfacing.

are more common following punch excision techniques. Cobblestoning is seen as elevation of the graft, persistence of depressed scars, and ring scars can occur due to improper technique **(Fig. 6)** and persistent hyperpigmentation of the grafts may be seen in darker skins. These subside spontaneously, but rarely can be persistent. PIH following resurfacing can occur in darker skins.

Sharply punched-out scars can also be effaced using an ablative CO_2 laser in the ultrapulse mode. The sharp edges of the scars are softened by shouldering and is then followed by fractional CO_2 laser.

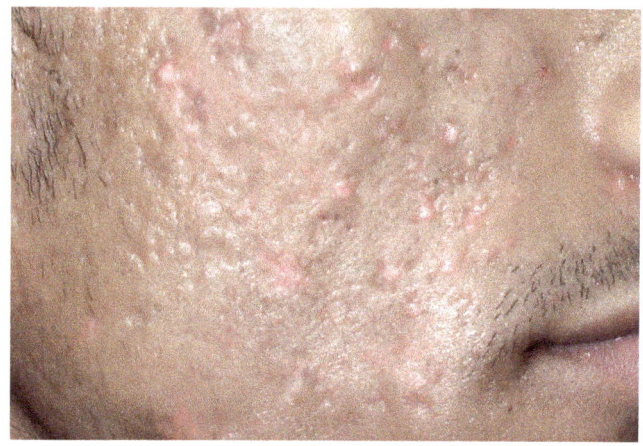

Fig. 6: Cobblestoning and ring scars.

CONCLUSION

Boxcar scars are sharply punched-out scars with vertical sharp edges. They are difficult to treat and require multiple modalities such as subcision and punch excision techniques followed by resurfacing.

REFERENCES

1. Khunger N. IADVL Task Force. Standard guidelines of care for acne surgery. Indian J Dermatol Venereol Leprol. 2008;74:S28-36.
2. Khunger N, Khunger M. Subcision for depressed facial scars made easy using a simple modification. Dermatol Surg. 2011;37:514-7.
3. Shah S, Alam M. Laser resurfacing pearls. Semin Plast Surg. 2012;26:131-6.
4. Goodman GJ. Treating scars: addressing surface, volume, and movement to expedite optimal results. Part 2: More-severe grades of scarring. Dermatol Surg. 2012;38:1310-21.

CHAPTER 17

Rolling Scars

Niti Khunger

IN A NUTSHELL

- Rolling acne scars are distensible and get effaced by applying the stretch test.
- Subcision followed by fillers or autologous fat transfer is the method of choice.
- Subcision combined with microneedling gives satisfactory results in mild scarring.
- Microneedling radiofrequency or fractional resurfacing with the carbon dioxide laser tightens the skin and improves the outcome.

INTRODUCTION

Rolling scars are shallow atrophic scars that are caused by tethering of the underlying dermis to the subcutaneous tissue by fibrous bands. They are wide scars, with relatively normal appearing skin surface. The clue to these type of scars is that these scars will get effaced and appear normal, if the skin is stretched **(Figs. 1A and B)**. Among the various types of acne scars, they are relatively easier to treat.

METHODS OF TREATMENT[1-3]

Rolling scars are best treated by a combination of subcision that breaks down the tethering dermal bands followed by fillers or fat transfer that raises the scars and improves appearance. The use of fillers gives instant results, though it is more expensive.

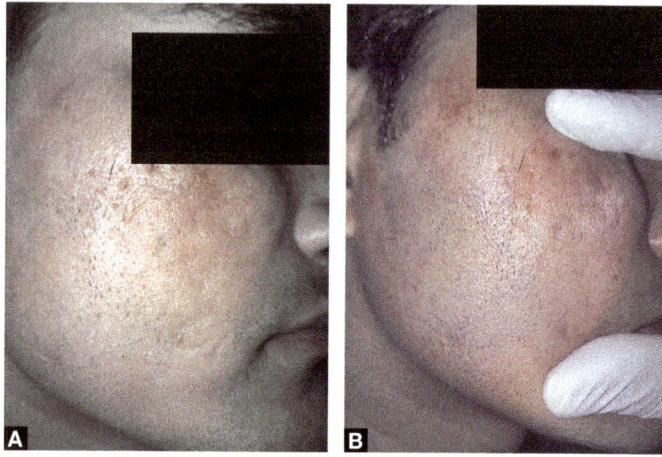

Figs. 1A and B: Stretch test.

The other simpler alternative is subcision combined with microneedling. Though microneedling is a useful technique for rolling scars, it requires at least three to five sittings to give satisfactory results. Fractional resurfacing with either carbon dioxide (CO_2) or erbium-doped yttrium aluminum garnet (Er:YAG) laser or the newer fractional radiofrequency machines is also an effective technique when combined with subcision.

A study compared the effect of 100% trichloroacetic acid (TCA) chemical reconstruction of skin scars (CROSS) with subcision in rolling acne scars in 20 patients with skin types III and IV.[4] The improvement was significantly better with subcision as compared to CROSS with fewer side effects.

INSTRUMENTS

- Hypodermic needle no. 20 or 18
- Hyaluronic acid filler (Juvéderm®, Juvéderm® Ultra, Restylane®, etc.)

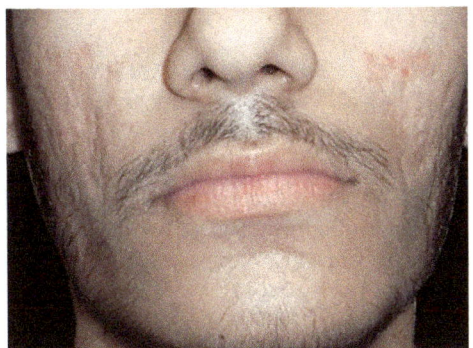

Fig. 2: Rolling scars with lipoatrophy.

- Instruments for autologous fat if planned
- Dermaroller 1.5-2 mm depth or dermastamp or dermapen
- Fractional CO_2 laser or fractional radiofrequency machine.

INDICATIONS

Rolling scars may not be very noticeable in the initial stages, but become more prominent with age, when the skin begins to sag. In the younger age group, they become prominent if the patient has a sudden loss of weight or healing of acne is followed by subcutaneous atrophy **(Fig. 2)**.

CONTRAINDICATIONS

Active inflammation, active infection—bacterial, viral, or fungal, and keloidal tendencies are relative contraindications. Patients on isotretinoin should also be carefully treated, though it is not an absolute contraindication.

LIMITATIONS

Though the treatment of rolling scars is the easiest among all atrophic acne scars, treatment may not be satisfactory if they are severe or numerous.

PRECAUTIONS

A detailed history including important points like keloidal tendency, diabetes, immune compromising conditions, history of herpes simplex, smoking, and degree of sun exposure are essential. Active infection should be controlled. Antiviral therapy with acyclovir or famciclovir beginning 2 days prior to the procedure and continued for 7-10 days until complete healing may be required in patients with a history of herpes simplex.

PREPROCEDURE PREPARATION

Sunscreens and topical retinoids are mandatory in all patients. Skin lightening agents like kojic acid, hydroquinone, and topical vitamin C serums are useful adjuncts, particularly in darker skins to minimize postinflammatory hyperpigmentation (PIH). These should be started at least 2 weeks before procedures.

TECHNIQUE

A proper informed consent regarding expected outcomes, downtime involved, and likely complications is mandatory. Adequate photographs in frontal and oblique views with standardized uniform lighting are essential.

Adequate subcision is the most important technique for rolling scars. It should precede a filler or fat transfer in order to avoid a lumpy, irregular appearance (**Fig. 3**). If the scars are not very prominent, fillers may not be required. Subcision followed by microneedling at the same session also gives good improvement. After the scars are marked, subcision is performed. It is then followed by microneedling in the same session. The sessions are repeated every 2-4 weeks till adequate response (**Figs. 4A and B**).

This is then followed by a final session of fractional resurfacing, which tightens the skin.

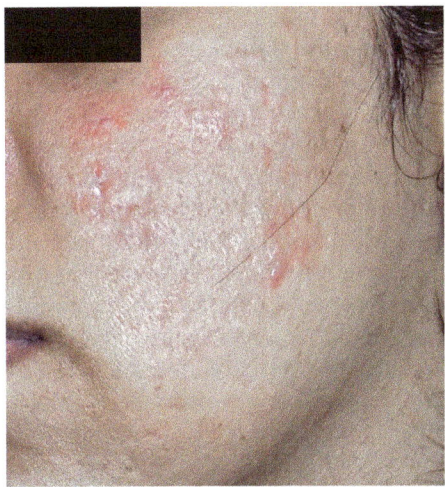

Fig. 3: Lumpy appearance after autologous fat transfer.

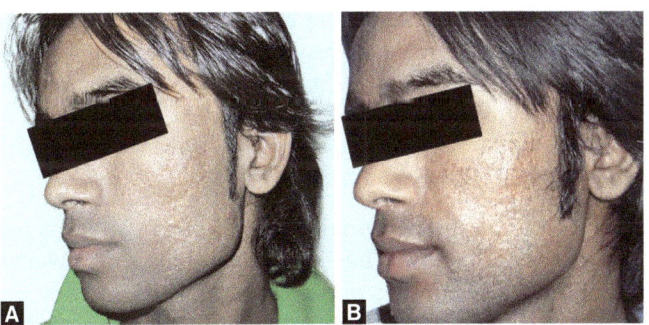

Figs. 4A and B: (A) Before treatment; and (B) After four sessions of subcision and one session of autologous fat.

Autologous fibroblasts injected intradermally have been reported to be successful for the treatment of moderate-to-severe distensible scars.[5] In this randomized multicenter, double-blind, and placebo-controlled trial, 99 subjects with distensible acne scars underwent three intradermal injections with 2 mL of autologous fibroblast suspension (10–20 million cells/mL) on one cheek and vehicle control (cell culture medium) on the other at 14-day intervals. The fibroblasts were obtained from three postauricular biopsies. Treatment with autologous fibroblast was associated with statistically significantly greater improvement in acne scar appearance than vehicle control based on the live subject and evaluator responder analysis and three independent photographic reviewer assessments. Side effects were mainly transient erythema and edema. However, treatment was well tolerated.[5]

Bipolar microneedling radiofrequency (MNRF) devices have also been reported to give satisfactory results after three to four sessions.[6]

POSTPROCEDURE CARE

Following subcision and fillers, the area should not be vigorously massaged to prevent movement of the filler. After microneedling and fractional resurfacing, sun exposure should be minimized to prevent PIH. Skin lightening agents should be used in darker skins.

COMPLICATIONS

Bruising, hematoma formation, and fibrous nodules can occur with subcision. These usually subside in 2 weeks. Rarely if fibrous nodules persist beyond 4 weeks, they can be treated with intralesional triamcinolone acetonide 2.5 mg/mL. Microneedling is usually a safe procedure with few complications. Persistent erythema and a sensitive skin can occur if the microneedling is done vigorously or too frequently. Withholding procedures till the skin comes back to normal, is usually sufficient. PIH is a common complication in darker skins following resurfacing. It should be treated with skin lightening agents or chemical peels if required.

CONCLUSION

Rolling acne scars are relatively easier to treat. Subcision followed by fillers or autologous fat transfer is the method of choice for multiple, large, or extensive rolling scars. Subcision combined with microneedling gives satisfactory results in mild scarring. Fractional resurfacing with the CO_2 laser or bipolar microneedling radiofrequency devices tightens the skin and improves outcomes.

REFERENCES

1. Fabbrocini G, Annunziata MC, D'Arco V, De Vita V, Lodi G, Mauriello MC, et al. Acne scars: pathogenesis, classification and treatment. Dermatol Res Pract. 2010;2010:893080.
2. Khunger N. IADVL Task Force. Standard guidelines of care for acne surgery. Indian J Dermatol Venereol Leprol. 2008;74:S28-36.
3. Goodman GJ. Treating scars: addressing surface, volume, and movement to optimize results: part 1. Mild grades of scarring. Dermatol Surg. 2012;38:1302-9.
4. Ramadan SA, El-Komy MH, Bassiouny DA, El-Tobshy SA. Subcision versus 100% trichloroacetic acid in the treatment of rolling acne scars. Dermatol Surg. 2011;37:626-33.
5. Munavalli GS, Smith S, Maslowski JM, Weiss RA. Successful treatment of depressed, distensible acne scars using autologous fibroblasts: a multi-site, prospective, double blind, placebo-controlled clinical trial. Dermatol Surg. 2013;39:1226-36.
6. Simmons BJ, Griffith RD, Falto-Aizpurua LA, Nouri K. Use of radiofrequency in cosmetic dermatology: focus on nonablative treatment of acne scars. Clin Cosmet Investig Dermatol. 2014;7:335-9.

CHAPTER 18

Linear and Lipoatrophic Acne Scars

Niti Khunger

IN A NUTSHELL

- ❖ The treatment of linear scars depends on their width. Narrow scars are treated with subcision followed by resurfacing with lasers.
- ❖ Wide scars are treated with subcision followed by fillers or autologous fat if the surface texture is normal or with excision and suturing if surface texture is abnormal.

INTRODUCTION

The process of scarring in acne is initiated when the microinflammatory comedone evolves into a larger inflammatory lesion and activates the mechanisms of wound healing. The morphology of the scar depends on the extent, depth, and degree of inflammation. Various types of acne scars have been described; however, linear scars have not been commonly reported in literature, though they are often observed. Linear scars result from a volume loss in the dermis or subcutaneous tissue.

There are three subtypes of linear scars—(1) narrow (<1 mm in width), (2) broad (>1 mm in width), and (3) lipoatrophic that are associated with lipoatrophy of the surrounding skin. Narrow linear scars appear as thin lines lying singly or connecting with each other **(Figs. 1A and B)**. They may be erythematous in the early stages or normopigmented, hypopigmented, or hyperpigmented in the later stages.

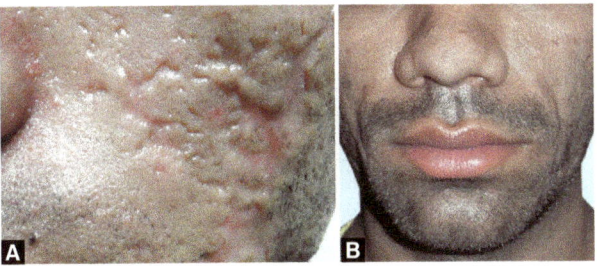

Figs. 1A and B: (A) Narrow linear hypopigmented atrophic scars; and (B) Narrow linear atrophic scars on both cheeks with a typical papular postacne scar on the nose.

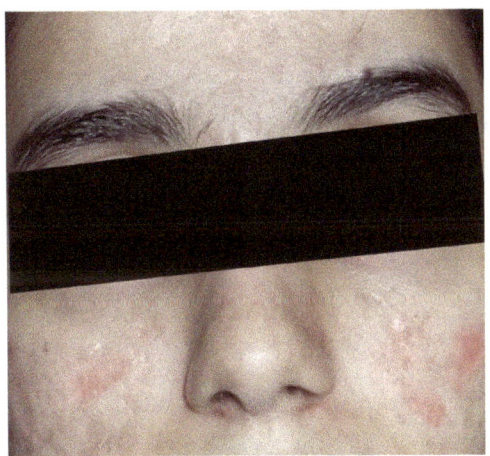

Fig. 2: Linear scar in the glabellar area.

They appear as linear atrophic lines that are commonly hypopigmented with relatively normal skin in between. They are commonly seen on the cheeks, but may also be seen in the glabellar region **(Fig. 2)**. Broad linear scars appear as wide linear dermal depressions, which often have atrophy of underlying subcutaneous fat, called as lipoatrophic linear scars **(Fig. 3A)**. These scars are more common in the lower cheeks parallel to the nasolabial folds and give a gaunt and prematurely aged appearance to the patients **(Fig. 3B)**. These

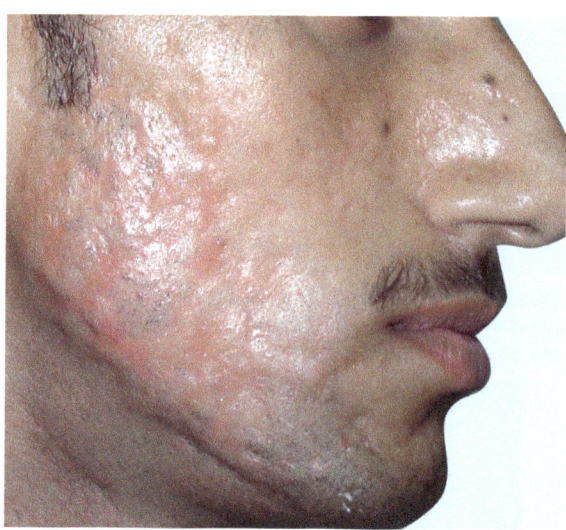

Fig. 3A: Lipoatrophic linear acne scars on the lower cheeks.

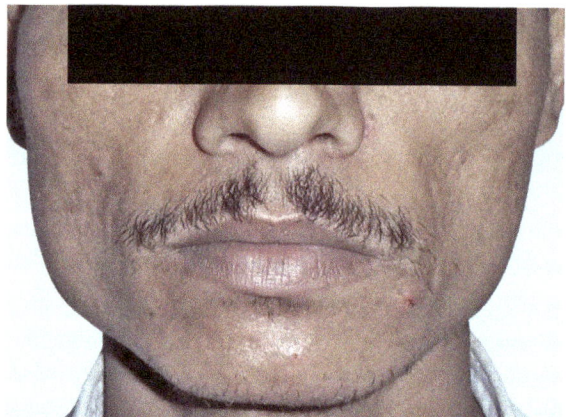

Fig. 3B: Lipoatrophic in nasolabial fold.

types of scars commonly occur following resolution of deep nodulocystic acne, which also destroys the subcutaneous fat.

METHODS OF TREATMENT

The method of choice for treatment of narrow linear scars is subcision, followed by nonablative laser resurfacing. These treatments target the dermal tissues and stimulate collagenization, which uplifts the scars.

Percutaneous collagen induction by microneedling is an alternative treatment, which also gives good results. However, the skin should be adequately stretched while microneedling to reach the bottom of the scars. Treatment has to be repeated every 2–4 weeks, till an optimal response is obtained **(Figs. 4A to C)**. Alternatively, the chemical reconstruction of skin scars (CROSS) technique may be useful, particularly in the hypopigmented linear scars.

The treatment of broad linear scars depends on the texture of the overlying epidermis. If the epidermis is relatively normal,

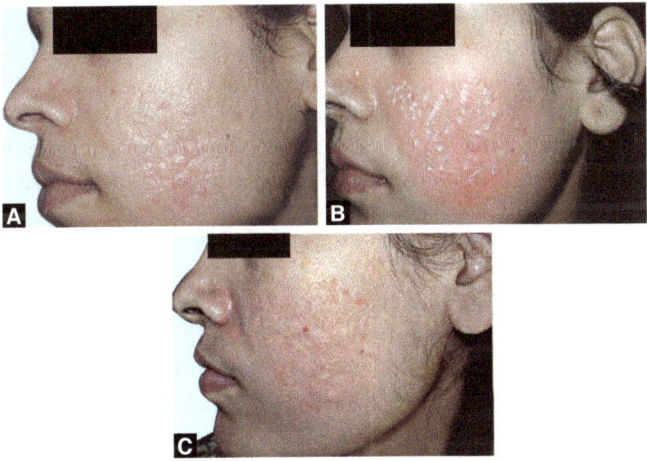

Figs. 4A to C: (A) Linear acne scars before treatment; (B) Subcision followed by CROSS techniques; and (C) Following five sessions of subcision and microneedling and later followed by one session of fractional CO_2 laser. (CROSS: chemical reconstruction of skin scars; CO_2: carbon dioxide)

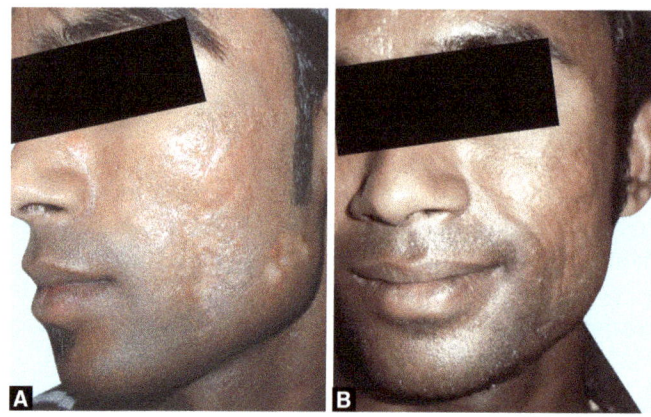

Figs. 5A and B: (A) Lipoatrophic linear scars; and (B) Lipoatrophic linear scars treated with four sessions of microneedling and one session of autologous fat transfer.

subcision followed by soft tissue augmentation with fillers or autologous fat is the treatment of choice **(Figs. 5A and B)**. If the overlying epidermis is atrophic, excision of the scar along the relaxed skin tension lines followed by suturing is the optimal method of treatment **(Figs. 6A to E)**. For deep lipoatrophic scars, fat grafting is the method of choice. Alternatively, a volumizing filler (Juvéderm Voluma®) may be used.

LIMITATIONS

The narrow linear scars, especially if hypopigmented are difficult to eliminate entirely. The broad linear scars can be made less conspicuous by excision and suturing along relax skin tension lines.

PRECAUTIONS

The method of treatment should be chosen with care as tissue augmentation with fillers or fat without proper placement will lead to the linear scars becoming more prominent. It is wiser to adequately undermine or subcise the scars so that the filler goes

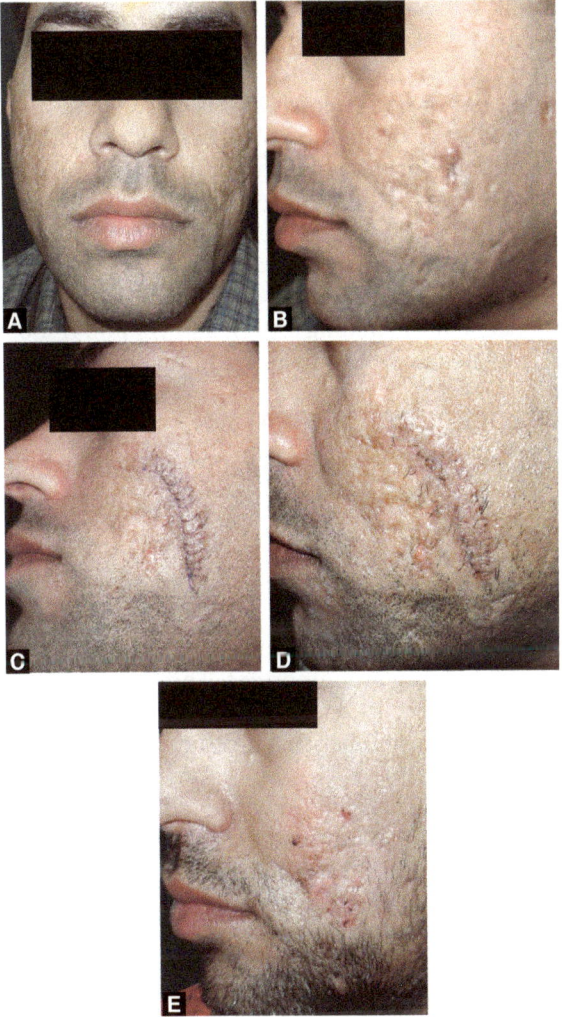

Figs. 6A to E: (A and B) Atrophic acne scars with poor skin texture; (C) Excision of scars along relaxed skin tension lines; (D) Following removal of sutures; and (E) Six months after treatment.

in smoothly rather than pushing it in with force. This will lead to the filler dispersing in the surrounding skin, causing ballooning.

In the glabellar region, extra care should be taken as there is a higher risk of skin necrosis in this area. Fillers should be avoided in this region because of higher risk of blindness.

The most important predictor of success in linear scars is the actual texture of the surface and degree of fibrosis in the scar. When more fibrosis is present and there are multiple scars criss-crossing in various directions, less correction is achieved with fillers. Patients with bleeding tendencies or on anticoagulants including aspirin and vitamin E should be carefully treated to avoid hematoma formation.

PREPROCEDURE PREPARATION

Acne should be adequately controlled. Patients with darker skins should be primed with sunscreens and hypopigmenting agents before resurfacing.

TECHNIQUE

- Informed consent and pretreatment photographs with indirect lighting are important. Three views should be taken—(1) front, (2) side, and (3) oblique views.
- Assess the sites, number, size, width and depth, and surface of the linear scars.
- Scrub the sites with spirit, povidone-iodine, and again spirit.
- Mark the scars requiring treatment with a marking pen with the patient in the sitting position. On lying down, many scars are effaced and may be missed.
- Infiltrate with local anesthesia. One percent lignocaine with adrenaline is preferred. If the area is extensive, a field block or nerve block is preferable. Topical anesthesia alone is usually not sufficient for these scars as they are deep, however it may be used to reduce discomfort of infiltration anesthesia.

Linear and Lipoatrophic Acne Scars

- Subcision is first done for all the linear scars by the modified technique described in Chapter 7. It is important to choose the size of the needle depending on the width of the scar. For narrow scars, no. 22- or 23-gauge hypodermic or Nokor needle should be used and 18 no needle can be used for wider scars. If the fibrotic bands are not released at one session, it is better to repeat subcision after 2 weeks before tissue augmentation. Subcision and undermining of scars should be repeated till fibrosis is reduced and there is smooth passage of the needle beneath the scar. Similarly, better success will be achieved after laser resurfacing if subcision is adequate. This can be gauged by stretching the skin. Adequate subcision will make the scars level with the surrounding skin on stretching it.
- Once adequate subcision is achieved, the next step depends on the predominant type of scars and the most prominent scars. Often it is observed that once the most prominent scar has been appropriately corrected, the other scars are not much disturbing to the patient.
- The wider linear scars and lipoatrophic scars should be treated with fillers or autologous fat. The choice of the agent depends on the surgeons experience and type of scars. Autologous fat is ideal because it is natural, nonimmunogenic, abundantly available, and perhaps the most permanent of all filling agents. Hyaluronic acid fillers are also popular because of easy availability, ease of injection, superior longevity, excellent safety profile, and low rate of hypersensitivity reactions because it is naturally present in the skin tissue. They are available as Restylane®, Restylane Fine Lines® and Perlane® (Medicis Aesthetics, Scottsdale, AZ), Hylaform®, and Juvéderm® Ultra Plus (Allergan, Irvine, CA). Poly-L-lactic acid (Sculptra, Dermik Laboratories, Bridgewater, NJ) is composed of crystalline, irregularly-sized microparticles of poly-L-lactic acid that is chiefly used for human immunodeficiency virus (HIV)-

related facial lipoatrophy. Calcium hydroxylapatite (CaHA) (Radiesse®, Bioform Medical, San Mateo, CA) is a synthetic filler that typically lasts 12–18 months and has been used for acne scars.[1,2]
- If the scar is very wide and the skin texture is abnormal or atrophic, excision followed by suturing along the relaxed skin tension lines is a better option as soft tissue augmentation will not improve surface texture.
- The narrow linear scars are best treated with fractional resurfacing.[3,4] If skin texture is relatively normal, nonablative resurfacing with 1,540 nm erbium glass laser gives a satisfactory response. However, this has to be repeated as results are slow. The advantage is that there is hardly any downtime. In case there are multiple linear scars as well as other boxcar scars, ablative fractional resurfacing with a carbon dioxide (CO_2) laser 10,600 nm is a better option.
- Microneedling is also a useful technique as it can induce collagenization and also improve the texture of the scars. At least three to four sittings are required at monthly intervals to achieve satisfactory results.
- Medium-depth chemical peels, phenol peels, and traditional electrical dermabrasion were popular in the past, but are now not frequently used because of the significant downtime and higher risk of pigmentary complications in darker skins.

POSTPROCEDURE CARE

Adequate sun protection and restarting the priming regimen are important.

COMPLICATIONS

Complications of subcision include hematoma and nodule formation. These usually subside spontaneously in 1–2 weeks. Complications with fillers include bruising and edema. Surface irregularities may occur if subcision has not been adequate and fibrous adhesions are not released. Visible papules and granuloma formation are other complications that can occur with fillers. Soft tissue augmentation with fat can also lead to irregular contours due to the adhesions. This can cause the scars to become even more prominent. Irregularities with fat transfer can be treated with intralesional triamcinolone acetonide 5 mg/mL and those with hyaluronic acid with injection hyaluronidase. Complications following fractional laser resurfacing include prolonged erythema, hyperpigmentation, hypopigmentation, demarcation lines, and scarring.

CONCLUSION

Postacne linear scars are common on the cheeks and glabella, caused by loss of dermal or subcutaneous tissue. They may be narrow or broad and are difficult to treat. Adequate subcision is the most effective treatment that is followed by fractional laser resurfacing or microneedling for narrow scars and soft tissue augmentation by fillers or autologous fat for broader scars.

REFERENCES

1. Goldberg DJ, Amin S, Hussain M. Acne scar correction using calcium hydroxylapatite in a carrier-based gel. J Cosmet Laser Ther. 2006;8:134-6.
2. Tzikas TL. Evaluation of the radiance FN soft tissue filler for facial soft tissue augmentation. Arch Facial Plast Surg. 2004;6:234-9.
3. Fulchiero GJ, Parham-Vetter PC, Obagi S. Subcision and 1320-nm Nd:YAG nonablative laser resurfacing for the treatment of acne scars: a simultaneous split-face single patient trial. Dermatol Surg. 2004;30:1356-9.
4. Chua SH, Ang P, Khoo LS, Goh CL. Nonablative 1450-nm diode laser in the treatment of facial atrophic acne scars in type IV to V Asian skin: a prospective clinical study. Dermatol Surg. 2004;30:1287-91.

CHAPTER 19

Papular Scars

Niti Khunger

IN A NUTSHELL

- ❖ Papular scars are not true papules but atrophic scars following destruction of dermal collagen and elastic tissue.
- ❖ They are common on the nose, chin, chest, and back. They can be treated with intralesional radiofrequency with an insulated wire electrode or nonablative fractional erbium glass laser or microneedle radiofrequency device.

INTRODUCTION

Scars following acne require customized treatment according to the type of scars. Hence, it is important to properly classify the scar in order to individualize treatment. Papular scars are skin colored or hypopigmented elevated lesions most common on the trunk, chin, and nose **(Figs. 1A and B)**.[1-3] They result from destruction of collagen and elastin fibers in the dermal tissues around the hair follicles. They are misnamed because they are not actually papules but appear as soft elevated lesions like anetodermas.

They should be differentiated from true hypertrophic scars which are also elevated. This can be done by stretching the skin. Papular scars will get effaced and disappear, whereas true hypertrophic scars remain elevated **(Figs. 2A and B)**. Papular scars are one of the most difficult scars to treat.[4,5]

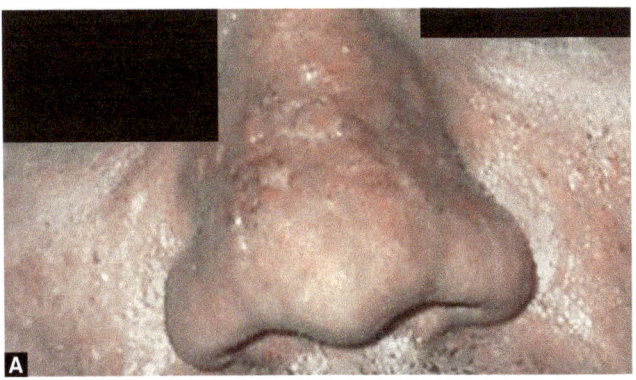
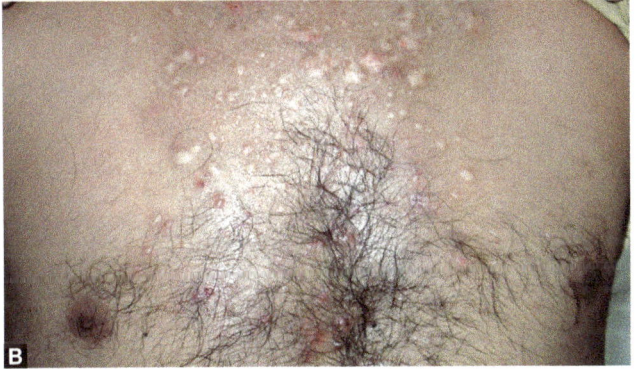

Figs. 1A and B: (A) Papular acne scars on the nose; and (B) Hypopigmented papular acne scars on the chest.

METHODS OF TREATMENT

There is no ideal treatment for papular scars and usually a multimodality approach is required.

Intralesional radiofrequency, nonablative lasers, and microneedling radiofrequency (MNRF) are most frequently used treatment modalities for papular scars.

Multiple treatment sessions may be required to achieve satisfactory results.

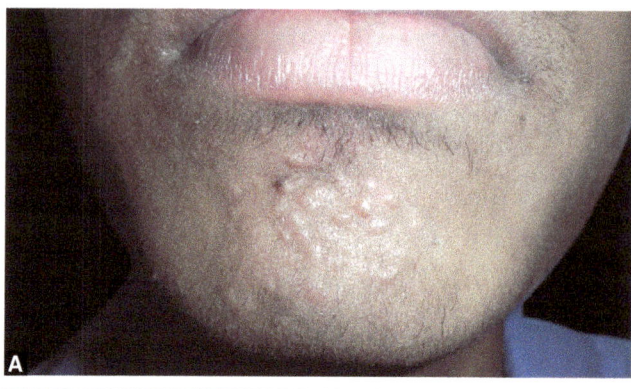
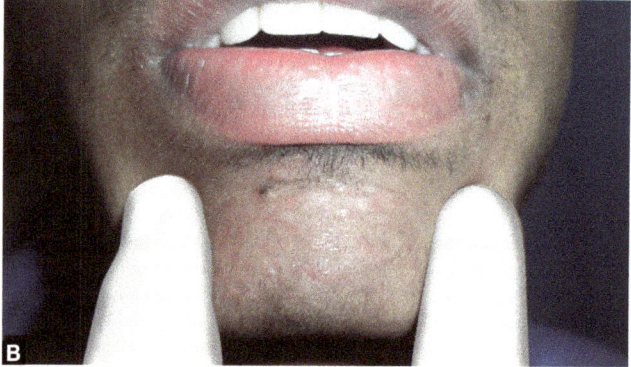

Figs. 2A and B: (A) Papular scars on the chin; and (B) Effacement of scars after stretching the skin.

INSTRUMENTS

- Radiofrequency machine
- Insulated wire electrode **(Fig. 3)**
- Nonablative fractional laser or fractional radiofrequency.

INDICATIONS

Papular scars causing cosmetic distress to the patient.

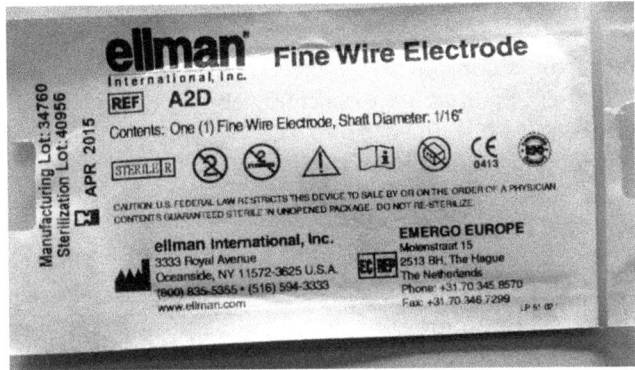

Fig. 3: Wire electrode of radiofrequency machine.

CONTRAINDICATIONS

High expectations of the patient. Since papular scars are difficult to treat, they require proper patient counseling and guidance.

LIMITATIONS

Response may be partial and repeat sessions may be required.

PRECAUTIONS

Postinflammatory hyperpigmentation (PIH) may occur following radiofrequency treatment.

PREPROCEDURE PREPARATION

Control of active acne is important. Sunscreens and topical retinoids, glycolic acid, kojic acid, or hydroquinone should be used 2 weeks prior to starting treatment, particularly in patients prone to PIH.

TECHNIQUE

- Informed consent and pretreatment photographs with indirect lighting are important. Three views should be taken—(1) front, (2) side, and (3) oblique views in a standardized manner.
- The sites, number, size, and depth of the papular scars should be assessed.
- After surgical scrubbing of the sites, the scars should be marked with a marking pen or with antibiotic cream with the patient in the sitting or standing position. On lying down, many scars are effaced and may be missed.
- Topical anesthesia is preferred as it does not efface the scars. However, it may not be sufficient in sensitive patients and a field block or regional nerve block may be given. It is better to avoid infiltration anesthesia, which will efface the scars.
- The power of the radiofrequency machine should be minimal. Ellman® power at 2 in the cut and coagulate mode is sufficient. Electrode should be single wire electrode, preferably insulated.
- The scar is approached perpendicularly and the wire electrode is inserted up to a depth of deep dermis **(Fig. 4)**.

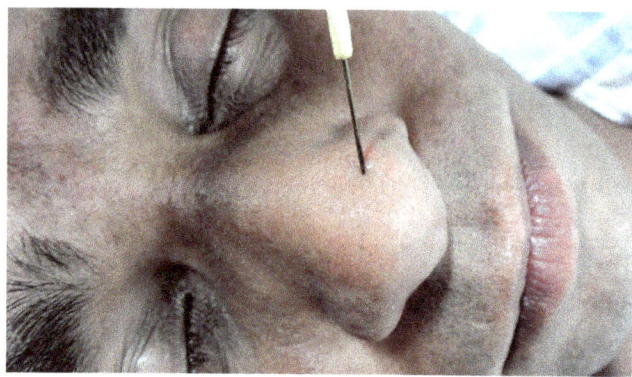

Fig. 4: Diagrammatic representation of intralesional radiofrequency.

The principle is that radiofrequency energy stimulates collagenization in the dermis, while causing contraction at the same time, making the scar less visible.
- Each scar is individually treated. This should be followed by adequate cooling of the skin.
- Sunscreens and skin lightening agents are continued till complete healing.
- If facilities are available, the erbium glass 1,540 nm nonablative fractional laser or MNRF is an alternative mode of treatment. The principle of treatment is the same.
- Multiple sessions of treatment may be required to achieve satisfactory results **(Figs. 5A to C)**.

POSTPROCEDURE CARE

No specific care is required, except sun protection and use of sunscreens. The procedure can be repeated at 2-4 weeks intervals.

COMPLICATIONS

Postinflammatory hyperpigmentation is common and responds to skin lightening agents.[1] Inadequate or unsatisfactory response can be seen, if collagenization has not been optimal. Depressed scars can occur following excessive tissue destruction.

CONCLUSION

Papular scars are difficult to treat and require methods that promote collagenization in the dermis. Intralesional radiofrequency with an insulated wire electrode or nonablative fractional erbium glass laser are the preferred modes of treatment.

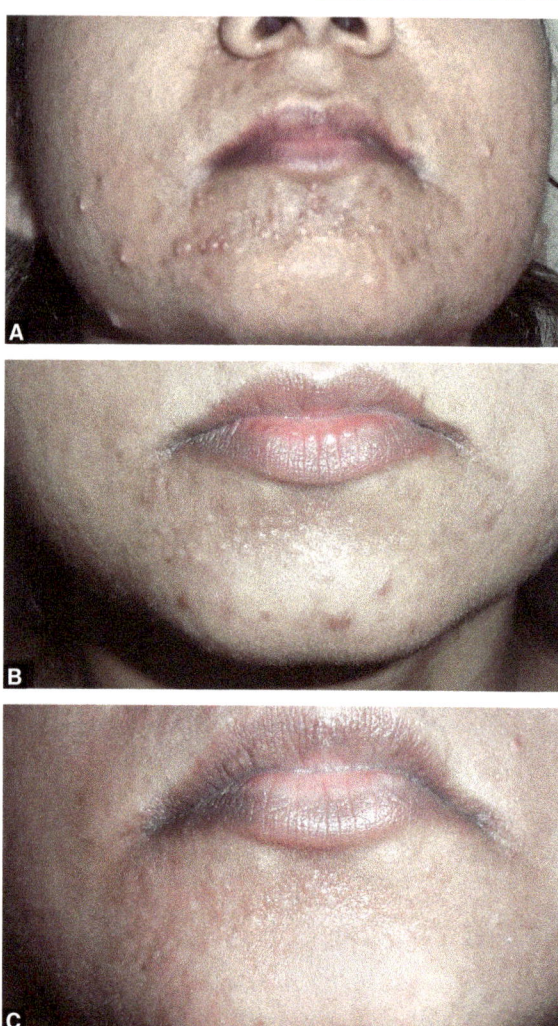

Figs. 5A to C: (A) Papulopustular acne on the chin; (B) Papular acne scars on the chin; and (C) Following two sessions of intralesional radiofrequency.

REFERENCES

1. Wilson BB, Dent CH, Cooper PH. Papular acne scars. A common cutaneous finding. Arch Dermatol. 1990;126:797-800.
2. Gan SD, Graber EM. Papular Scars: An addition to the acne scar classification scheme. J Clin Aesthet Dermatol. 2015;8:19-20.
3. Ali FR, Kirk M, Madan V. Papular acne scars of the nose and chin: An under-recognised variant of acne scarring. J Cutan Aesthet Surg. 2016;9:241-3.
4. Chan HH, Manstein D, Yu CS, Shek S, Kono T, Wei WI. The prevalence and risk factors of post-inflammatory hyperpigmentation after fractional resurfacing in Asians. Lasers Surg Med. 2007;39:381-5.
5. Lee SJ, Kim JM, Kim YK, Seo SJ, Park KY. The pinhole method using an erbium: YAG laser for the treatment of papular acne scars. Dermatol Ther. 2017;30:e12512.

CHAPTER 20

Keloids, Hypertrophic, and Bridging Scars

Niti Khunger

IN A NUTSHELL

- ❖ Hypertrophic scars and keloids following acne are more common in males, predominantly on the back, chest, shoulders, deltoid, and the mandibular region.
- ❖ Aggressive and appropriate treatment of acne is important to prevent occurrence of new lesions.
- ❖ The key to successful treatment therapy is prolonged treatment with antiacne agents, particularly topical retinoids and topical silicone gel along with low strength intralesional steroids as required.

INTRODUCTION

The chronic prolonged inflammation in acne leads to scarring. Hypertrophic scarring occurs when the scar is raised above the skin level, but stays within the confines of the original lesion. These scars are common on the back, chest, shoulders, deltoid, and the mandibular region **(Fig. 1)**. They are more common in males as compared to females. The initial lesion may be an innocuous papule or pustule, which is only noticed when the lesion becomes hypertrophic.

When the scars extend beyond the borders of the original lesion and develop irregular claw-like borders, they are termed as keloidal scars. These scars can be very persistent, extensive, and disfiguring and be associated with pruritus and pain.

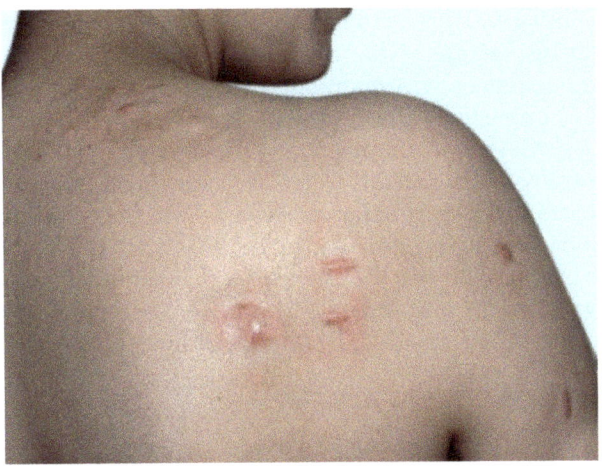

Fig. 1: Hypertrophic scars on the back.

PATHOPHYSIOLOGY AND PREVENTION OF SCARS

Hypertrophic scars and keloids occur due to an abnormal wound healing process where tissue repair and its regulatory mechanisms are impaired. The wound healing phase consists of an initial inflammatory phase, which lasts for 48–72 hours, followed by the proliferative phase which lasts for 3–6 weeks, followed by a maturational or remodeling phase that can last for several months. A multitude of signaling molecules, including growth factors such as transforming growth factor-β (TGF-β), platelet-derived growth factor (PDGF), vascular endothelial growth factor (VEGF), mitogen-activated protein (MAP) kinases, matrix metalloproteinases (MMPs), and tissue inhibitor of metalloproteinases (TIMPs), regulate this complex process of wound healing on the molecular level.[1] In hypertrophic scars, the collagen synthesis is approximately three times greater than in normal skin and 20 times greater in keloids. In addition, the ratio of type I to type III collagen is also high. The most important consideration in patients presenting with hypertrophic scars and keloids is prevention of further lesions. The principle of prevention is to treat inflammation early. Appropriate management of acne lesions is also important, however small or minor the lesion may be. Delay in treatment potentiates the development of scars. In a study of 185 patients with severe scarring, Layton et al.[2] reported that hypertrophic and keloidal scars on the truncal region were more common in males. Though 85% of patients with hypertrophic scar were affected with nodular acne, in 15% only superficial inflammatory lesions were observed. Hence, keloids can occur even with minor inflammatory lesions.

METHODS OF TREATMENT

Once hypertrophic scars or keloids are formed, the principles of treatment remain the same. The methods of treatment include the following.

Nonsurgical Conservative Therapy

- Silicon-based products
- Intralesional steroids (ILS)
- Cryotherapy
- Pulsed dye laser
- Surgical excision followed by ILS
- Preparations containing *Allium cepa*.

Hypertrophic scars may improve naturally during the process of scar maturation. However, the advantage of using nonsurgical therapies is that they can accelerate this process and improve the subjective symptoms, making the patient more comfortable. Keloids require active treatment.

INDICATIONS

- Hypertrophic scars are not improving or at cosmetically important sites
- Keloids causing pain or functional disturbances.

Keloids, Hypertrophic, and Bridging Scars

CONTRAINDICATIONS

Topical steroids should be avoided to prevent aggravation of acne and development of new lesions. Aggressive treatment with ILS should also be avoided to prevent atrophy, particularly on the face.

LIMITATIONS

The limitations of treating keloids should be clearly explained to the patient. The scars will not completely go away and chances of recurrence are high.

PRECAUTIONS

If the acne is active, the treatment of acne should be continued to prevent newer lesions. Isotretinoin should be given, even if patient has mild acne. If there is active infection, systemic antibiotics should be given first to prevent aggravation of acne that can occur with isotretinoin.

CHOICE OF TREATMENT

Treatment should be begun with silicon gels under occlusion or silicon sheets. If lesions are significantly raised, intralesional triamcinolone acetonide 10 mg/mL (0.4 mL) combined with injection 5-fluorouracil (5-FU) 50 mg/mL (0.6 mL) should be given. Intralesional radiofrequency or cryotherapy can be used to debulk the lesions if there are multiple or extensive lesions. For early red lesions, pulsed dye laser 585 nm or intense pulsed light (IPL) may be used.

POST-TREATMENT CARE

After initial treatment, when the lesions have completely flattened, close follow-up is essential. Topical silicone gel products and pressure by using adhesive tapes help in reducing recurrences. Prophylactic low strength ILS 2.5 mg/mL should be administered once a month for 6 months after the lesions have flattened out **(Figs. 2A and B)**.

COMPLICATIONS

Skin atrophy, scarring, and hypo- or depigmentation **(Fig. 3)** can occur following ILS. These complications usually improve over time.

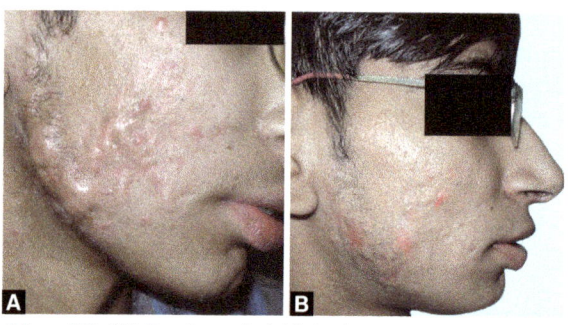

Figs. 2A and B: (A) Persistent keloids in the mandibular area following acne; (B) Improvement following intralesional triamcinolone acetonide combined with 20 mg/mL hyaluronidase.

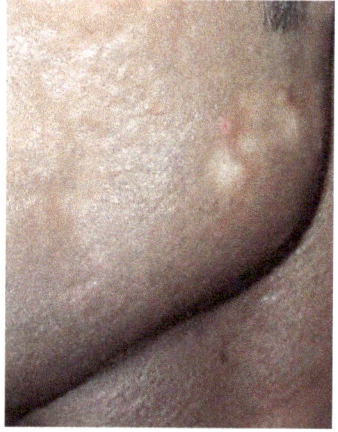

Fig. 3: Hypopigmentation following intralesional steroids.

BRIDGING SCARS

Bridging scars occur following healing of severe acne. They appear as fibrous strings overlying scarred skin or as multiple linear scars joined together by epithelial tracts (**Figs. 4A to C**). They often contain foul-smelling products of sebum. The best method is to excise the tracts, evacuate the contents, and completely excise the scarred tissue. This is to be followed up suturing along relaxed skin tension lines (RSTLs).

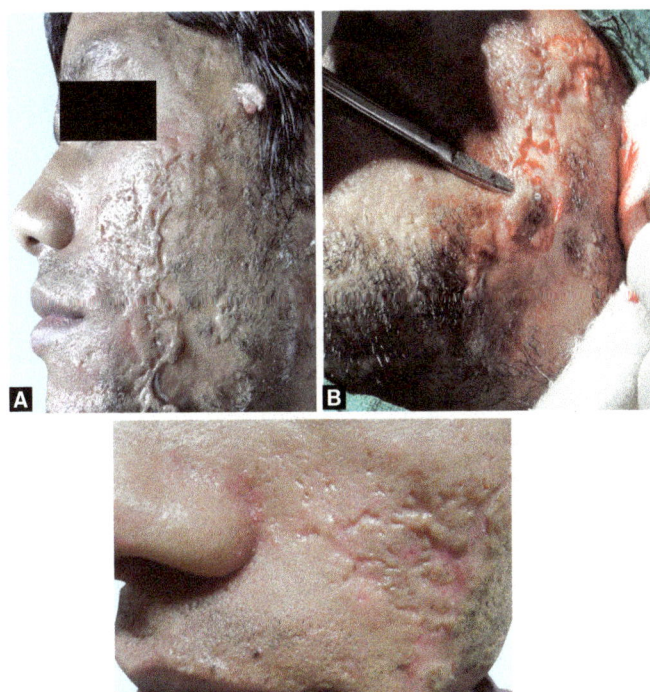

Figs. 4A to C: Bridging scars on the cheeks.

CONCLUSION

Treatment of hypertrophic scars and keloids following acne is a laborious task as lesions are often widespread, multiple, and occur on cosmetically important sites such as the face. The best method is prevention with aggressive antiacne treatment. When scars and keloids have occurred, the treatment should be conservative. Intralesional steroids with 5-FU are the mainstay of therapy. This can also be combined with cryotherapy. Prolonged follow-up with maintenance therapy with silicon gel and occlusive therapy can help to prevent recurrences.

REFERENCES

1. Wolfram D, Tzankov A, Pülzi P, Piza-Katzer H. Hypertrophic scars and keloids—a review of their pathophysiology, risk factors, and therapeutic management. Dermatol Surg. 2009;35:171-81.
2. Layton AM, Henderson CA, Cunliffe WJ. A clinical evaluation of acne scarring and its incidence. Clin Exp Dermatol. 1994;19:303-8.

CHAPTER 21

Acne Scars in Darker Skin Types: Special Precautions

Mukta Sachdev, Ayushi Khandelwal

IN A NUTSHELL

- Darker skin types include skin types IV, V, and VI.
- They are at greater risk of developing pigmentary abnormalities and hypertrophic or keloid scars.
- Adequate sun protection, priming the skin before procedures and postprocedure care with hydroquinone and retinoids can minimize risk of complications.
- Parameters for ablative lasers must be at lower fluencies and fractional ablative laser therapy is safer.
- Radiofrequency as an energy-based treatment is advantageous as it is blinded to skin phototypes.

INTRODUCTION

Racial or ethnic differences exist in perceptions of beauty, the prevalence of specific cosmetic concerns, as well as optimal approaches to treatment. Most important is the need to avoid treatment-associated complications such as pigmentary alterations and keloid scarring, which have a greater risk in darker skin patients.[1] In this era of globalization, it is reasonable to anticipate that dark-skinned patients (Fitzpatrick skin types IV–VI) will be treated world over and hence the physician must be aware of management of procedures in all skin types.

The current Fitzpatrick skin type classification denotes six different skin types, skin color, and reaction to sun exposure which ranges from very fair (skin type I) to very dark (skin type VI) depending upon whether the patient burns at the first average sun exposure or tans at the first average sun exposure. Fitzpatrick skin typing has a proven diagnostic and therapeutic value and is widely used for estimating ultraviolet (UV), PUVA (psoralen and ultraviolet A), and laser treatment doses.[2]

CHARACTERISTICS

Darker skin types or "skin of color" which include Fitzpatrick skin phototypes (SPTs) IV–VI is characterized by increased epidermal melanin and labile melanocytes. Hence, pigmented skin tends to absorb about 40% more laser energy than nonpigmented skin and thermal injury can extend beyond targeted areas.[3] This poses special challenges for the use of laser and light-based therapies, which are associated with a greater risk of dyspigmentation and scarring. Therefore, careful selection of device and treatment parameters and experience are required to minimize complications. Whereas early-generation lasers for resurfacing were generally contraindicated for individuals with Fitzpatrick SPTs IV–VI, advances in the past decade have given rise to a range of devices that can be safely used in darker skin. Longer wavelength lasers such as the 810 nm and 1,064 nm neodymium-doped yttrium aluminum garnet (Nd:YAG); fractional lasers; and radiofrequency devices have all been used safely for pigmentary abnormalities and laser resurfacing in darker skin. In this context, understanding structural and functional differences of darker skin types, particularly how they contribute to nuances in the approach to laser and light-based procedures is of increasing importance to the practitioner.

The leading indications for laser or light-based procedures in patients with SPT V and VI are laser hair removal, resurfacing for the treatment of acne scarring and photorejuvenation, dyschromias, removal of pigmented lesions, skin tightening and tattoo removal.[4] Whereas considerable published data exist on the use of lasers and light therapies in Asian populations with SPT III and IV, studies involving individuals of African ancestry (black subjects) and/or those with SPT V and VI are limited. This represents a significant knowledge gap given the growing diversity of the patient population seeking laser or light-based procedures and the greater risk of disfiguring pigmentary complications in patients with darker skin.

CLINICALLY RELEVANT STRUCTURAL AND FUNCTIONAL DIFFERENCES

Structural and functional differences observed among darkly pigmented skins compared with lightly pigmented populations have been reported. Key biological characteristics to consider when performing laser or light-based aesthetic procedures in dark skin types include:[5]

- Increased epidermal melanin
- Larger melanosomes that are more singly dispersed and widely distributed within epidermal keratinocytes
- Labile melanocyte responses
- Reactive fibroblasts

These features, in turn, contribute to differences in the frequency of specific dermatological disorders, and the safety of laser or light-based procedures. Increased melanin content, packaging and epidermal distribution of melanin confer greater protection against deleterious effects of UV radiation. Labile melanocyte responses contribute to an increased prevalence of pigmentary disorders. Of particular relevance to laser or light procedures, the tendency for injury or inflammation to incite alterations in pigment production is associated with a greater risk for postprocedure hyper- or hypopigmentation in individuals with SPT IV-VI. Racial differences exist in the frequency of keloids, with the highest prevalence being observed in populations of African ancestry. This is probably due to genetic factors that contribute to increased fibroblast reactivity among individuals at risk. Therefore, a greater overall risk of keloids and hypertrophic scars associated with iatrogenic dermal injury is observed in ethnic populations. With the above characteristics in mind, minimization of epidermal and dermal injury through careful selection of treatment modality and settings as well as the use of pre- and post-treatment precautions are paramount when performing laser or light-based procedures in dark-skinned patient populations.

SPECIAL PRECAUTIONS

It is very important to be cautious in laser skin resurfacing procedures in patients with Fitzpatrick skin types III–VI because of the well-known and well-documented side effects that may occur in this group, including hyperpigmentation, hypopigmentation and scarring.

Hyperpigmentation occurs from 6 weeks to 6 months after laser ablation in almost 100% of dark-skinned patients. Although transient in most patients, it can persist from 9 months to a year. Treatment for this condition is bleaching with hydroquinone. Hypopigmentation may occur 6 months after laser abrasion.[1] Although incidence of hypopigmentation is much less than that of hyperpigmentation, hypopigmentation may result in permanent hypopigmented scars. In dark-skinned people, these scars are much more obvious and difficult to conceal.

Take a careful pretreatment history, including the patient's previous exposure to trauma, dermabrasion, or chemical peels. These factors carry increased risk for hypopigmentation. Scarring is a consideration with laser resurfacing. Darker skin types are more predisposed to the formation of hypertrophic and keloid scars.[1] Most complications with procedures in darker skins can be avoided with adequate knowledge and judicious use **(Table 1)**.

TABLE 1: Prevention and treatment of complications in darker skins.

Complication	Prevention	Treatment of complication
Hyperpigmentation—occurs from 6 weeks to 6 months after laser ablation in almost 100% of dark-skinned patients. Although transient in most patients, it can persist from 9 months to a year	• Pretreatment with bleaching agents like hydroquinone • Regular use of sunscreen	• Topical depigmenting creams • Sunscreen • Sunprotection
Hypopigmentation may occur 6 months after laser abrasion. Incidence of hypo-pigmentation is less than hyperpigmentation	• Take a careful pretreatment history, including the patient's previous exposure to trauma, dermabrasion, or chemical peels • These factors carry increased risk for hypopigmentation	• Tacrolimus • Pimecrolimus
Scars	• Scarring is a consideration with laser resurfacing. • Darker skin types are more predisposed to the formation of hypertrophic and keloid scars	• Silicone gel/sheet • Topical steroid • Intralesional steroid

TREATMENT CONSIDERATIONS FOR DARK SKIN TYPES

Pre- and post-treatment sun protection (sun-protective behaviors, broad-spectrum sunscreen SPF ≥30) is essential to prevent postinflammatory hyperpigmentation (PIH).

Preoperative treatment or priming includes 4% hydroquinone with 0.1% tretinoin for a minimum of 4–6 weeks before the procedure. Once re-epithelialization has occurred, combine post-treatment regimen of bleaching and blending with hydroquinone and tretinoin. Consider topical corticosteroids post-treatment (to reduce inflammation), especially when significant postprocedure erythema or edema are noted.

Wavelength: Longer wavelengths are associated with less epidermal absorption and therefore greater safety in patients with higher SPT.

Treatment parameters: Employ settings that minimize extent of epidermal and dermal injury (typically more conservative than in lighter skins).

It should be emphasized that SPT I–III, often require a greater number of sessions, either because of lower fluences and lower treatment densities (microthermal zones per cm^2) for fractional laser resurfacing.[6] Judicious epidermal cooling, e.g., slower treatment speeds when using lasers with contact cooling; pausing between passes of resurfacing lasers to reduce bulk heating and ice packs post-procedure help to minimize complications.

Lasers and Energy-based Devices

Traditional laser resurfacing using ablative CO_2 or erbium:yttrium aluminum garnet (Er:YAG) lasers are associated with high rates of severe pigmentary abnormalities and scarring in dark-skinned patients.[6] As such, patients with SPT V and VI were generally excluded from having such procedures due to the unfavorable risk to benefit ratio. The development of nonablative and fractional lasers has broadened the scope of safe and effective treatment options for patients with darkly pigmented skin. While these newer technologies are safe and effective in all skin types, pigmentary abnormalities remain a notable risk after the first treatment and for 4 weeks after each treatment.[1] Allowing time for skin cooling between individual passes is also a preferred strategy when treating higher SPT, lowering the risk of PIH secondary to thermal injury.

Several published studies in East Asian subjects (SPT III and IV) report favorable efficacy in the treatment of acne scarring, surgical scars and photoaging, with a considerable risk for PIH. There are no published studies of fractional CO_2 lasers in patients with SPT VI and therefore these devices should be used with caution as well as careful consideration of the high risk of hyperpigmentation when treating this population. Pretreatment conditioning and post-treatment prophylaxis with bleaching agents is strongly recommended when fractional ablative lasers are considered for darker skin types. Nonablative resurfacing with a short-pulsed 1,064-nm Nd:YAG laser has been studied in patients with SPT V and VI and is associated with a low risk of adverse events. The microsecond-pulsed Nd:YAG and the 1,550-nm erbium-doped fractional laser are frequently used lasers in skin of color.

The 1,550-nm laser is a mid-infrared erbium doped laser (Fraxel SR 1500, Solta Medical Inc.) that is indicated for all skin types but most studies have been done in SPTs I–IV. This therapy is used in phototypes IV and above but caution should be taken because an increased density of microthermal zones (MTZ) of destruction can lead to PIH in darker skin types. Kono and Chan et al. in their study documented that the use of higher densities (MTZ/cm^2), even with the use of lower fluences, increased the risk of developing hyperpigmentation in Asians with minimal increase in clinical efficacy and patient satisfaction seen. In darker phototypes, regional treatment can be appropriate for selective disorders such as acne scarring or melasma. Ablative and fractional lasers have evolved significantly over time and the current devices are not only more effective but safer. Ablative full-face resurfacing is best avoided on darker skins owing to a significant risk of hyperpigmentation and scarring. Fractional resurfacing, on the other hand, has gained popularity for the treatment of acne scars due to its favorable safety profile.

Prolonged redness may occur after resurfacing of the skin, especially with ablative lasers. Temporary fragility of skin and peeling can occur up to a month. Strict photoprotection and moisturizers are helpful in managing these issues. PIH may occur in 26–36% of the patients undergoing laser resurfacing.[7] Demarcation lines (areas of contrast in between the lased and nonlased skin) may be avoided by peripheral feathering of the laser beam into the borders of the treated areas.

Radiofrequency as an energy-based treatment is advantageous as it is blinded to SPTs.

Chemical Peeling and Dermabrasion

Textural concerns and pigmentary alterations or dyschromias are a leading aesthetic concern among patients with skin of color. Patients with Fitzpatrick skin types I–III tolerate resurfacing procedures with minimal risk of pigmentary complications. They may develop prolonged postoperative erythema but are less likely to develop the pigmentary sequelae. In patients with Fitzpatrick skin types IV–VI, the risk of pigmentary change is higher with deeper wounding beyond the upper one-third of the reticular dermis that can be achieved with dermabrasion and deep chemical peels. The higher the type and the degree of pigmentation, the greater is the risk of PIH.[8]

While chemical peels can ameliorate hyperpigmentation and textural changes, they also have the ability to induce new areas of hyperpigmentation and, in the case of deep peels, they can induce hypertrophic scarring and keloids. Therefore, chemical peeling in darker phototypes IV–VI for acne scars should be preceded with caution. The risk of complications seen from peels increases with the depth of the insult created. Superficial peels therefore impart the lowest risk of complications; however, resultant hyperpigmentation can still be seen. Deep phenol peels, though effective for acne scars, should be avoided.[9,10] Cutaneous side effects are hypopigmentation, hyperpigmentation, hypertrophic and keloid scarring, and prolonged erythema.

CONCLUSION

Today, more patients are expressing the desire to minimize acne scars and as such aesthetic concerns and cosmetic procedures are pervading everyday life. Now more than ever the patient population wanting these procedures is becoming increasingly diverse. Therefore, it is imperative to address the unique concerns and differences that the skin of color populations possess. Controlled studies in the skin of color population help to elucidate the specific ways to maximize outcomes, while minimizing risks. When performing procedures on darker SPTs, the physician must take into account the increased risk of dyschromia and aberrant scarring or keloid formation and therefore seek to minimize epidermal and dermal injury. Since each patient is inherently different regardless of which SPT, the ideal technique must be tailor-made in order to optimize results.

REFERENCES

1. Taylor SC. Cosmetic procedures—Chemical peels. In: Treatments of Skin of Color, 1st edition. Philadelphia: Saunders; 2011.
2. Sachdeva S. Fitzpatrick skin typing: Applications in dermatology. Indian J Dermatol Venereol Leprol. 2009;75:93-6.
3. Griffin AC. Laser resurfacing procedures in dark-skinned patients. Aesthet Surg J. 2005;25(6):625-7.
4. Chan HH. Effective and safe use of lasers, light sources, and radiofrequency devices in the clinical management of Asian patients with selected dermatoses. Lasers Surg Med. 2005;37:179-85.

5. Taylor SC. Skin of color: biology, structure, function, and implications for dermatologic disease. J Am Acad Dermatol. 2002;46(Suppl 2):S41-62.
6. Alexis AF. Lasers and light-based therapies in ethnic skin: treatment options and recommendations for Fitzpatrick skin types V and VI. Br J Dermatol. 2013;169(Suppl. 3):91-7.
7. Graber EM, Tanzi EL, Alster TS. Side effects and complications of fractional laser photothermolysis: experience with 961 treatments. Dermatol Surg. 2008;34(3):301-5; discussion 305-7.
8. Sarkar R. Medium-depth chemical peels and deep chemical peels. In: Grimes PE (Ed). Aesthetics and Cosmetic Surgery for Darker Skin Types. Philadelphia, PA: Lippincott Williams & Wilkins; 2008. pp. 170-8.
9. Garg VK, Sinha S, Sarkar R. Glycolic acid peels versus salicylic-mandelic acid peels in active acne vulgaris and post-acne scarring and hyperpigmentation: a comparative study. Dermatol Surg. 2009;35(1):59-65.
10. Al-Waiz MM, Al-Sharqi AI. Medium-depth chemical peels in the treatment of acne scars in dark-skinned individuals. Dermatol Surg. 2002;28(5):383-7.

CHAPTER 22

Acne Scars: Complications of Treatment and their Management

Shehnaz Arsiwala

IN A NUTSHELL

- ❖ Complications occur more commonly with aggressive treatment modalities such as medium depth and deep peels and ablative laser resurfacing.
- ❖ Prolonged hyperpigmentation is the most common complication seen in darker skins.
- ❖ The key to preventing complications is to combine minimally invasive modalities.
- ❖ Priming and counseling the patient throughout the treatment period is important.

INTRODUCTION

The demand for treatment of acne scarring is on the rise. In spite of the availability of multiple treatment modalities, obtaining visible correction remains a challenge. The challenge is more while treating darker skin types, as the risk of complications is higher. One has to tread a balanced path while handling acne scars in darker skin types where the optimal outcome outweighs the risk of adverse effects. Often the physician has to under treat acne scars and perform repeat procedures in order to minimize side effects. The traditional treatment modalities, including deep dermal phenol peels, dermabrasion, ablative laser resurfacing, and surgical scar revision techniques, are limited options in skin types IV through VI due to increased risks of hyper- and hypopigmentation.

PROBLEMS IN DARKER SKINS

The issues while handling darker skin types are:
- Prolonged inflammation with deeper interventions
- Persistent pigmentary changes
- Unpredictable outcomes

In order to prevent complications, techniques which may result in lower efficacy are often preferred over aggressive procedures, which can cause pigmentary complications. Hence, for darker skin types, techniques have to be chosen carefully and individualized to optimize efficacy and minimize side effects. Acne scars show certain clinical characteristic features that have to be kept in mind in order to achieve satisfactory results **(Box 1)**.

Evaluating Patients at Risk

Multiple interventional modalities can be used either as standalone techniques or in combination or in sequential ways to improve the outcome. The efficacy and tolerability of prior interventions and the degree of patient's compliance with the recommended therapies are some of the relevant factors influencing treatment. Thus, the framework of evaluating a patient at the potential risk of developing a complication from a procedure must include the following factors.

Grade, Depth and Severity of the Scars

Scars which are mild in grade, superficial and focally distributed have less chance of developing a complication to

> **Box 1:** Peculiar features of acne scars.
> - Varied morphology of scars
> - Distributed in different anatomical locations of the face
> - Exhibit variable appearance in different areas
> - Each area may have multiple types of scars
> - May have secondary features like erythematous and pigmented base
> - Coexisting active acne may be superimposed

an intervention compared to deeper, severe, pigmented panfacial scars. For mild scars not very visible at a social distance, procedures like microdermabrasion or superficial peels with minimum complication risks suffice. Deeper and severe scars visible at a social distance require medium-depth modalities, like laser resurfacing or scar revision techniques, often in combinations with more number of sittings.

Distribution of Scars

Scars on the forehead and nose may have a less favorable outcome than on the cheeks or chin and being on the projectile part of face also carry a higher risk of pigmentary alterations than on cheeks, jawline, etc. Scars on the chest and back are less amenable to modalities used for acne scars on the face. The risk of complications rises especially after deep peels or laser resurfacing on nonfacial areas as the number of appendages are less and there is slow recovery.

Type of Scars

A patient may often have mixed types of scars and one needs to evaluate the predominant scar type before choosing a treatment mode. Deep boxcar scars often need either medium-depth or deep peels, CO_2 laser combined with erbium:yttrium aluminium garnet (erbium:YAG) resurfacing, high-strength trichloroacetic acid (TCA) dot peels or punch grafting, etc., as compared to superficial and rolling scars of grade 1 or 2. Combination treatments work better. The more deeper and invasive the intervention, higher is the chance of an untoward effect.

Skin Type, Sex and Age of the Patient

The darker skin types are at greater risk for hyperpigmentation. A skin though on lighter side but not sun protected and unprimed is also at a substantial risk of complication, especially dyspigmentation. This is true for interventions involving medium-depth chemical peels and laser resurfacing techniques.

A tanned skin is at a very high risk for pigmentary adverse effects even with superficial peels and this risk rises fourfold with a deeper intervention like a deep peel or a laser resurfacing and such interventions should be undertaken after adequate priming methods only.[1]

Epidermal melanin produced by ultraviolet (UV) light exposure may interfere with laser treatment and increase the risks for scarring, hypopigmentation, or hyperpigmentation. To check for tanning, it is wise to compare the color of the potential treatment site to that of a nonexposed skin site, similar to the buttock or axilla. If a tan is present, treatment should be delayed until the tan has faded as much as possible in the treatment area.[1]

A dry sensitive skin is more prone to a complication especially with peels and more so with an inflammatory peeling agent. An oily skin has lesser chances of irritation and even retinoid dermatitis in the priming phase than a dry skin. The author finds that the skin in males is thicker and oilier and has less chances of irritation to an interventional scar procedure like peeling or microdermabrasion or laser resurfacing as compared to female skin.

A more mature skin is dry, irregularly textured than a younger skin. In author's experience during the recovery phase, a mature skin has slower re-epithelialization rate than a younger skin and so potential for complications are more in a mature skin than in a young patient. Patients with reduced numbers of adnexal skin structures, such as those with scleroderma, burn scars, or history of prior ionizing radiation to the skin, are not good candidates for ablative resurfacing. Patients with keloidal tendency are a relative contraindication to aggressive interventions, while those on topical steroids, allergic potential, photosensitizing medications, previous surgeries, smoking, and outdoor activities should be dealt with utmost caution to avoid complications.

Patient Compliance

The mind frame of the patient is an important factor which needs attention. The minor adverse effects of treatment are always easy to handle by the clinician through adequate counseling in a compliant patient, as against a very anxious demanding patient who may have unrealistic expectation and will not tolerate minimal and transient side effects. It is important not to promise excellent results and always underplay the expected outcome.

Patient Expectations

An unrealistic patient will never be happy with even an optimum result and one has to decide to work on these patients by thorough counseling and information about pros and cons of every treatment modality offered. The details of the procedure and requirement of patient adherence to priming and postprocedure care should be emphasized. Also, recovery time for laser intervention or dermabrasion is much more than for chemical peels and should be explained.

Pretreatment photographs are mandatory for tracking the outcome of the treatment.

CHOICE OF TREATMENT MODALITY

The treatment modality chosen to improve the scars is dependent on the risk of side effects. A treatment mode like microdermabrasion or microneedling causes minimal side effects, but at the same time, is ineffective for scars of higher grades. A superficial depth chemical peel carries less risk of pigmentary changes post-treatment as compared to medium-depth peel. Deep peels are largely avoided in darker skin due to a strong potential for hypo- or hyperpigmentation. The more inflammatory the peeling agent greater is the risk of pigmentary change. A salicylic acid peel has lower risk of pigmentation as compared to a TCA peel. Ablative lasers are more pigment generating during the postprocedure phase as compared to the nonablative lasers. The fractionated lasers are very popular as they offer partial ablation with minimal thermal damage, minimal downtime and less adverse effects. Long pulse lasers are better suited for skin of color than short pulse mode. Fractional erbium laser resurfacing has a lesser risk of pigmentary changes as compared to the CO_2 laser.[2]

Combination of Procedures

No single modality of treatment may suffice to improve acne scars completely. Hence, the current trend is to combine or rotate treatment techniques. This is true for patients with deep boxcar, deep rolling and ice pick scars where chemical peels, fractional resurfacing lasers, microneedling and subcision are combined or rotated. One should choose a technique best suited to scar types and least risk of complications, e.g., while treating boxcar scars and ice pick scars, it is better to combine a chemical reconstruction of skin scars (CROSS) TCA peel with a fractional resurfacing method rather than a full-face TCA peel with fractional laser resurfacing. Evaluating risk of combinations helps long term in preventing complications.

Stage of Scar Intervention

The stage at which the scars are being treated is important for clinical outcome and avoiding complications. Interventions in the early stages have better outcomes as compared to mature atrophic scars (**Box 2**).

> **Box 2:** Stages of evolution of acne scars.
> - Initially erythematous
> - Later purplish or bluish in color
> - Late scars are atrophic either pigmented or skin colored

Acne Scars: Complications of Treatment and their Management

The current trend is to treat scars in the early phase to prevent long-term atrophic changes and progression. Prevention and anti-scar treatment have to be initiated in a number of cases while patient is on anti-acne regimen, immediately after the acne resolves. The ability of a person to scar after acne depends on patient's inflammatory profile while healing. Nonspecific robust inflammatory infiltrate with quick resolution are the nonscarring patients. Those patients who exhibit more specific but ineffectual inflammatory response with prolonged angiogenesis are the scarring patients.[2]

Thus, if the interventions are sought with any physical therapies, it seems reasonable to target either the poorly resolved inflammatory response or the poorly resolving angiogenesis.[3] Treating early will help in preventing the progressive scarring of the healing lesions in inflammatory acne.[2,3]

A history of previous treatments like laser skin resurfacing, peels, etc., is noteworthy because these procedures could potentially slow the wound healing process due to the presence of fibrosis.[4,5]

Aggressive interventions should be avoided or cautiously done in high-risk patients (**Box 3**).

Box 3: Relative contraindications for aggressive treatment.

Avoid aggressive intervention in patients with:
- Keloid tendency
- Active severe acne
- Unrealistic expectations
- Active herpes simplex or bacterial infections
- Isotretinoin recipient in last 6 months
- Unstable vitiligo and psoriasis
- Associated photoaggravated skin diseases
- Salicylic peels during pregnancy, lactation and in patients with sensitivity to aspirin
- Phenol peels in cardiac patients

BASIC PRECAUTIONS AND AVOIDING COMPLICATIONS

The basic principle of minimizing complications is avoiding aggressive interventions in high-risk patients **(Box 3)**.

Pretreatment Preparation Phase

After basic evaluation of the scar type, skin type and decision to conduct an interventional approach to scars, one needs to carry out basic pretreatment regimen to prime the patient. Whatever the chosen modality, peels to lasers, one needs to prep and prime the skin to make it conducive to treatment. The author follows a general pattern of must-do list before executing the treatment. This not only helps to build up patient compliance but also helps the physician to prepare the skin for an aggressive procedure. The threshold of skin is gauged and it also helps to unmask any hidden or unexpected dangers.

For example, while priming with a sunscreen, unmasking of a photosensitive skin may be expressed due to photosensitizing potential of the sunscreen. Similarly, priming with retinoids may unmask a dry sensitive skin which may reflect a retinoid dermatitis, thus enabling the physician to defer the intervention.

Acne Control

Overenthusiastic approach to treating scars while active severe acne exists should be avoided. When active acne is nearly controlled, chemical peels work on residual acne as well as target postacne pigmentation and early mild scars. An attempt to conduct laser resurfacing or microneedling while residual acne is present increases the risk of further acne flare and new scarring and one needs to be vigilant in control and maintenance of acne clearance before seeking deeper interventions. The author currently uses superficial chemical peels with salicylic, mandelic or glycolic acid as priming before fractional laser resurfacing. It helps to alleviate residual acne as well as eliminate superficial pigment in scars, thus making the skin more amenable to fractional laser resurfacing for moderate-to-deep scars.

Sun Control

Broad-spectrum sunscreens with good ultraviolet A (UVA) and ultraviolet B (UVB) coverage are recommended before and throughout the treatment period. Patients with darker skin types and tanned patients are advised to apply hydroquinone-containing compounds (2–4%), topical retinoids like tretinoin or adapalene, kojic acid, arbutin or other lightening agents preoperatively to minimize the risk of postinflammatory hyperpigmentation (PIH). Broad-spectrum sunscreen with SPF of 15 or above and UVA coverage is started well in advance (about 3 months). Sunscreens with photosensitizing property in certain patients can be unmasked before the procedures undertaken. The newer photostable broad-spectrum sunscreen agents containing a physical block are commonly prescribed.[1,6]

Isotretinoin and Photosensitizing Drugs

The patients on oral retinoid therapy should not undergo intervention for deep acne scars such as deep chemical peels and ablative resurfacing for 6 months following discontinuation of the medication, as they have an increased risk of keloid formation. However, superficial chemical peels and fractional laser resurfacing are relatively safer and may be performed with all precautions. Photosensitizing drugs should be withheld at least 6 weeks before a procedure for acne scars is undertaken.[6]

History of Herpes Simplex

There is an increased risk of reactivation of herpes simplex following a procedure, which can disseminate to the treated area and cause scarring. If the treating physician decides to perform the procedure, the risk and benefit should be explained to the patient and the procedure should be performed after proper informed consent and only after a course of oral acyclovir.[1,7-10]

Lightening Agents

Priming reduces wound healing time and also decreases risk of PIH before any intervention. Priming determines patient tolerance and establishes patient compliance. Choosing a right and specific priming agent is essential in order to improve the result and minimize side effects for any modality of treatment for acne scars.

- Hydroquinone (2-4%) is gold standard—especially for peels and fractional laser resurfacing in pigmented scars (dual combinations can be used).
- Retinoids (tretinoin, adapalene, tazarotene) are ideal primers in acne and scars, and can be combined with kojic acid, arbutin or glycolic acid. Triple combination should be avoided.
- Glycolic acid is best primer for peels for scars with fine lines and textural improvement, particularly in more older patients.
- Priming is undertaken for 2-4 weeks before peels. Retinoids are discontinued 4-7 days before peels and restarted 4-5 days after.

Test patch: A test patch helps to determine the laser treatment parameter or peel strength for an individual; this is true for chemical peels and lasers. It is also helpful in medicolegal situations. In particular, it is advisable for all beginning practitioners to perform laser/peel test spots in all patients prior to treating full face, since skin type and color do not always match. For peels, patch test should be done for salicylic acid, lactic acid/glycolic acid peels. In darker skin, resorcinol is not commonly used due to irritation potential and is largely replaced by citric acid which is a peel booster.

INTRA-TREATMENT VIGILANCE

Right Technique

Conducting an intervention with the right technique depends on the acumen and skill of the clinician. An improperly or hastily conducted procedure or performed by inexperienced staff or underqualified personnel often leads to significant adverse effects. While performing laser resurfacing, stacking mode gives a better result on deep scars compared to a multiple passes mode according to the author's experience. An overenthusiastic coating after coating of a TCA peel without adequate interval in-between coats often always leads to inadvertent patchy absorption and deep peeling, with subsequent epidermolysis, inflammation and pigmentary side effects. A free glycolic acid, high-strength peel has to be terminated at the right end point. Appropriate end points are essential to ensure optimum outcome. While performing subcision of adherent scars avoiding very aggressive sweeping moments along with adequate pressure immediately afterwards often prevents a hematoma and cyst formation.

Right Peel Strength

Complexities of formulations, pH, molecular size, combinations, mechanism of action and compatibility issues for each peel demand consideration while choosing an appropriate peeling agent.

Starting with right strength of peels is important, especially while working with glycolic acid. In sensitive skin, gel peels can be used to minimize irritation and then worked up with free acid peels. Optimum combinations, compatibility and pH should be kept in mind while performing peels. Optimal combinations with low risks of inflammation are good to start with.

Selecting the Appropriate Laser Parameters

Fluence: It is always preferable to begin with the lowest energy fluence and then work up the energy in subsequent sittings. Darker the skin, lesser energy should be used initially. Fluence may be increased if response is suboptimal. If epidermal debris is significant, the fluence should be lowered. Multiple stacking mode works better for acne scars rather than multiple pass method while treating with erbium:YAG fractional ablative resurfacing. Long pulse mode is better for dark skin types than short pulse mode. Larger spot sizes allow deeper penetration and produce less tissue splatter.[4]

Postprocedure Phase

Broad-spectrum sunscreens with good UVA/UVB coverage are recommended before and throughout the treatment period. Immediately after treatment, the treated area appears erythematous and inflamed. Apply ice packs till burning sensation subsides, then apply a layer of antibiotic such as mupirocin and cover with gauze in patients undergoing dermaroller, laser or peels. Patient is instructed to clean the area with copious amount of water and apply the ointment twice daily till the skin heals which can take around 5-10 days. Oral antibiotics may be used, if considered essential, by the treating physician, but are not mandatory. Anti-inflammatory agents may be needed while treating large areas. Patient should be instructed to avoid sun exposure and use of cosmetics on the treated area. Treatments are scheduled at an interval of 6-8 weeks. Postprocedure bleaching agents may be used, but only after the crust subsides.[6,10]

Adequate Counseling in the Post-treatment Phase

Adequate post-treatment counseling is mandatory to improve patient compliance and adherence to treatment protocols.

HOW TO MINIMIZE RISKS OF COMPLICATIONS WITH SPECIFIC MODALITIES OF TREATMENT?

Microdermabrasion

Microdermabrasion benefits comedogenic acne as well as improves the texture and quality of the skin in grade 1–2 acne scars.

Microdermabrasion before phytic peels which are slow-release glycolic peels and TCA peels are to be avoided due to potential risk of deeper inadvertent peel absorption and postinflammatory pigmentary changes. Temporary stripping of treated area, bruising, burning, photosensitivity and pain are transient. Acne flare, milia, secondary bacterial infection, persistent erythema edema and PIH arise after aggressive microdermabrasion[11] (**Fig. 1**).

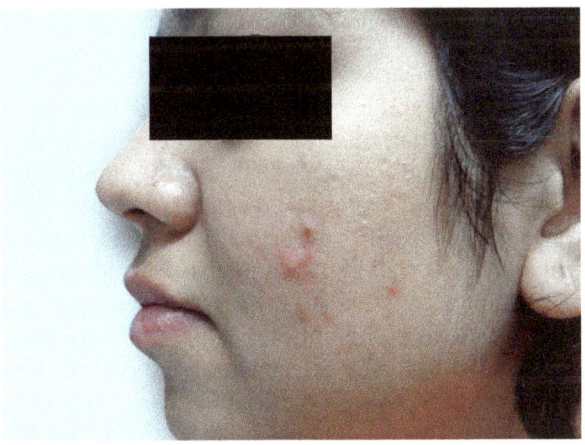

Fig. 1: Focal pustular acne after microdermabrasion.

Dermabrasion

Full-face dermabrasion, though once very popular for treatment of severe and extensive acne scars, is no longer done since the current trend is for use of ablative fractional lasers like erbium and CO_2. The downtime for recovery with these newer techniques runs in days as compared to full-face dermabrasion where patient has to be homebound for period of many weeks. The full-face dermabrasion has very high potential for side effects like persistent edema, erythema, prolonged healing time, hyperpigmentation, hypopigmentation as well as lines of demarcation. Milia formation is also reported with dermabrasion.[12,13]

Cryosurgery

Primarily used for hypertrophic scars and keloids with either liquid nitrogen or CO_2. Blistering, crusting is seen commonly, while secondary bacterial infection can be seen rarely in the postprocedure phase. Atrophy and hypopigmentation are the delayed phase side effects. Depigmentation after cryotherapy is often long lasting and permanent.

Chemical Peels

Both the positive and negative results of the peel are based on the concentration, duration, skin type, prior medical or surgical intervention, location, sun exposure preprocedure and postprocedure, concomitant medications, and other factors.

Amidst the peeling agents, salicylic acid is the least inflammatory followed by TCA and glycolic acid. Resorcinol, Jessner's and phenol peels are the most inflammatory peels.

Limitations of standalone glycolic peels are inability to use high-strength free acid peels as the potential risk of complication increases on darker pigmented skin **(Fig. 2)**. Slow release and combination of alpha-hydroxy acids (AHAs) with other peels like beta-hydroxy acids (BHAs) have slowly

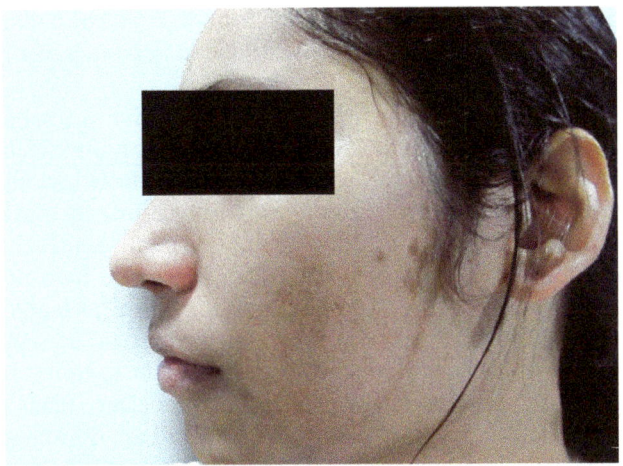

Fig. 2: Postinflammatory hyperpigmentation after high-strength glycolic peels.

replaced traditional glycolic peels. Newer glycolic acid peels are formulated with strontium nitrate to reduce the irritation potential.

Mandelic acid has antibacterial properties and is safer for dark skin types. Gel based combination peels have lesser free acid availability and hence lower incidence of side effects and are safer for sensitive skin types.

The medium-depth peels are primarily considered to be TCA solutions. TCA causes epidermal coagulative necrosis and protein precipitation along with dermal collagen necrosis and regeneration. Recent studies have shown that injury to the reticular dermis heals with scarring.[14] The increased risk associated with the use of TCA for deeper peels is definitely not recommended. High-strength TCA may lead to scarring or pigmentary changes, but not as frequently when used at lower concentrations and hence lower-strength TCA peels are preferred for Indian and darker skin. Also, focal use of high-strength TCA has lesser risk of pigmentary side effects than full-face TCA peels. In newer modified formulations, hydroquinone and kojic acid are added instead to lower the risk of hyperpigmentation.

The peels considered to be deep are often phenol (carbolic acid) or croton oil based. These can certainly be more effective but carry an even greater potential for side effects including acne, milia, dermatitis, pigmentary alteration, secondary infection, atrophy, or scarring. Phenol peel requires full cardiopulmonary monitoring and intravenous hydration because of potential direct cardiac toxicity that leads to decreased myocardial contraction and electrical activity.[13] While using resorcinol and phenol, direct toxicity and pigmentary changes should be borne in mind. Deep peels are generally avoided in the pigmented skin and are now largely replaced by fractional resurfacing modalities.

Sheer vigilance is of utmost value during peel procedure as most of the adverse effects result from poor priming, noncompliance, wrong peeling agent, etc. Treating skin of color demands additional consideration as one has to focus on preventing pigmentary altercations, so adequate priming and achieving right depth of peel is essential.

Peel complications are highest with phenol peels which fortunately are rarely done for acne scars in darker skins. Salicylic acid peels are relatively safer. High-strength free acid glycolic peels are associated with tendency to epidermolysis, PIH and irritation as compared to lower-strength or gel-based or combination peels which have low-strength compatible formulations.[14-17]

Flare of acne can occur after glycolic acid and salicylic-mandelic acid peels (**Fig. 3**). Erythema and hyperpigmantation are also common with high strength TCA peels beyond 25% (**Fig. 4**).

USEFUL STRATEGIES WHILE CONDUCTING PEELS

A peeling agent must yield optimum result creating minimal inflammation and no pigmentary adverse effects (**Box 4**).

Acne Scars: Complications of Treatment and their Management

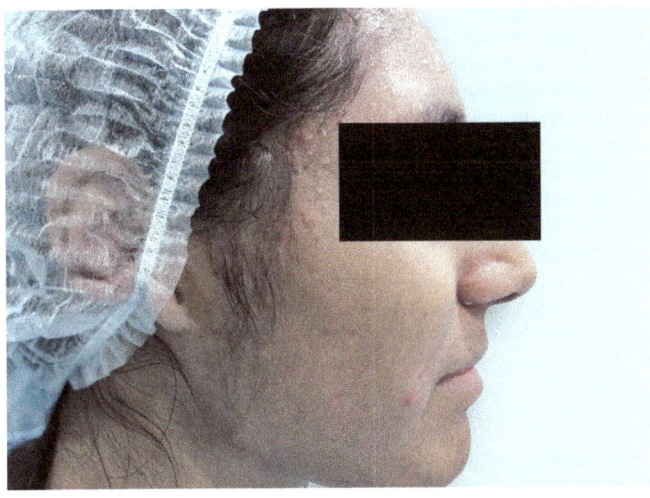

Fig. 3: Flare after salicylic–mandelic acid peels.

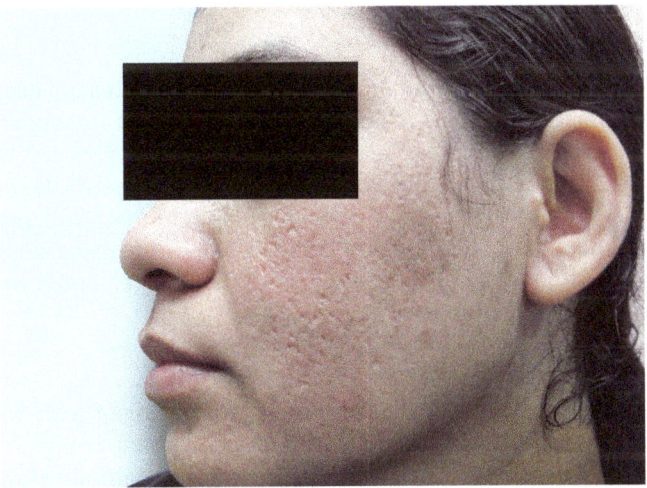

Fig. 4: Erythema and hyperpigmentation after trichloroacetic acid peels.

> **Box 4:** Minimizing risks with chemical peels.
>
> - When starting peels, stay on limited basic peel types and concentrations—salicylic acid, glycolic acid, and mandelic acid are good starting peels before adding trichloroacetic acid, combination, sequencing and switching peels
> - Minimize risks by choosing least potent agent and combine or sequentially use compatible agents to optimize results
> - Work with gels and upgrade to liquid peels with higher free acid availability
> - Antioxidants like oral vitamin C, oral beta-carotene, citric acid, mandelic acid, ascorbic glucoside, ferrulic acid, phloretin, and phytic acid help to control inflammation to a certain extent
> - Document photographic records for comparison and monitoring results between peel sessions—form the learning curve!

A peeling agent must yield optimum result at optimum strength! Create minimal inflammation and no pigmentary adverse effects. For achieving this, one must have a controlled stage of inflammation **(Table 1)**.

Microneedling

Microneedling procedure is often associated with acne flare, edema, and erythema, which is transient. Sometimes secondary bacterial infections and reactivation of herpes simplex may be seen. This can be easily managed by acyclovir prophylaxis and adequate post-treatment antibiotics. Sometimes accidental cutaneous implantation of needle can occur, though this is not seen with usage of this technique by qualified personnel and good quality equipment.

Lasers Resurfacing

Ablative lasers bring about excellent resurfacing of scars but are associated with sequelae, which make them unpopular to use and are nearly given up. Pigmentary complications especially in Asian skins are a drawback. Side-effect profile after erbium:YAG laser resurfacing is similar but less severe and

Acne Scars: Complications of Treatment and their Management

TABLE 1: Complications of interventional procedure for acne scars.

Interventional procedure	Mild complications	Moderate complications	Severe complications
Micro-dermabrasion	• Edema • Erythema	• Acne flare • Hyper-pigmentation	–
Chemical peels	• Edema • Erythema • Transient Hyper-pigmentation • Irritation • Dryness	• Persistent hyper-pigmentation • Contact dermatitis • Bacterial infections • Reactivation of herpes • Acneiform eruptions	• Hypo-pigmentation • Hypertrophy/Keloids
Fractional ablative lasers	• Pain • Edema • Erythema • Irritation • Dryness	• Prolonged erythema • Milia • Acne flare • Contact dermatitis	• Infections • Hyper-pigmentation • Persistent Hypo-pigmentation • Hypertrophy/Keloid
Nonablative lasers	• Edema • Erythema	Prolonged erythema	–
Microneedling	• Pain • Edema • Erythema	• Infections—(herpes, bacterial) • Acne	–
Subcision	• Pain • Edema • Erythema • Puncture marks	• Hematoma • Infections • Acne flare	• Cyst formation • Deep bacterial infections • Keloid

Contd...

Contd...

Interventional procedure	Mild complications	Moderate complications	Severe complications
Punch techniques (elevation, grafting, flotation)	• Pain • Edema • Erythema	• Hyperpigmentation • Acne flare • Infections • Graft rejection	• Cobblestoning • Ring scars
Fillers	• Needle marks and bruising • Erythema • Edema pain	• Acneiform eruption • Lumpiness • Infection • Migration	• Allergic reactions • Granuloma formation • Vascular occlusion • Tyndall effect

more transient than CO_2 laser resurfacing which causes deep partial thickness skin injury. With ablative mode in CO_2 laser, the edema and erythema may last for 3–4 months, and with short-pulse erbium:YAG laser, it lasts for 2–4 weeks. Time for re-epithelialization with CO_2 laser is 8–10 days as compared to 5 days with erbium:YAG laser.[18] Postprocedure phase requires intensive topical skin therapy and attendant risk of surface yeast, viral and bacterial super infection.[19] Hyperpigmentation is common after CO_2 laser resurfacing and can last up to 3–6 weeks. Demarcation lines in the periorbital area more in darker skin types. With erbium:YAG lasers, this incidence is less and hyperpigmentation resolves faster with lightening and bleaching creams, and light peels.

Hypopigmentation after ablative lasers is often longstanding and recalcitrant but is seen lesser than hyperpigmentation and often with aggressive treatments.[19,20]

A potentially serious complication is reactivation of herpes simplex as well as bacterial infections as scarring becomes inevitable. Worsening of scars may be seen with aggressive laser parameters, especially while resurfacing nonfacial areas, due to sparse pilosebaceous units and slow re-epithelialization.

Combination of CO_2 and erbium:YAG laser resurfacing helps better in deeper scars by causing finer tissue ablation and better collagen contraction and remodeling.[20]

Fractional Lasers

Fractional lasers are a balance between ablative and nonablative laser modalities. Microthermal zones of ablated tissue are extruded through the epidermis and surrounding untreated zones facilitate quick re-epithelialization and remodeling.

Pain management is most significant and usage of surface anesthetic creams is mandatory. Analgesics are often needed to reduce patient discomfort. Postprocedure, the patient has edema and erythema which is transient. Edema generally lasts for 2-4 days. The risk of edema increases with higher energies and topical steroids for a short course may be added for the same. Tightness and dryness of skin is felt at 1-3 days with desquamation and sometimes crusting if treated with higher fluence **(Fig. 5)**. Though largely safer, fractional lasers are no exception for PIH and a 10-12% incidence has been reported commonly in darker skin types. Prelaser priming agents as well as peels are a key to minimizing these. Bulk heating by treating very large areas at a high fluency is best avoided and cooling between passes is beneficial. Treatment of more than 30-40% of the skin in a single session may lead to adverse sequelae.[21,22]

Mild complications of Er:YAG laser resurfacing include milia, acne exacerbation, contact dermatitis, or perioral dermatitis. Moderate complications include localized viral, bacterial **(Fig. 6)** and candida infection, prolonged erythema, transient post-treatment hyperpigmentation, and delayed hypopigmentation. The most severe complications include fibrosis, hypertrophic scarring, disseminated infection, and the

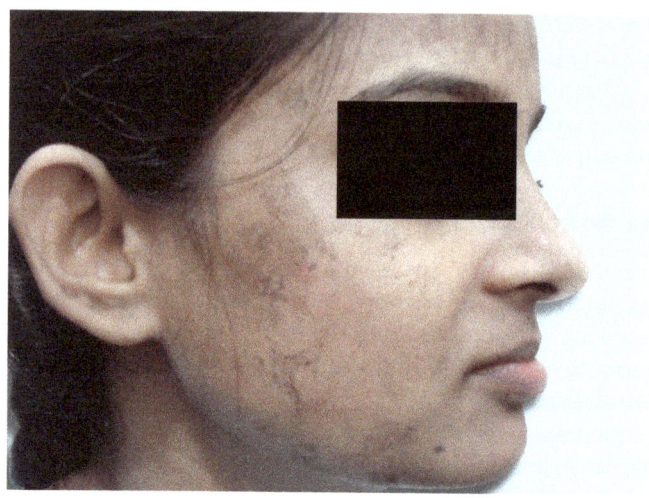

Fig. 5: Post fractional resurfacing laser exfoliation phase at 4 days.

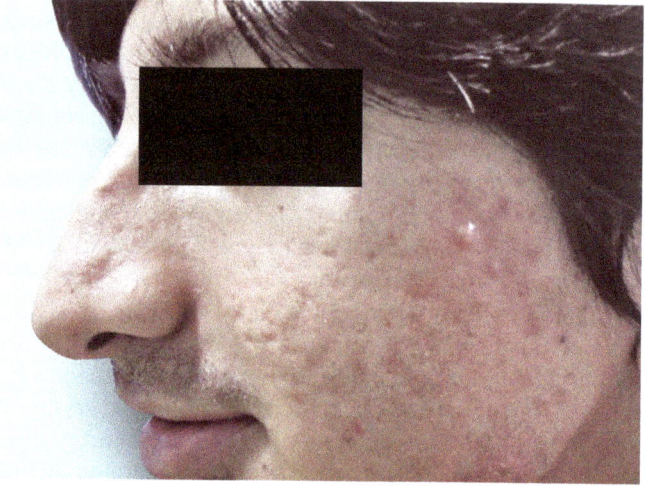

Fig. 6: Pustular folliculitis after fractional Er:YAG resurfacing laser.

development of ectropion. Diligent evaluation of the patient is necessary during the re-epithelialization phase of healing. This is important because a delay in recognition and treatment of complications can have severe deleterious consequences such as permanent dyspigmentation and scarring.[23]

Nonablative Lasers

These lasers heat the papillary and reticular dermis without any epidermal damage. Deep dermal heat activates fibroblast proliferation and collagen remodeling; hence, it is also called as subsurface resurfacing or laser toning. Though they exhibit modest improvement compared to ablative and fractional lasers, the safety profile is much better with minimal downtime.[24]

Uncontrolled epidermal heating with inadequate cooling can lead to complications like epidermal blistering, burns, loss of barrier function, dyspigmentation and scarring. An optimum epidermal temperature is 40–48°C which correlates with a dermal temperature of 50–55°C. Complications occur if temperature shoots to 60–65°C.[24] Too much cooling can cause inflammation, cryonecrosis, hyperpigmentation and scarring if done aggressively. Gel cooling may be messy and also the gel coats the laser head and collects debris. Though nonablative fractional lasers offer larger safety margin than ablative fractional therapies, dyspigmentation is a worry and often lower fluencies and multiple treatments are needed for darker skin types.[25]

Melanin absorption of laser energy can result in epidermal damage and also decrease the energy meant for dermal chromophores. Since absorption coefficient of melanin decreases as wavelength increases, the near-infrared and infrared wavelengths provide best nonablative rejuvenation for darker skin.[26] Infections like herpes reactivation can occur and can be avoided with antiviral therapy in patients at risk.

Nonablative fractional resurfacing is effective and safe in Asians. By reducing the number of passes and the total treatment density, the risk of PIH can be reduced. Meanwhile, clinical efficacy can be maintained by increasing the total number of treatment sessions.[27-30]

Dermatosurgical Procedures—Subcision

Breaking the attachments in the adherent scars helps to release the scar skin from its deeper structures. The subsequent hematoma which forms helps in reorganizing and regeneration of the connective tissue. Immediately after subcision, some amount of blood oozing is common and more if a large bevel needle is used. The bleeding is valuable as it prevents reattachment, and organization of the ecchymoses helps neocollagenosis. Bruising, swelling, cyst formation and secondary infection are sequelae to subcision.

Subcision can be immediately followed by dermaroller therapy or a filler injection and the combination of these techniques culminates in aesthetically pleasing results of the treatment for grade 3-4 scars. Sometimes combining subcision with microneedling may produce an acne flare and double up chances of secondary infection. Often hematoma may be significant and may get secondarily infected too. Adequate oral and topical antibiotics and anti-inflammatory agents in the postprocedure phase are helpful **(Fig. 7)**.

Scar Revision Techniques: Punch Grafting, Punch Flotation and Punch Excision

The ice pick, boxcar, and rolling scars can be managed by revision techniques. Although uncommon, there is the potential for bruising, hypertrophy, cysts from pilosebaceous unit disruption, infection, or worsening of the scar. Cobblestoning and ring scar formation are seen after punch grafting and flotation techniques. Laser resurfacing after punch excision of

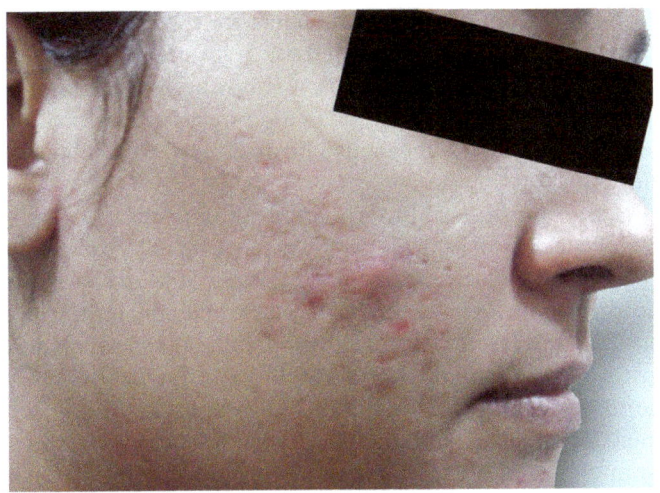

Fig. 7: Cystic acne 1 week after subcision.

scars is a suitable option for refining after revision techniques. The noted advantage is that punch excision eliminates the deeper scars and allows for only superficial laser treatment with fewer passes. So, if surgery is done, laser resurfacing may also be a consideration because the chance of unwanted side effects could be reduced.[31]

Fillers

Injectable fillers can enable short, medium, or long-term correction of acne scars.

Cross-linked hyaluronic acid (HA) fillers are often used to fill scars in acne and are best used for macular and rolling scars. HA products can be injected directly beneath individual pitted or boxcar scars, or be used to buttress areas of rolling scars. HA fillers have very low allergenic potential as they are not species or tissue specific.[32]

Silicon and polyacrylamide fillers are used for long-term correction but have an increased risk of granuloma formation. Undermining the adherent scars with subcision followed by fillers is a common technique and produces an aesthetically pleasing outcome but can also be associated with increased side effects.

Large-particle semipermanent fillers such as calcium hydroxylapatite have a longer persistence up to 1 year and are appropriate for larger areas of rolling scars. Thicker fillers must be injected no higher than the dermal subcutaneous junction.

True adverse effects of fillers include allergic reactions, granuloma formation and rarely vascular occlusion or compromise. Tyndall effect is a bluish tint resulting from injections that are too superficial. Overcorrection or persistent lumpiness and infection are other adverse effects. Examples of transitory reactions, including needle marks, bruising, erythema or edema, acneiform eruptions, transient lumpiness and sterile abscesses, may also be seen.[33,34] Migration of the filler, secondary infection and biofilms, granuloma formation and technique-related necrosis are reported too.[35]

Microneedle Radiofrequency

This technique is currently used for grade 3–4 boxcar scars. It delivers radiofrequency energy into the dermis at predetermined depths through insulated or noninsulated needles. Microneedle radiofrequency devices are chromophore-independent in contrast to most lasers that target specific chromophores. This allows significantly higher penetration into the skin and safer treatment of darker skin types. An advantage of fractional radiofrequency is that it causes less epidermal disruption by only 5%, compared with 10–70% of that of fractional ablative laser systems.[36] The healing process is faster with minimal downtime. Therefore, this technique may be an alternative choice of facial rejuvenation and atrophic scars, especially in patients with darker skin complexion.[36] Common adverse effects are erythema and edema which are transient and last for 2-4 days. Epidermal burns, needle footprints, PIH and infections are complications that may occur.

The disadvantages of this technology are that it is painful and requires topical anesthesia. In addition, there is high cost of consumables.[37]

Platelet-rich Plasma

Platelet-rich plasma is now used as a standalone procedure or in combination with ablative, nonablative fractional resurfacing lasers and microneedle radiofrequency technique. Common side effects seen are pain, erythema, bruising, and infections—bacterial or viral. However, no serious infections are reported and it is used as an adjuvant therapy to facilitate faster wound repair.[38-40]

MANAGEMENT OF COMPLICATIONS

Side effects and complications from various interventional procedures are varied and depend on patient selection, skill of physician, and pre- and postoperative care. Once complications arise, they have to be managed specifically **(Table 2)**.

TABLE 2: Management of complications.

• Edema • Erythema	Mild topical steroids/tacrolimus
Pain	Analgesics
• Acne flare • Acneiform eruptions	• Topical antibiotics/retinoids • Oral antibiotics
Hyperpigmentation	• Topical lightening agents (dual or triple combinations)

Contd...

Contd...

	• Sun protection • Light superficial peels • Antioxidants
Hypopigmentation	Tacrolimus/Pimecrolimus
• Irritation • Dryness	• Bland emollients/sunscreen agents • Topical steroids
Infection	• Bacterial—topical and oral antibiotics, guided by culture reports if severe • Viral—oral acyclovir or valacyclovir • Candida—topical/oral antifungals
Lumpiness	Molding and ice compresses/injection hyaluronidase/incision and expression
• Cobblestoning • Ring scars	Fractional laser resurfacing
Allergic reactions/ Granuloma formation	Oral steroids and immunosuppressive agents
Keloid/hypertrophic scar	Topical or intralesional steroids/silicone gel sheet/cryotherapy

Postprocedure Erythema

Transient complications include edema and erythema **(Figs. 8A to D)**. This usually resolves with time; usually in 3–4 days with superficial peels, 4–10 days with medium-depth peels, a week with fractional erbium laser resurfacing and up to 10 days to 2 weeks with fractional CO_2 resurfacing. Prolonged erythema is a signal of deeper intervention and impending scarring. Mild potent topical steroids or tacrolimus may be used for erythema with irritation for a short period. Prolonged erythema usually resolves with this method. Erythema which persists may need a more potent steroid, sunscreen and a

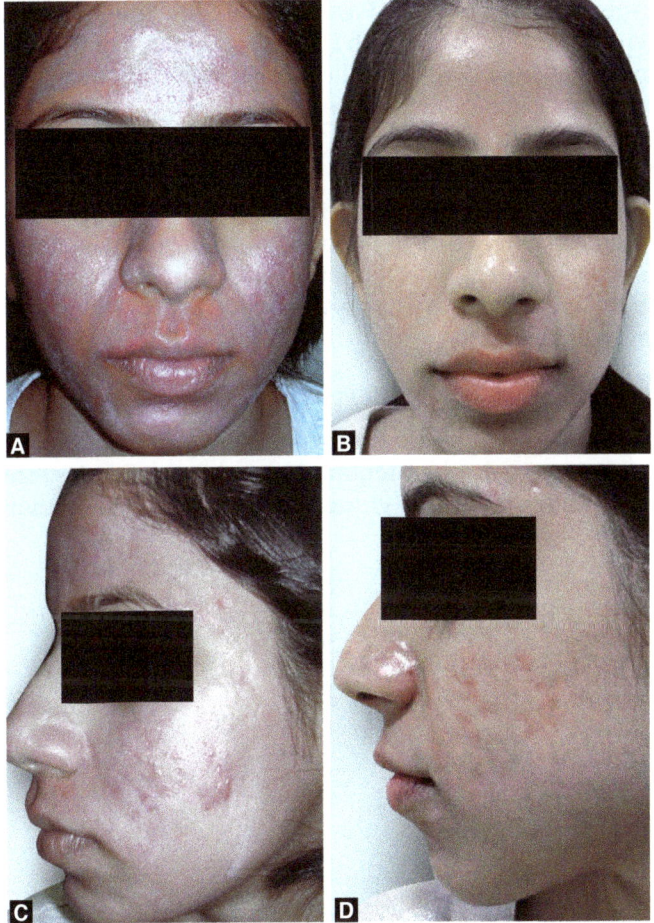

Figs. 8A to D: (A to C) Immediate post fractional Er:YAG laser resurfacing-induced erythema and edema; (D) Six months after Er:YAG fractional laser resurfacing.

mild bleaching cream as prolonged erythema can lead to hyperpigmentation[19,36-40] **(Figs. 9 and 10)**. Bland emollients in sensitive patients along with sunscreens suffice in most post-treatment situations. Topical calamine lotion has a soothing effect and can be used post-treatment.[19,37-42]

Pain

Pain control is important to improve patient comfort and compliance. It occurs in the postoperative phase after laser resurfacing, deep peels, microneedling and scar revision techniques. It can be minimized by use of ice pack compresses and painkillers.

Infection

Bacterial infections are treated by topical antibacterials in mild cases and, when required, systemic antibiotics. The ideal method is to be guided by culture and sensitivity

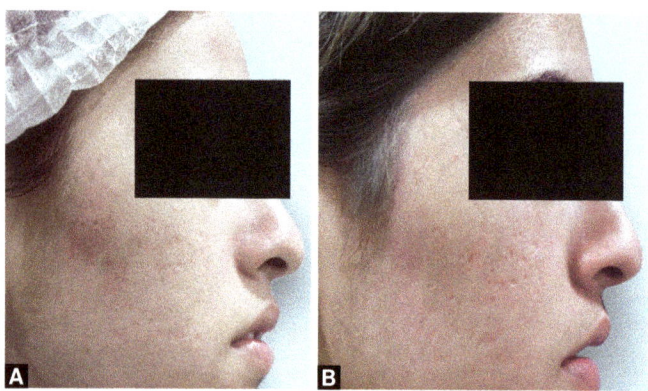

Figs. 9A and B: (A) Focal postinflammatory erythema after fractional Er:YAG laser resurfacing; (B) Clearance after topical hydrocortisone in 10 days.

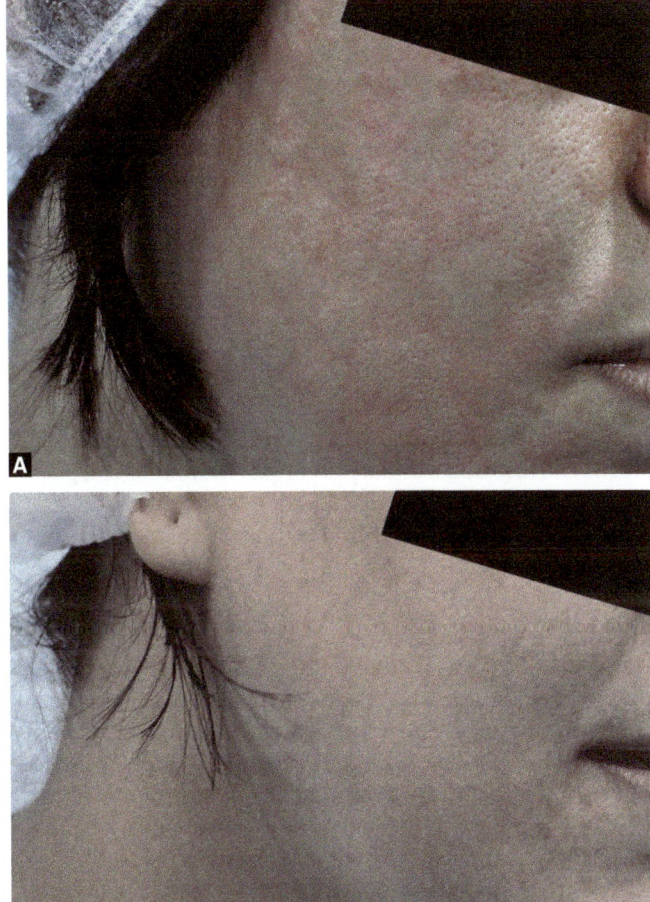

Figs. 10A and B: (A) Post carbon dioxide laser immediate post; (B) Post carbon dioxide laser resolution of edema.

reports especially when infections seem extensive and deeper. Emphasis should be laid on topical wound care in the post-treatment phase. Prophylactic antibiotics and antivirals should be given in susceptible patients and any sign of infection should be treated aggressively as it may lead to scarring. Oral antiviral agents should be used in case of herpes reactivation if no prophylaxis was given.[19,39-44] *Candida* superinfection may occur in patients on topical steroids or diabetics and should be treated with oral and topical antifungal agents.[19,40-44]

Pruritis

It is often seen after laser resurfacing or certain peels like retinol or salicylic peel, usually in the re-epithelialization phase. With salicylic acid peels, pruritis associated with urticaria should be watched for in patients who could be sensitive to salicylates. Pruritis can also be secondary to contact dermatitis to a peeling or priming agent.

Pruritis can be treated by topical mild steroids or antihistamines.

Acne Flare

A flare in acne is encountered if residual active acne persists while a procedure is undertaken. Acne flare may be seen after microdermabrasion and laser resurfacing. Adequate coverage with antibiotics, oral and topical, helps to resolve this issue. Topical retinoids in the priming phase help to prevent acne flare. Milia and acneiform eruption were largely seen with full-face dermabrasion, which is now replaced by fractional laser resurfacing techniques. Milia require extraction with a 26-number needle or light electrocautery.

Hyperpigmentation

It is the most common complication seen with almost all types of procedures used for acne scars from chemical peels to laser resurfacing techniques. The risk of hyperpigmentation is more in darker skin individuals. The PIH is difficult to treat and sometimes persistent due to prolonged sun exposure in the subtropics.[19,41-45]

Emphasis is made on sun avoidance, sun protection and lightening agents. While using fillers, minimizing the number of needle punctures to the skin can reduce the risk of hyperpigmentation. The use of ice before and during treatment, the use of hydrogen peroxide instead of alcohol to clean the skin and retreating darker skin with skin bleaching agents is the key to reduce PIH.[41] Once PIH sets in hydroquinone, retinoids or glycolic acid or even peels like retinol or kojic acid peels are used by the author in the postprocedure and intertreatment intervals. Also, it is sensible not to continue the treatment modality aggressively and defer further treatment till the PIH resolves. The current trend is to use triple combination of retinoids, hydroquinone and mometasone 0.1% or fluocinolone acetonide (class VI steroid) 0.01%. Procedurewise the risk of hyperpigmentation is much lesser with microdermabrasion and microneedling as well as superficial chemical peels than with laser resurfacing and medium-depth peels. With lasers, PIH is higher with ablative CO_2 laser due to deep thermal damage than fractional CO_2 laser. Fractional erbium laser is much safer than CO_2 laser as the water absorption coefficient is 16 times more; hence, thermal damage is much less. The longer wavelength is much safer for darker skin types. Hyperpigmentation can be treated with hydroquinone topically in strength of 2-5%, kojic acid, arbutin, azelaic acid, vitamin C and other lightening agents **(Fig. 11)**.

Hypopigmentation

Transient hypopigmentation can occur due to elimination of epidermal melanin. Laser resurfacing procedures can cause hypopigmentation both due to epidermal elimination as well as thermal damage to the melanocytes **(Fig. 12)**. In

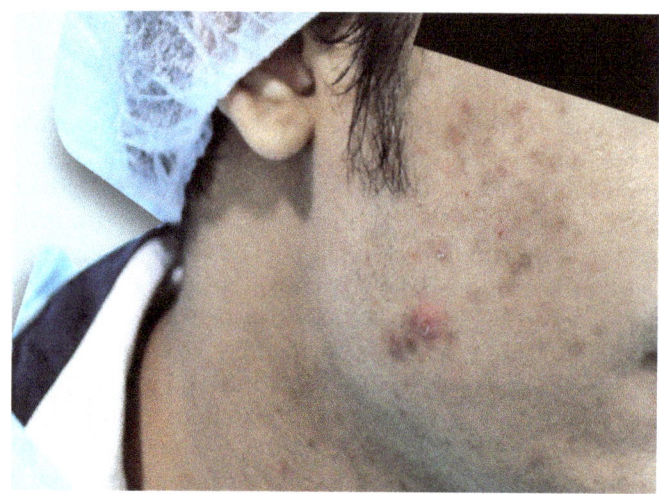

Fig. 11: Postinflammatory hyperpigmentation after fraction.

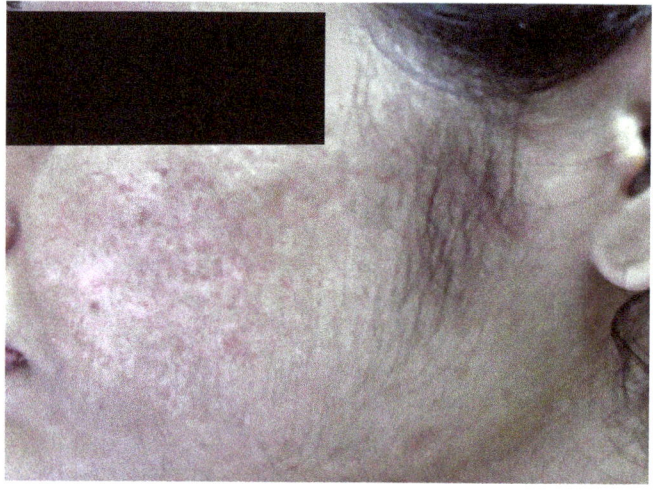

Fig. 12: Hypopigmentation after fractional carbon dioxide laser resurfacing.

deeper procedures, damage to the basal cell layer occurs leading to secondary hypopigmentation. Phenol peels cause toxic damage to melanocytes and may lead to permanent irreversible hypopigmentation or depigmentation. Mild and transient hypopigmentation may be seen with superficial peels, laser resurfacing and usually resolves with time. Deep peeling especially TCA and phenol and aggressive lasers can give rise to persistent hypopigmentation in the postprocedure phase and is often difficult to handle. Sometimes hypopigmentation resolves in 2–3 months but often it persists and may require treatment with topical tacrolimus. Further intervention should be immediately withheld once hypopigmentation is encountered.

Demarcation Lines

These are often encountered at the junction of treated and untreated areas with TCA peels and laser resurfacing, especially with CO_2 lasers. It can also be seen with focal or spot dermabrasion. This is more evident in dark-skinned patients particularly in the preauricular, infraorbital, jawline and neck areas. These can be avoided by feathering at margins during treatment.[19,40-44]

Delayed Healing

Delayed healing can occur due to infection, contact dermatitis, previous interventions, and patients on isotretinoin within last 6 months. Aggressive wound care management helps one to overcome this issue.

Keloid Formation

A patient with keloid tendency should be identified and is a contraindication for treatment. Such patients often show jawline areas with keloid, nodular keloids and hypertrophic bridging scars. Intralesional steroid injections or 5% fluorouracil can be used for hypertrophic scars as well as silicon sheeting or gels. Cobblestoning and ring scars are encountered in patients who undergo punch grafting and excision.[19,41-45]

Lumpiness and Granuloma Formation

These can be seen after fillers. Adequate post-filler molding and ice compresses, and antibiotic cream with or without topical steroid help to manage transient side effects and mild infections. Incision and expression may be required for lumpiness or biofilm formation with oral antibiotics. Granuloma formations are difficult to treat and may warrant use of oral steroids and immunosuppressives in severe cases.

Worsening of Scars

Worsening of scars is uncommon and may be seen with aggressive interventions like laser resurfacing and deep peels, if interventions are sought while patient is on isotretinoin or an infection (bacterial or viral) complicates the procedure. The temple, mandible and jawline, cheeks, upper lip, etc., are areas prone to this. Worsening of ice pick scars can also occur after CROSS therapy with high-strength TCA, due to improper application. Hypertrophic scars especially in jawline zone can set in with atrophic shiny skin. Topical steroids along are helpful to a certain extent in early hypertrophic scars.[41-46]

Toxicity

This is rarely encountered while conducting peels with salicylic acid, resorcinol and phenol. Salicylic acid applied to large areas especially on the trunk can manifest features of salicylism on systemic absorption such as tinnitus, dizziness, abdominal cramps and deafness. Copious amount of water intake is to be advised to prevent salicylism. Resorcinol can cause toxicity in the form of headache, diarrhea, dizziness, drowsiness, bradycardia and dyspnea. Restricting areas of application prevents this.[42-50] Phenol can cause cardiotoxicity, especially arrhythmias. Cardiac status monitoring and intravenous hydration need to be maintained. Discontinuing the peel and IV lignocaine administration is required if arrhythmia develops.[46-51]

CONCLUSION

Acne scars need to be addressed with multimodality treatments. In patients with skin of color, the risks of complications with procedures increase. The most common complication is pigmentary alterations. Strict sun protection, adequate priming, right modality of treatment either as standalone or combination and good postoperative regimen enables one to get substantial results without side effects. Newer fractional lasers and peel techniques in rotation lower the risk of complications. These modalities must be pursued with utmost caution in darker skin types. The responsibility lies on the clinician to be aware of all the complications of various techniques and be able to manage mild to most severe adverse effects when they happen.

REFERENCES

1. Aurangabadkar S, Mysore V. Standard guidelines of care: Lasers for tattoos and pigmented lesions. Indian J Dermatol Venereol Leprol. 2009;75(Suppl 2):S109-24.
2. Goodman GJ, Baron JA. The management of post acne scarring. Dermatol Surg. 2007;33:1-14.
3. Holland DB, Jeremy AH, Roberts SG, Seukeran DC, Layton AM, Cunliffe WJ. Inflammation in acne scarring: a comparison of the responses in lesions from patients prone and not prone to scar. Br J Dermatol. 2004;150:72-81.
4. Cole RP, Widdowson D, Moore JC. Outcome of erbium:yttrium aluminium garnet laser resurfacing treatments. Lasers Med Sci. 2008;23(4):427-33.

5. Cohen JL, Babcock MJ. Ablative fractionated erbium:YAG laser for the treatment of ice pick alar scars due to neodymium:YAG laser burns. J Drugs Dermatol. 2009;8(1):65-7.
6. Nouri K, Lanigan SW, Rivas MP. Laser treatment for scars. In: Goldberg DJ, Dover JS, Alam M (Eds). Procedures in Cosmetic Dermatology: Laser and Lights, Volume 1, 1st edition. Philadelphia: Elsevier; 2005. pp. 67-74.
7. Barlow RJ, Hruza GJ. Lasers and light tissue interactions. In: Goldberg DJ, Dover JS, Alam M (Eds). Procedures in Cosmetic Dermatology: Lasers and Lights, Volume 1, 1st edition. Philadelphia: Elsevier; 2005. pp. 1-11.
8. O'Shea DC, Callen WR, Rhodes WT. Introduction to Lasers and their Applications. Menlo Park (CA): Addison-Wesley Publishing Co.; 1978.
9. Anderson RR, Parrish JA. Selective photothermolysis: precise microsurgery by selective absorption of pulsed radiation. Science. 1983;220:524-7.
10. Kilmer SL, Garden JM. Laser treatment of pigmented lesions and tattoos. Semin Cutan Med Surg. 2000;19:232-44.
11. Savardekar P. Microdermabrasion. Indian J Dermatol Venereol Leprol. 2007;73:277-9.
12. Orentreich D, Orentreich N. Acne scar revision update. Dermatol Clin. 1987;14:261-76.
13. Roenigk HH Jr. Dermabrasion: state of art. J Dermatol Surg Oncol. 1985;11:306-14.
14. Lee JB, Chung WG, Kwahck H, Lee KH. Focal treatment of acne scars with trichloroacetic acid: chemical reconstruction of skin scars method. Dermatol Surg. 2002;28:1017-21.
15. Landau M. Advances in deep chemical peels. Dermatol Nurs. 2005;17:438-41.
16. Khunger N, Arsiwala S. Combination and sequential peels. In: Khunger N (Ed). Step-by-Step Chemical Peels. New Delhi: Jaypee Brothers Medical Publishers; 2008. pp. 201-18.
17. Kubba R, Bajaj AK, Thappa DM, Sharma R, Vedamurthy M, Dhar S, et al. Acne in India: guidelines for management. IAA consensus document. Acne scars. Indian J Dermatol Venereol Leprol. 2009; 75(Suppl 1):52-3.
18. Bhutani T, Batra S. Ablative devices. In: Alam M, Gladstone H, Tung RC (Ed). Cosmetic Dermatology, Volume 2. Philadelphia: Elsevier; 2009. pp. 113-30.

19. Alster TS. Cutaneous resurfacing with CO_2 and erbium: YAG lasers: preoperative, intraoperative, and postoperative considerations. Plast Reconstr Surg. 1999;103:619-32;discussion 633-4.
20. Goldman MP, Marchell N, Fitzpatrick RE. Laser skin resurfacing of the face with a combined CO_2/Er:YAG laser. Dermatol Surg. 2000;26:102-4.
21. Polnikorn N, Goldberg DT, Suwachinda A, Ng SW. Erbium:YAG laser resurfacing in Asians. Dermatol Surg. 1998;24:1303-7.
22. Rahman Z, Alam M, Dover JS. Fractional laser treatment of pigmentation and texture improvement. Skin Therapy Lett. 2006; 11(9):7-11.
23. Cho SI, Kim YC. Treatment of atrophic facial scars with combined use of high-energy pulsed CO_2 laser and Er:YAG laser: a practical guide of the laser techniques for the Er:YAG laser. Dermatol Surg. 1999;25(12):959-64.
24. Manstein D, Herron GC, Sink RK, Tanner H, Anderson RR. Fractional photothermolysis: a new concept for cutaneous remodeling using microscopic patterns of thermal injury. Lasers Surg Med. 2004;34:426-38.
25. Handley JM. Adverse events associated with nonablative cutaneous visible and infrared laser treatment. J Am Acad Dermatol. 2006; 55:482-9.
26. Kaidbey KH, Agin PP, Sayre RM, Kligman AM. Photoprotection by melanin—a comparison of black and Caucasian skin. J Am Acad Dermatol. 1979;1:249-60.
27. Chan NP, Ho SG, Yeung CK, Shek SY, Chan HH. The use of non-ablative fractional resurfacing in Asian acne scar patients. Lasers Surg Med. 2010;42(10):710-5.
28. Alam M, Dover JS. Treatment of acne scarring: ablative resurfacing. Skin Therapy Lett. 2006;11(9):7-9.
29. Lipper GM, Perez M. Nonablative acne scar reduction after a series of treatments with a short-pulsed 1,064-nm neodymium:YAG laser. Dermatol Surg. 2006;32:998-1006.
30. Alster TS, Tanzi EL, Lazarus M. The use of fractional laser photothermolysis for the treatment of atrophic scars. Dermatol Surg. 2007;33:295-9.
31. Grevelink JM, White VR. Concurrent use of laser skin resurfacing and punch excision in the treatment of facial acne scarring. Dermatol Surg. 1998;24:527-30.
32. Bisaccia E, Saap L, Kadry R, Scarborough D. Noninvasive procedures in cosmetic dermatology. Skin Aging. 2007;15:38-40.

33. Alam M, Dover JS. Management of complications and sequelae with temporary injectable fillers. Plast Reconstr Surg. 2007;120(Suppl 6): 98S-105S.
34. Vedamurthy M; IADVL Dermatosurgery Task Force. Standard guidelines for the use of dermal fillers. Indian J Dermatol Venereol Leprol. 2008;74:S23-7.
35. Hirch RJ, Cohen JL. Soft tissue augmentation. Cutis. 2006;78:165-72.
36. Hruza G, Taub AF, Collier SL, Mulholland SR. Skin rejuvenation and wrinkle reduction using a fractional radiofrequency system. J Drugs Dermatol. 2009;8:259-65.
37. Park JY, Lee EG, Yoon MS, Lee HJ. The efficacy and safety of combined microneedle fractional radiofrequency and sublative fractional radiofrequency for acne scars in Asian skin. J Cosmet Dermatol. 2016;15(2):102-7.
38. Abdel Aal AM, Ibrahim IM, Sami NA, Abdel Kareem IM. Evaluation of autologous platelet-rich plasma plus ablative carbon dioxide fractional laser in the treatment of acne scars. J Cosmet Laser Ther. 2018;20:106-13.
39. Garg S, Baveja S. Combination therapy in the management of atrophic acne scars. J Cutan Aesthet Surg. 2014;7:18-23.
40. Gawdat HI, Hegazy RA, Fawzy MM, Fathy M. Autologous platelet rich plasma: topical versus intradermal after fractional ablative carbon dioxide laser treatment of atrophic acne scars. Dermatol Surg. 2014;40:152-61.
41. Alster TS, Lupton JR. Prevention and treatment of side effects and complications of cutaneous laser resurfacing. Plast Reconstr Surg. 2002;109:308-16.
42. Alster TS, West TB. Resurfacing of atrophic facial acne scars with a high-energy, pulsed carbon dioxide laser. Dermatol Surg. 1996;22(2):151-4;discussion 154-5.
43. Alster TS, Nanni CA. Famciclovir prophylaxis of herpes simplex virus reactivation after laser skin resurfacing. Dermatol Surg. 1999;25(3):242-6.
44. Khunger N. Complications. In: Khunger N (Ed). Step-by-Step Chemical Peels. New Delhi: Jaypee Brothers Medical Publishers; 2008. pp. 280-98.
45. Khunger N. Acne scar revision. In: Khunger N, Sachdev M (Eds). Practical Manual of Cosmetic Dermatology and Surgery. Pune: Mehta Publishers; 2010. pp. 231-52.
46. Odunze M, Cohn A, Few JW. Restylane and people of color. Plast Reconstr Surg. 2007;120:2011-6.

47. Duffy DM. Avoiding complications with chemical peels. In: Rubin MG (Ed). Chemical Peels: Procedures in Cosmetic Dermatology. Philadelphia: Elsevier Inc.; 2006. pp. 137-70.
48. Fanous N. A new patient classification for laser resurfacing and peels: predicting responses, risks, and results. Aesthetic Plast Surg. 2002;26(2):99-104.
49. Rubin MG. Complications. In: Rubin MG (Ed). Manual of Chemical Peels—Superficial and Medium Depth, 1st edition. Philadelphia: JB Lippincot Co.; 1995. pp. 130-53.
50. Grimes PE. The safety and efficacy of salicylic acid chemical peels in darker racial-ethnic groups. Dermatol Surg. 1999;25:18-22.
51. Landau M. Cardiac complications in deep chemical peels. Dermatol Surg. 2007;33(2):190-3.

CHAPTER 23

Imaging Techniques for Acne Scars

Niti Khunger

IN A NUTSHELL

- ❖ Documenting acne scars not only helps in tracking progress, but is also useful for conducting scientific studies as improvement can be subtle and gradual.
- ❖ Digital photography is a standard technique, but change in the position or lighting can give erroneous and variable results.
- ❖ Ultrasound imaging and various 3D imaging tools are emerging technologies.
- ❖ Dermoscopy and reflectance confocal microscopy are recent advances.

INTRODUCTION

There is a dire need for good and consistent imaging techniques to document acne scars. Improvement after minimally invasive techniques can be subtle and gradual and often patients forget what they looked like initially. Documenting the scars not only helps in tracking progress, but is also useful for conducting scientific studies.

PHOTOGRAPHY

Digital photography is the most basic essential imaging technique for acne scars. It gives a global picture, is easily available and cost effective. Three views, frontal, right and left oblique are the basic requirements. Additional views and

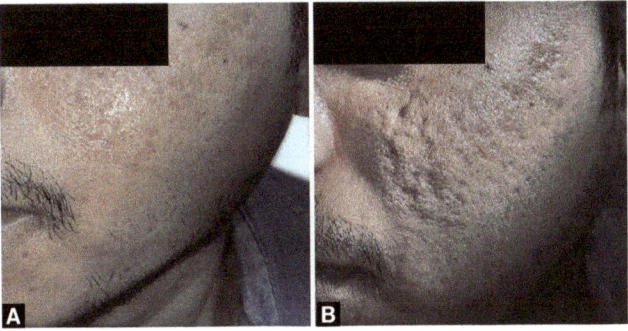

Figs. 1A and B: Effect of lighting on appearance of acne scars. (A) Direct light; (B) Indirect light.

close-ups may be taken as required. For detailed imaging of individual scars, a camera in the macro mode or a macro lens in an single-lens reflex (SLR) camera with a focal length of 60–100 mm is appropriate.[1] Acne scars look prominent because of the shadowing effect, where light plays a great role in their appearance. Hence, comparative photographs before and after treatment should be taken with standardized positioning, lighting and distance. This is very essential for acne scars as slight change in the position or lighting can give erroneous results **(Figs. 1A and B)**.

HIGH FREQUENCY ULTRASOUND[2,3]

Ultrasound imaging is a noninvasive technique that uses various acoustic properties of biologic tissues, obtaining one-dimensional images (A-mode) or two-dimensional images (B-mode). Ultrasound of the skin is best performed by equipment using high frequencies of 22 MHz. In B-mode imaging, normal skin shows an epidermal entrance echo, the dermal layer, and the subcutaneous layer and provides an objective measurement of skin thickness up to 8 mm in depth **(Fig. 2)**. (EasyScan Echo®, Business Enterprise, Trapani, Italy).

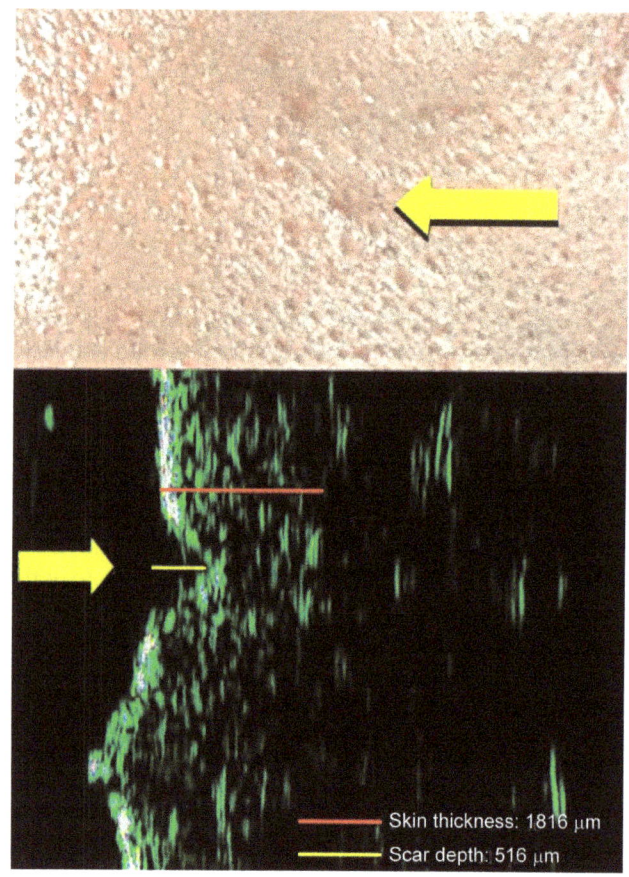

Fig. 2: Ultrasound image of an atrophic scar at 22 Mz.

The various types of acne scars, atrophic and hypertrophic can be well visualized.

OPTICAL IMAGING DEVICES

Three-dimensional imaging is a recent measuring method in dermatology. It uses optical projections, a high-resolution video camera, and computer software to rapidly generate images and measurements of skin topography.

A variety of imaging devices are now available with their software to give a topographic measurement of acne scars.[4-10] Some examples include the Primos®[5], Visia®, Antera®[6], stereoimage optical topometer (SOT)[7] system that uses a pair of images taken using two video cameras to produce a three-dimensional (3D) image. Petukhova et al.[9] compared the Goodman grading system on the basis of high resolution photographs and found that the interrater agreeability differed according to the level of training among the graders. It was good for board-certified dermatologists but moderate for dermatology residents. They used a 3-dimensional facial modeling device (Clarity 3D Research Ti System, BrighTex Bio-Photonics, San Jose, CA), which is based on the principle of three-angled cameras reconstructing a topographic map of the acne scars. The system gave a quantitative volumetric measurements for each scar, which they concluded was a more objective method of scar measurement. Petit et al.[10] evaluated 31 patients with acne scars with a 3D imaging system using the LifeViz® Micro system and analyzed images with MountainsMap® software. They were able to quantify the scar volume loss with good repeatability and concluded that this can be integrated into an automated workflow in the treatment of acne scars.

Optical Coherence Tomography

Optical coherence tomography (OCT) is a 3D imaging, real-time, noninvasive technique that produces cross-sectional morphological images of tissue microstructures in vivo with a reasonable field of view (millimeters) and a micron-level imaging resolution analogous to histology.[11] It is slowly gaining popularity due to its relatively high resolution (up to 1 μm), deep imaging depth (1-3 mm), and real-time image acquisition. Baran et al.[11] used a commercial OCT system (SL1310V1-10048, Thorlabs Inc.) to evaluate facial acne and acne scarring by optical microangiography and showed that acne scarring involves microvascular changes and fibrosis in the initial acne lesion that leads to scarring. Ortiz et al.[12] reported that laser-based acne treatment methods modify the subdermal microvasculature and lead to improvement that can be evaluated by OCT.

DERMOSCOPY

Dermoscopy is a noninvasive tool that allows visualization of cutaneous lesions in vivo up to the beginning of the reticular dermis. It is not a simple magnifying glass, but a more complex instrument that allows the superimposition of the skin layers. Though it is mainly used for visualization of pigmented lesions, the scope of dermoscopy has expanded rapidly including inflammatory lesions such as psoriasis, cutaneous infestations, and nail and hair disorders. There are limited studies in the use of dermoscopy in acne and acne scars.[13]

REFLECTANCE CONFOCAL MICROSCOPY

This is an exciting new technique that gives detailed high-resolution images of the skin in vivo. The vivascope uses a 830-nm diode laser to give a near histologic image including the epidermis and dermis. The advantage of the newer techniques is that they are noninvasive and patient friendly. Campos et al.[14] recently published their findings on the use of reflectance confocal microscopy (VivaScope® 1500 Reflectance Confocal Microscopy—RCM, Lucid, United States) in the evaluation of epidermal thickness, enlarged pores and comedones in their evaluation of oily skin in acne. Fabbrocini et al.[15] assessed the efficacy of one session of microneedling in acne scars using reflectance confocal microscopy and concluded that confocal microscopy can better define the changes induced on the skin by skin needling.

CONCLUSION

There is a dire need for standardized imaging techniques for acne such as changes can often be subtle. Various 3D imaging tools that can accurately reflect the depth of scars and texture are evolving techniques.

REFERENCES

1. Bhatia AC. The clinical image: archiving clinical processes and an entire specialty. Arch Dermatol. 2006;142(1):96-8.
2. Lacarrubba F, Patania L, Perrotta R, Stracuzzi G, Nasca MR, Micali G. An open-label pilot study to evaluate the efficacy and tolerability of a silicone gel in the treatment of hypertrophic scars using clinical and ultrasound assessments. J Dermatol Treat. 2008;19:50-3.
3. Naouri M, Atlan M, Perrodeau E, Georgesco G, Khallouf R, Martin L, et al. High-resolution ultrasound imaging to demonstrate and predict efficacy of carbon dioxide fractional resurfacing laser treatment. Dermatol Surg. 2011;37(5):596-603.
4. Lee JW, Kim BJ, Kim MN, Choi YH, Kim K, Hwang E. A new method for evaluating postacne scarring. Skin Res Technol. 2012;18(3):384-5.
5. Friedman PM, Jih MH, Skover GR, Payonk GS, Kimyai-Asadi A, Geronemus RG. Treatment of atrophic facial acne scars with the 1064-nm Q-switched Nd:YAG laser. Six-month follow-up study. Arch Dermatol. 2004;140(11):1337-41.
6. Fisk NA, Jensen K, Knaggs H, Ferguson S. The clinical utility of a hand-held computerized optical imaging system at assessing skin discoloration. J Cosmet Dermatol. 2010;9(2):103-7.
7. Kyrgidis A, Becker M, Zampeli V, Fauger A, Sayag M, Zouboulis CC. Multimodal clinical imaging assessment of the outcome in mild-to-moderate acne: A prospective study. Dermatology. 2019;235:471-7.
8. Kim JE, Lee OS, Choi J, Son SW, Oh CH. The efficacy of stereoimage optical topometry to evaluate depressed acne scar treatment using cultured autologous fibroblast injection. Dermatol Surg. 2011;37:1304-13.

9. Petukhova TA, Foolad N, Prakash N, Shi VY, Sharon VR, O'Brecht L, et al. Objective volumetric grading of postacne scarring. J Am Acad Dermatol. 2016;75:229-31.
10. Petit L, Zugaj D, Bettoli V, Dreno B, Kang S, Tan J, et al. Validation of 3D skin imaging for objective repeatable quantification of severity of atrophic acne scarring. Skin Res Technol. 2018;24:542-50.
11. Baran U, Li Y, Choi WJ, Kalkan G, Wang RK. High resolution imaging of acne lesion development and scarring in human facial skin using OCT-based microangiography. Lasers Surg Med. 2015;47:231-8.
12. Ortiz A, Van Vliet M, Lask GP, Yamauchi PS. A review of lasers and light sources in the treatment of acne vulgaris. J Cosmetic Laser Therapy. 2005;7:69-75.
13. Chae WS, Seong JY, Jung HN, Kong SH, Suh HS, Choi YS. The consideration of dermoscopic findings during atrophic acne scar treatment: a pilot study. Korean J Dermatol. 2015;53(1):23-29.
14. Maia Campos PMBG, Melo MO, Mercurio DG. Use of advanced imaging techniques for the characterization of oily skin. Front Physiol. 2019;10:254.
15. Fabbrocini G, Ardigò M, Mordente I, Ayala F, Cacciapuoti S, Monfrecola G. Confocal Microscopy Images to Monitor Skin Needling in the Treatment of Acne Scars. J Clin Exp Dermatol Res. 2015;6:301.

CHAPTER 24

Camouflage Techniques for Acne Scars

Niti Khunger, Kumar Abhishek

IN A NUTSHELL

- ❖ Skillful camouflage makeup can be life changing, covering scars, red and pigmented spots of acne.
- ❖ Cosmetic camouflage techniques include color and contour correction.
- ❖ Primers, foundations, and concealers are useful in camouflaging the atrophic acne scars.
- ❖ Brimonidine gel is temporarily useful in erythematous acne scars.

INTRODUCTION

Acne scars are common sequelae to acne, and have significant cosmetic and psychological impact on the patient. Particularly adolescents are worst affected by the disfigurement caused due to acne and the scars. Acne scarring has significant negative impact on the quality of life in adults also.[1] This can be reduced to a great extent by camouflage by makeup which makes scars less obvious. The use of makeup has been traced back to mankind's earliest days. It was used as a decorative product with the intent to frighten enemies, possibly attract a mate or assist in retelling the story of the hunt and fortunes of war. Makeup is an illusionary product only; it has no lasting effect and, as a general rule, it does not affect the general health of the skin.

Cosmetic camouflage is the technique to use makeup to diminish the appearance of disfiguring skin lesions, making the skin appear relatively normal. Specialized products are applied in a systematic way that can rapidly disguise areas of visible scars. They are generally waterproof and allow adherence to variably textured skin, including diseased or scarred skin. When skillfully applied, they can significantly impact the quality of life and give self-confidence to a distressed patient.[2-4]

Before starting camouflage therapy, the following things must be considered:
- Patient's medical and psychological history
- History of allergies to any external application agent
- History of any concomitant application which can alter the effect of the makeup
- Indication for which camouflage is being used.

INDICATIONS

Cosmetic camouflage can reduce the appearance of acne and its scars and should be offered to patients who have psychosocial distress. Scars are a personal matter and are significant, no matter big or small, if they are causing significant distress. Camouflage is especially useful when quick or immediate results are desired such as before marriage or social functions. Though commonly used by females, they can also be recommended to male patients, particularly on special occasions like marriage. In a patients with body dysmorphophobic disorder, camouflage is a good technique to avoid repeated surgeries demanded by patients.[5]

CONTRAINDICATIONS

They should be used judiciously in patients with sensitive skin as they can cause irritant dermatitis, particularly when removing the makeup. They are relatively contraindicated in patients who have concomitant eczema, psoriasis, contact dermatitis, open wounds, fungal, bacterial or viral infections on the relevant areas.[6] They should also be avoided immediately following surgery until all wounds, stitches, and scabs have completely healed and the skin has re-epithelialized.

TYPES OF MEDICAL MAKEUP FOR SCARS[6-9]

Medical makeup is of three types. It can be subtle coverage, which is light application that moderately covers and is localized to the scars. It can be camouflage makeup, which is useful for correcting color changes, and corrective makeup which is useful for correcting deformities and contour changes.

Subtle Coverage

This is a light application of makeup that partially corrects the scar and is localized to the scar. A sponge applicator is used.

Camouflage Makeup

This utilizes the color theory to hide color changes such as erythema, hyper- and hypopigmentation. It is useful for erythematous and hyperpigmented macular scars as well as active acne.

Corrective Makeup

This is used to correct irregularities and can be used to diminish the appearance of atrophic and raised keloidal acne scars. It utilizes the principle of light and dark technique for correction of scars. It is done by highlighting, filling the gaps, contouring and planning to give the appearance of smooth skin.

MAKEUP PRODUCTS FOR ACNE SCARS

In patients with active acne, they should be noncomedogenic. An ideal product should be available in a variety of colors to suit all skin types, have a good adhesive property so that it is longwearing and not be rubbed off easily, be water resistant, and give a mattifying effect. It should be hypoallergenic, formulated without any potential irritants and sensitizing ingredients, and be well tested for heavy metals.

Primer

It is the first product that is applied in the makeup product. It can be liquid or creamy.

Foundation

A cosmetic used to color and smooth out the face. It can be in liquid, powder, or cream form. It usually contains titanium dioxide and iron oxides.

Concealer

It increases the effect of foundation. It is more opaque, adherent and waterproof.

Powder

Powders include talc and titanium dioxide in increasing amounts.

Manganese carbonate buffers the oil, while kaolin increases the control of the oil. Manganese stearate increases its adhesiveness to the skin.[1]

TOOLS

Good brushes in small pointed and large sizes, sponge applicators, cotton swabs and cotton pads are essential

Camouflage Techniques for Acne Scars

tools. They should be kept clean after every use. An airbrush system consisting of an airbrush gun suitable for makeup and a compressor with a PSI setting as low as 5 is optional and desirable, but not mandatory.

TECHNIQUES

There are basically five steps to applying a good camouflage makeup:[10]

Cleansing

Cleansing the skin is an important step so that the makeup is long lasting. The cleanser should be mild, either rinse-off or rinse-free and gentle so that it preserves the barrier function of the skin. It should be gently massaged on the face and neck to remove dirt and previous makeup. The cleanser is then rinsed with a warm wash cloth. An alcohol-free toner on a cotton pad is used to remove excess cleanser, if any.

Moisturization

This is essential for patients with dry skin or in patients with acne where the skin has become dry due to application of anti-acne medication. The moisturizer should be light, creamy, water-based and noncomedogenic. If the skin is oily, the shine should be removed with a toner or astringent as the makeup will not set well on oily skin.

Color Correction

This is done by optical correction using the right color concealer. It is an important step and will reduce the amount of makeup required and give an even skin tone. It is done according to the theory of complementary colors, that is opposite colors cancel each other **(Fig. 1)**. Hence, the color of the concealer is a complementary color to the scar. It is applied by dabbing with fingers or by using a sponge. A coral or orange color neutralizes bluish, purplish and hyperpigmentation spots and softens dark brown skin areas, like dark circles, bruises, capillaries and hyperpigmented scars. A green color neutralizes reddish discolorations like redness, rosacea, recent scars, red active acne lesions and persistent erythematous macules.

Color of the facial makeup should be tested on the jawline and not on the wrist or the back of the hand as the skin here can have a different color. A little should be applied and gently blended with the fingertip. The ideal color should seem to disappear into the skin. The makeup should be applied by layering till the color is even.

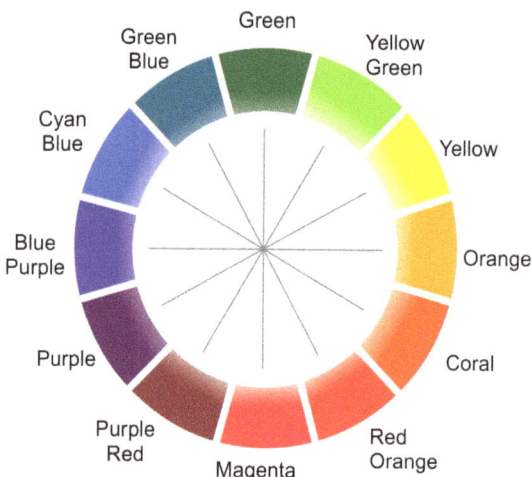

Fig. 1: Color wheel for choosing color-correcting makeup. Applying one color over its opposite color on the wheel will create an optical effect of neutralizing the underlying color and thus providing camouflage.

Contour Correction

This is done for depressed or raised scars. Depressed or atrophic scars are corrected by a technique called as highlight makeup. It is based on the principle that lighter shades give an optical illusion of lifting up. Using a pointed brush, a highlight concealer that is one to two shades lighter is applied focally to the depressed scar. Alternatively, a pencil stick can be used in the indented areas. A similar technique can be used for ice pick scars and large pores.

Raised scars are corrected by a technique called as contour makeup. Dark colors give the optical illusion of recession where they are applied; hence, a raised scar becomes less prominent. Contouring is using a shade of makeup that is slightly darker than the surrounding skin, providing the illusion of a smoother appearance. The same technique can also be used to help camouflage puffy or edematous areas to reduce the illusion of swelling.

Application of the Foundation

This is an important step to blend the scars with surrounding normal skin. The foundation shade should be a shade lighter or closest to the normal complexion. The foundation texture should be based on the type of scars. A stick foundation that is more opaque is used for severe scars and a fluid foundation is used for mild-to-moderate scars. The foundation is applied by dabbing with the fingertips or a sponge and then blended with the entire skin.

SETTING OR FIXING THE MAKEUP

The makeup is then set or fixed by applying a face powder that is of the normal skin tone by gently dabbing it on skin with a brush. Finally, a refreshing spray may be sprayed over the makeup to finish off and prevent any makeup thickness from showing, thereby giving a very natural dewy look to the skin. Any excess product is removed by gently dabbing with a paper tissue.

Other Makeup

After concealing imperfections or scars, the makeover can be completed with other color makeup products such as blushers, glitter, eyeshadow, etc. which are specifically formulated for sensitive skin. Some foundations have added sunscreens which are useful to prevent or reduce hyperpigmentation and erythema. Foundations containing cosmeceuticals for active acne and pigmentation may be useful.

MAKEUP REMOVAL

It is important to remove all makeup from the face or other body areas where camouflage makeup was applied before sleeping. This is done by using a gentle creamy makeup remover, that is effective in removing makeup, yet does not disturb the skin barrier function.

SIDE EFFECTS

Usually medical makeup causes no adverse effects. However, patients with sensitive skin may experience irritation, itching and breakouts. The products must be stopped and then singly applied to see the culprit. Alternatively, a different brand may be used.

BRIMONIDINE GEL

Brimonidine 0.5% gel causes temporary vasoconstriction and may be used in reducing erythema of scars for a short duration of time. Hence, it can be used as a camouflaging agent in those who have erythematous acne scars.[11] The effect appears within 1 hour and lasts for about 3 hours. However, it can cause rebound redness, hence must not be used routinely.

CONCLUSION

Camouflage is an art of optical illusion and requires skill, knowledge and experience. It is an effective, adjunctive therapy and can greatly benefit patients suffering from psychosocial distress caused by unsightly acne scars. It is a value addition, particularly in this social age of Facebook, selfies and Instagram photos and should be offered to patients disturbed by their scars. Use of camouflaging agents is a cheap, result-oriented yet short-lasting measure to enhance the appearance of the acne scars. Not only can it improve the appearance, but it also improves the quality of life of the affected individual.

REFERENCES

1. Chuah SY, Goh CL. The impact of post-acne Scars on the quality of life among young adults in Singapore. J Cutan Aesthet Surg. 2015;8(3):153-8.
2. Westmore GM. Camouflage and makeup preparations. Clin Dermatol. 2001;19:406-12.
3. Holme SA, Beattie PE, Fleming CJ. Cosmetic camouflage advice improves quality of life. Br J Dermatol. 2002;147:946-9.
4. Levy LL, Emer JJ. Emotional benefit of cosmetic camouflage in the treatment of facial skin conditions: personal experience and review. Clin Cosmet Investig Dermatol. 2012;5:173-82.
5. Thanveer F, Khunger N. Screening for body dysmorphic disorder in a dermatology outpatient setting at a tertiary care centre. J Cutan Aesthet Surg. 2016;9:188-91.
6. Mee D, Wong BJ. Medical makeup for concealing facial scars. Facial Plast Surg. 2012;28:536-40.
7. Draelos ZK. Cosmetic camouflaging techniques. Cutis. 1993;52:362-4.
8. Viera MH, Amini S, Huo R, Valins W, Berman B. Cosmetic camouflage for scars. J Cosmet Dermatol. 2009;22:260-4.

9. Westmore MG. Camouflage and makeup preparations. Clin Dermatol. 2001;19:406-12.
10. Bionike. Camouflage makeup: what it is and how to apply it. [online] Available from: https://www.bionike.it/en/your-needs/maquillaje-y-camuflaje-corrector/camouflage-makeup-what-it-and-how-apply-it. [Last accessed on December, 2019].
11. Reinholz M, Heppt M, Tietze JK, Ruzicka T, Gauglitz GG, Schauber J. Photoletter to the editor: Topical 0.5% brimonidine gel to camouflage redness of immature scars. J Dermatol Case Rep. 2015;3:87-8.

CHAPTER 25

Newer Techniques: Fractional Microneedle Radiofrequency for the Treatment of Acne Scars

Anuj Pall

IN A NUTSHELL

- Microneedling radiofrequency (MNRF) combines the technique of microneedling with radiofrequency energy that is delivered between the needles to amplify collagen and elastin production.
- It is an effective technique for acne scars with minimum downtime and side effects, particularly in darker skin patients.
- Bipolar radiofrequency is highly beneficial for treating acne scars.
- MNRF can be combined with subcision, platelet rich plasma and fractional lasers for better results.
- Latest technologies in acne scar management are electro-optical synergy, functional aspiration controlled electrothermal stimulation and nanofractional radiofrequency.

INTRODUCTION[1,2]

Fractional radiofrequency (RF) is a technology that emits electromagnetic current into the skin generating microthermal wounds along with deep dermal heating. In microneedling radiofrequency (MNRF), energy is conducted between the alternating rows of positive and negative electrode pins which initiates collagen remodeling. The advantage of MNRF over fractional lasers is that MNRF is effective in all skin types with a low risk of skin burns and postinflammatory hyperpigmentation (PIH). The depth of the microneedles can be adjusted from 0.5 to 3 mm based on the depth and type of scars, whereas the maximum depth which can be achieved safely with fractional lasers is 1–1.5 mm. RF energy is specifically focused at the tip of electrodes, resulting in minimum trauma to the epidermis. This leads to far less downtime and pain for the patient as compared to conventional fractional CO_2 laser.

EQUIPMENT[2]

Microneedling radiofrequency devices consist of a handheld applicator with a disposable single-use treatment tip. The tip contains 25–49 microneedle electrodes in 1 cm^2 area **(Fig. 1)**. In noninsulated microneedles, RF energy is delivered directly to a certain depth of dermis through the whole length of microneedles **(Fig. 2)**. In insulated needle, the microneedle electrodes are nonconductive except for the distal 0.3 mm **(Fig. 3)**. Because the shaft of the needles is insulated, there is no electrothermal damage to the epidermis as compared to the noninsulated needles.

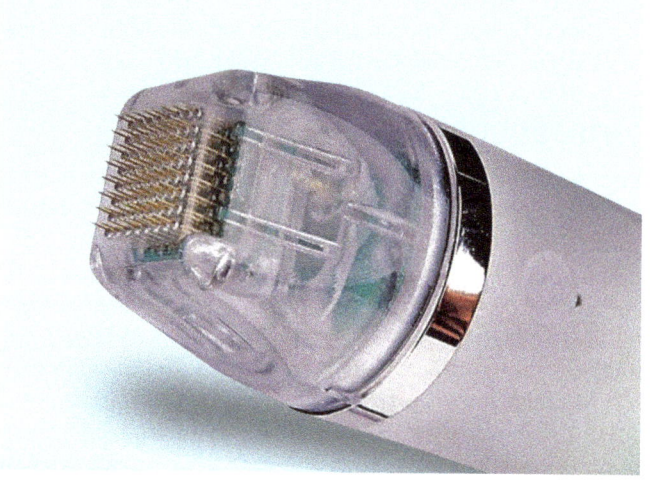

Fig. 1: Microneedling radiofrequency probe with microneedles.

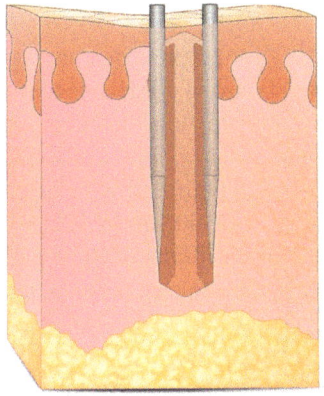

Fig. 2: Noninsulated needles.

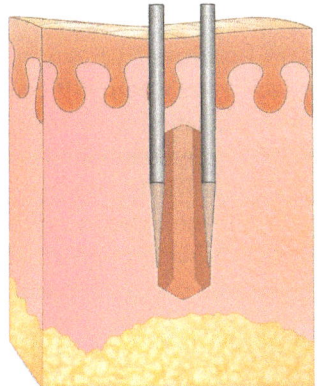

Fig. 3: Insulated needles.

MONOPOLAR AND BIPOLAR RADIOFREQUENCY[3]

Monopolar RF current is applied between electrodes and a grounding plate. On the other hand, bipolar RF energy is confined between two electrodes. Bipolar RF creates limited coagulative necrosis zone around needle in contrast to monopolar RF which causes wider and deeper denaturation zone. The main advantage of monopolar system is that it can achieve high penetration of emitted current and is considered to be the best for skin tightening. On the other hand, bipolar RF is more effective for treating acne scars, open pores and surgical scars.

COMBINATION TREATMENTS

Microneedling radiofrequency can be combined with subcision, gel-based chemical peels, mesosolutions, hyaluronic acid, fractional lasers and platelet-rich plasma (PRP). PRP is typically injected into the skin at regularly spaced intervals after MNRF procedure, which releases growth factors that accelerate soft tissue regeneration.[4]

NEWER ADVANCEMENTS[5,6]

Nanofractional RF works with tiny pins which create microdermal wounds. It enables ablation of epidermis along with coagulation of the dermis, resulting in more effective skin resurfacing with minimal downtime.

Bipolar RF devices are frequently combined with light-based technologies, termed electro-optical synergy (ELOS). The ELOS system uses the synergistic effects of light and RF-based devices. Preheating with light energy reduces the tissue's impedance. The lower impedance makes the tissue more susceptible to the RF component.

Functional aspiration controlled electrothermal stimulation (FACES) is another system used with the bipolar device that uses a vacuum to maximize and control penetration of the electric current.

INDICATIONS

All types of acne scars can be treated **(Figs. 4A and B)**. In addition, it has also been found to be effective in treating skin laxity, open pores, fine lines and wrinkles.

CONTRAINDICATIONS

Contraindications to MNRF procedure are skin infection, bleeding disorder, pregnancy, keloidal tendency, skin

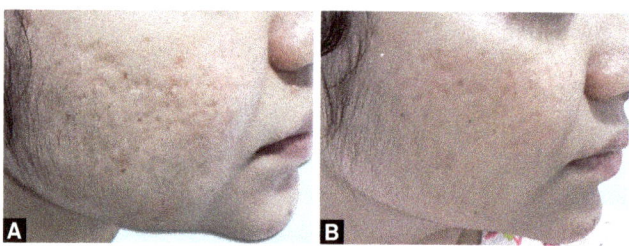

Figs. 4A and B: (A) Before treatment; (B) After four sessions of microneedling radiofrequency treatment.

malignancy, pacemaker devices, vascular stents or metal implants.

PROCEDURE

Before the procedure, an informed consent and pretreatment photographs are taken. Patients may be advised oral valacyclovir in case of herpes simplex in the past. Topical anesthetic cream under occlusion is applied an hour before the procedure. Depending on the type of acne scar, desired depth of the needle (1.5 mm or 2 mm) is adjusted and treatment is performed. Multiple passes are usually given depending on the severity of scars.

Chandrashekar et al.[7] used the MNRF device on 31 patients with acne scars, including 15 male and 16 female patients with type III-V skin. Patients underwent 4 sessions at 6-week intervals. The needle depth varied according to the scar type and site. For ice pick scars and mixed scars, the needle depth was kept at 3.5 mm on the first pass, 2.5 mm on the second pass and 1.5 mm on the third pass with minimal or no overlapping. This was reduced to 1.5 mm on the forehead, temple area and bony prominences. The energy settings depend on the machine, but it should be reduced with lesser depth, to prevent epidermal injury and coagulation. They used 25-30 W at 1.5 mm, 30-35 W at 2.5 mm and 35-40 W at depths of 3.5 mm. At 3 months of follow-up after the last treatment, 58% of the patients had moderate improvement, 29% had minimal improvement, 9% had good improvement and 3% showed very good improvement according to the Goodman and Baron's global quantitative acne scarring system. All patients had treatment related pain and transient erythema. Five had PIH and two patients showed track marks of the needle probe.

Faghihi et al.[8] compared MNRF with subcision versus MNRF alone in a split-face study in 12 patients with II-IV Fitzpatrick skin type. Two weeks after subcision on one side,

MNRF treatment was done on both cheeks and repeated at 4-week intervals for two more sessions. They reported better patient satisfaction in the combination side. Elawar and Dahan[9] used electronically controlled noninsulated MNRF device (Intensif applicator, EndyMed, Caesarea, Israel) and reported satisfactory treatment in acne scars, texture and pore size after 2-5 treatment sessions at 1 month intervals (76-100% improvement was seen in 5.26% of patients, 51-75% improvement was seen in 57.89% of patients and 36.84% saw 26-50% improvement). They observed that emission of RF energy that is delivered over the entire noninsulated needle length allows heating of larger volumes of dermal tissue as compared to insulated needles. Similar results were reported by Pudukadan[10] with noninsulated needles. Tatlıparmak A et al.[11] combined fractional carbon dioxide laser and fractional MNRF in 72 patients and reported greater improvement with increased number of sessions.

PRECAUTIONS

Keep cleaning blood and fluid with sterile gauze during the treatment to avoid sliding of probe especially on the nose and bony prominences. High RF energy should be avoided on the areas such as forehead and temple where underlying bones are close to the skin surface.

POST-TREATMENT CARE

After treatment, the patient is advised to apply topical antibiotic for 2-3 days. Patients are instructed to avoid sun exposure and to apply sunscreen with SPF 30. Downtime is limited to only about 1-2 days of a sunburn-like sensation and slight redness.

COMPLICATIONS

Mild pain, temporary redness and crusting are common side effects seen during and post procedure. Patients taking

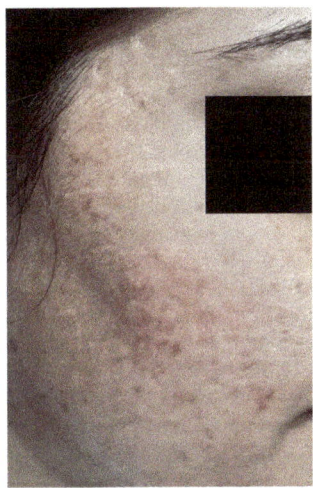

Fig. 5: Shoe marks—an uncommon side effect of MNRF.

isotretinoin experience more bleeding during the treatment than a normal person. Bruising usually occurs around the eyes when needle length of 0.8 mm or more is used. A rare side effect is persistence of marks post MNRF treatment **(Fig. 5)**. They usually resolve after 3-6 months. There is a report of temporary greater auricular nerve paresthesia after radiofrequency microneedling treatment.[12]

CONCLUSION

Fractional bipolar RF is an excellent treatment modality for acne scars with advantages of patient safety, shorter downtime and less adverse events, especially in Asian skin.

REFERENCES

1. Fabbrocini G, Annunziata MC, D'Arco V, De Vita V, Lodi G, Mauriello MC, et al. Acne scars: pathogenesis, classification and treatment. Dermatol Res Pract. 2010;2010:893080.

2. Cho SI, Chung BY, Choi MG, Baek JH, Cho HJ, Park CW, et al. Evaluation of the clinical efficacy of fractional radiofrequency microneedle treatment in acne scars and large facial pores. Dermatol Surg. 2012;38:1017-24.
3. Lolis MS, Goldberg DJ. Radiofrequency in cosmetic dermatology: a review. Dermatol Surg. 2012;28(11):1765-76.
4. Saeed MY, Elethawi AMD, Al-Ani ZT, Abdullah RA. Application of fractional microneedling radiofrequency and autologous platelet-rich plasma in managing facial acne scars. Br J Med Res. 2016;14(2):1-18.
5. Taub AF, Garretson CB. Treatment of acne scars of skin types II to V by sublative fractional bipolar radiofrequency and bipolar radiofrequency combined with diode laser. J Clin Aesthet Dermatol. 2011;4(10):18-27.
6. Werschler WP, Herdener RS, Ross VE, Zimmerman E. Critical considerations on optimizing topical corticosteroid therapy. J Clin Aesthet Dermatol. 2015;8(Suppl 8):S2-8.
7. Chandrashekar BS, Sriram R, Mysore R, Bhaskar S, Shetty A. Evaluation of microneedling fractional radiofrequency device for treatment of acne scars. J Cutan Aesthet Surg. 2014;7:93-7.
8. Faghihi G, Poostiyan N, Asilian A, Abtahi-Naeini B, Shahbazi M, Iraji F, et al. Efficacy of fractionated microneedle radiofrequency with and without adding subcision for the treatment of atrophic facial acne scars: A randomized split-face clinical study. J Cosmet Dermatol. 2017;16:223-9.
9. Elawar A, Dahan S. Non-insulated fractional microneedle radiofrequency treatment with smooth motor insertion for reduction of depressed acne scars, pore size, and skin texture improvement: a preliminary study. J Clin Aesthet Dermatol. 2018;11:41-4.
10. Pudukadan D. Treatment of acne scars on darker skin types using a noninsulated smooth motion, electronically controlled radiofrequency microneedles treatment system. Dermatol Surg. 2017;43(Suppl 1):64-9.
11. Tatlıparmak A, Aksoy B, Shishehgarkhaneh LR, Gökdemir G, Koç E. Use of combined fractional carbon dioxide laser and fractional microneedle radiofrequency for the treatment of acne scars: A retrospective analysis of 1-month treatment outcome on scar severity and patient satisfaction. J Cosmet Dermatol. 2020;19(1):115-21.
12. Niamtu J 3rd. Temporary Greater Auricular Nerve Paresthesia After Radiofrequency Microneedling Treatment. Dermatol Surg. 2019 Aug 12.

CHAPTER 26

Combination Treatments for Acne Scars

Niti Khunger

IN A NUTSHELL

- Combining therapies leads to better outcomes as compared to individual treatments.
- Procedures can be combined simultaneously, which reduces downtime and costs or at different times, which reduces the risk of adverse effects.
- Subcision can be combined with CROSS (chemical reconstruction of skin scars) technique or microneedling to kick start the regenerative process.
- Fractional resurfacing lasers can be combined with subcision, CROSS, platelet-rich plasma (PRP) and fat transfer.
- PRP combined with other modalities leads to faster healing and skin recovery.
- Fillers should not be combined with lasers in the same session and should be done after laser resurfacing.
- Planning a tailored treatment plan for each patient after detailed discussion is more likely to result in improvement and patient satisfaction.

INTRODUCTION

There are varied morphologies of acne scars and no single treatment can effectively address all types of scars. Hence, different techniques are utilized for individual types of scars. In combination therapy, distinct techniques are utilized either at the same time or at different times to treat acne scars. The choice and order of combination depends on the predominant scar type, the downtime involved, and schedule and preference of the patient. For example, in a patient with rolling scars, due to get married shortly in a week's time, will benefit from a combination of gentle subcision followed by a filler.

ADVANTAGES OF COMBINATION TECHNIQUES

Combining techniques can lead to better efficacy and shorten the duration of treatment, with fewer sessions.[1] It also reduces the total downtime involved, reduces cost and saves multiple trips to the physician's office. It is also advantageous to the physician as it optimizes treatment and leads to greater patient benefit.

CURRENT TRENDS

Management of acne scars is one of the most common procedures sought by patients in a dermatosurgery or esthetic practice. Hence, the physician should be well versed with several techniques in order to optimize treatment. The current trends are to have a minimally invasive approach, which leads to reduced downtime and minimizes risk of side effects. The older techniques of full-face resurfacing by dermabrasion or phenol peels or CO_2 laser ablation, though effective in a single session had long downtimes for skin recovery and a huge risk of adverse effects, particularly in dark skin patients. These are almost given up now and the current trend is to combine minimally invasive techniques like subcision, microneedling, CROSS (chemical reconstruction of skin scars), fractional laser resurfacing, fractional microneedle radiofrequency, fillers and autologous fat transfer. With the advent of these simple techniques, it has become possible for a beginner who may not have the finances to invest in machines like lasers to treat patients **(Table 1)**. Though lasers are very effective and easy to handle, they require not only initial investment, but also

TABLE 1: Minimally invasive techniques for acne scars.

Type of scars	Without machines	With machines
Erythematous scars	Topical agents, chemical peels	Pulsed dye laser, intense pulsed light, blue light, green light, red light
Hyperpigmented scars	Topical agents, chemical peels	Q-switched Nd:YAG laser 1,064 nm
Ice pick scars	Subcision, CROSS, minipunch grafting	FAST technique with CO_2 laser
Rolling scars	Subcision, micro-needling, fillers, fat transfer, PRP	Fractional CO_2 laser, fractional Er:YAG laser, fractional MNRF
Boxcar scars	Subcision, punch excision techniques, microneedling, PRP	CO_2 laser, fractional MNRF

(CROSS: chemical reconstruction of skin scars; Er:YAG: erbium-doped yttrium aluminum garnet; MNRF: microneedling radiofrequency; Nd:YAG: neodymium:yttrium aluminum garnet; PRP: platelet-rich plasma)

regular maintenance. In addition, machine models quickly get outdated, hence one needs to keep investing in latest machines with better technologies.

PLAN OF TREATMENT

Assessment

The plan of treatment should begin with a thorough assessment of the acne, type and severity of acne scars, general health of the patient, and the healing capacity of the patient, hyperpigmented, hypertrophic or delayed. Assessing the mental status of the patient is important as a patient with body dysmorphophobic disorder will always be a dissatisfied patient. The plan of treatment, timeline, cost of therapy and likely complications and how to deal with them are the most important part of management. A well-informed patient is more likely to be compliant with postprocedure instructions and less likely to complain. It is a good idea to grade the scars and document the detailed findings as patients often forget what they looked like before treatment. Serially grading the scars gives an objective assessment (for details see Chapter 3). Photographs are a must and should be taken with standard angles and lighting.

Priming

Priming the patient with topical agents is the next essential step. Active acne should be controlled; topical agents should be chosen according to the skin type and patient preference. There is no single formula which fits all. The basic priming regimen includes a sunscreen, skin lightening agent, topical retinoid and/or alpha hydroxyl acid like glycolic acid. The physician must ensure that the priming agents are being tolerated and regularly used by the patient, especially male patients who are generally not comfortable with using facial products. Patients with sensitive skin and dark skin patients, prone to hyperpigmentation, need special care. (For details in priming see Chapters 4, 6 and 22).

Macular Scars

The erythematous and hyperpigmented scars should be treated first as they are easier to treat and give a quick visible change to the appearance. Persistent erythematous scars can be treated with a combination of sunscreens, topical anti-inflammatory agents like nicotinamide 4%, salicylic acid 2% or adapalene 0.03% and chemical peels containing salicylic and mandelic acid, every 2–4 weeks. If response is inadequate, it can be combined with intense pulsed light (IPL), or pulsed dye laser, if facilities are available. Persistent hyperpigmented scars respond to a combination of chemical peels with Q-switched Nd:YAG (neodymium:yttrium aluminum garnet) laser. The chemical peels have a synergistic effect as they prevent or reduce the risk of postinflammatory hyperpigmentation (PIH). Fractional CO_2 lasers combined with chemical peels also give synergistic results, but the energy settings must not be aggressive and the patient must be adequately primed.

Atrophic Scars

The choice of technique depends on the type of scars, severity, number, size, surface and depth of the scars **(Table 1)**. Subcision is a basic technique useful for all atrophic scars. This can be synergistically combined with other techniques in the same sitting or prior. *Ice pick scars* can be treated with a combination of subcision, CROSS technique and fractional laser or microneedling radiofrequency (MNRF). These can be done at the same session or at different sessions. Subcision is done first. The mild edema makes the scars more prominent. This is followed by CROSS technique. Fractional laser, ablative or nonablative, or MNRF is done next. Kang et al.[2] evaluated a combination treatment of subcision, dot peeling (TCA CROSS) and nonablative fractional resurfacing using a 1,550 nm laser, done at monthly intervals for 4 sessions in 10 patients. They reported that acne severity scores decreased by 55%, and 8 out of 10 patients experienced significant (50–75%) or marked (>75%) improvement in their scars. No significant adverse effects such as PIH were noted. *Rolling scars* can be treated with a combination of subcision followed by microneedling or fractional laser or MNRF, particularly if there is skin laxity, as fractional CO_2 laser or MNRF have a tightening effect. If quick results are required, with no downtime, subcision followed by hyaluronic acid filler is a better technique. In patients with extensive rolling scars, poor skin texture or those that cannot afford fillers, combination with subcision and autologous fat transfer is a better option. Fat transfer improves skin texture as well as gives a filling effect. There are several reports of the combination of platelet-rich plasma (PRP) with other techniques such as microneedling, fractional laser resurfacing and fat transfer with added benefit. Microneedling is often combined with PRP to optimize treatment. In a split-face study in 35 patients with acne scars, Ibrahim et al.[3] reported that addition of PRP to microneedling led to faster recovery, though efficacy was similar. Chawla[4] compared microneedling in combination with PRP versus microneedling and topical vitamin C in 30 patients with acne scars at monthly intervals for 4 sessions. Better results were observed with microneedling combined with PRP. PRP has also been combined with fractional laser therapy, with added advantage.[5-8] Lee et al.[5] treated 14 patients with acne scars with fractional ablative CO_2 laser resurfacing and compared it with combination of intradermal PRP on one side versus saline on the other side, in a split-face study. Erythema and edema was significantly reduced on the PRP treated side versus saline at day 4. Clinical improvement of acne scars was also significantly greater on the PRP treated side versus saline 4 months after the last treatment. Similar results were reported by Faghihi et al.[6] in 16 patients with acne scars (Fitzpatrick skin type II–IV) and Abdel et al.[7] in 30 patients. In another study, Gawdat et al.[8] compared the efficacy of topical versus intradermal PRP in combination with fractional CO_2 laser in 30 patients with facial atrophic acne scars with Fitzpatrick skin types III to V. In group 1, fractional CO_2 laser was followed by intradermal PRP (volume 0.2 mL injected 1.5 cm apart) on one half of the face and intradermal saline on the other half. In group 2, combination of fractional CO_2 laser with intradermal PRP was compared with topical PRP (volume 2 mL) on the other side. Patients were evaluated after three treatment sessions at monthly intervals. Combination of ablative fractional CO_2 laser and PRP showed significantly better results than ablative fractional CO_2 laser alone ($P = 0.03$), 3 months after the last session and no significant difference was observed between topical and intradermal PRP ($P = 0.10$). They concluded that the combination of PRP and ablative fractional CO_2 laser produced a significantly better response, quicker recovery and fewer side effects. Fat grafting has also been combined with PRP to enhance results. Nita et al.[9] reported a synergy using fat grafting, CO_2 laser and PRP in the treatment of scars. The addition of PRP to the fat is reported to give better results as it is said to improve fat survival.[10] Fat grafting can also be combined with laser ablative or nonablative resurfacing to optimize treatment. The lasers should ideally be done prior to fat grafting. Tenna et al.[10] treated 20 patients with acne scars in combination with PRP. Ten patients additionally received fractional CO_2 laser treatment. They reported improvement in both the groups with no significant difference between the two groups. Sezgin and Ozmen[11] combined microneedling with fat grafting in the treatment of scars and reported better results in the combination.

Boxcar scars can be treated with a combination of subcision, punch excision techniques and fractional CO_2 laser to optimize results and reduce downtime. Hwang[12] combined punch excision with fractional laser and long-pulsed Er:YAG resurfacing on the same day in 15 patients and compared this with sequential combination therapy with three sessions of punch excision followed by laser resurfacing at a later date in 5 control patients. Simultaneous combination therapy showed greater improvement in acne scars as compared to sequential combination therapy, with fewer adverse effects and more convenience as there were lesser number of office visits.

Fillers can also be combined with fractional lasers. In an interesting study, Farkas et al.[13] studied filler and laser interactions in live porcine abdominal skin. Following a hyaluronic acid filler, the area was treated 2 weeks later with various lasers. On histopathological examination, microthermal zones of both fractional Er:YAG laser and fractional CO_2 laser column penetrated deeply enough to interact with hyaluronic acid deposits in the skin, though there was no obvious clinical extrusion of filler. Hence, the authors recommend that when superficial filler is planned with aggressive deep laser resurfacing, it is better to treat with the laser before the soft tissue filler and to stagger the procedures in order to maximize the effect.

COMBINATION TRIPLE LASER TECHNIQUE

The author uses the triple laser technique as a combination therapy for boxcar scars with sharp edges and ice pick scars. In this technique, the sharp edges of the scar are first shouldered and minimized with the CO_2 laser in the ultrapulse mode. The pinpoint scars are targeted with the CO_2 laser in the normal pulsed mode. Then the entire scarred area is carpeted with the CO_2 laser in the fractional mode, all in one sitting (results to be published).

COMPLICATIONS

Complications can occur if very aggressive parameters are used in combination treatments. Transient erythema, edema and pain are common and can be managed conservatively. PIH is the most common complication in dark skin patients and can be avoided by proper priming of the skin 2-4 weeks prior. The CROSS technique has the highest potential to cause PIH. Prolonged erythema and potential scarring can be avoided by using lower fluencies, less aggressive therapy especially in prone areas such as the mandibular region.

CONCLUSION

Combination of techniques provides a synergistic effect in the treatment of acne scars. The choice of combination treatment should be individualized to the type of scars, skin texture, skin type and patient preference as regards downtime. CROSS and subcision should be combined on the same day to reduce the downtime period and also as the initial treatment to prime the regenerative capacity of the skin. CO_2 laser sculpting of the atrophic edges will also reduce downtime in deep scars with sharp edges. Addition of PRP to microneedling or resurfacing or fat grafting provides added benefit. An individualized approach tailored to the patient provides optimal results and there is no single therapy that suits all.

REFERENCES

1. Fife D, Zachary B. Combining techniques for treating acne scars. Curr Derm Rep. 2012;1:82-8.
2. Kang WH, Kim YJ, Pyo WS, Park SJ, Kim JH. Atrophic acne scar treatment using triple combination therapy: dot peeling, subcision and fractional laser. J Cosmet Laser Ther. 2009;11(4):212-5.
3. Ibrahim MK, Ibrahim SM, Salem AM. Skin microneedling plus platelet-rich plasma versus skin microneedling alone in the treatment of atrophic post acne scars: a split face comparative study. J Dermatolog Treat. 2018;29:281-6.
4. Chawla S. Split face comparative study of microneedling with PRP versus microneedling with vitamin C in treating atrophic post acne scars. J Cutan Aesthet Surg. 2014;7:209-12.
5. Lee JW, Kim BJ, Kim MN, Mun SK. The efficacy of autologous platelet rich plasma combined with ablative carbon dioxide fractional resurfacing for acne scars: a simultaneous split-face trial. Dermatol Surg. 2011;37:931-8.
6. Faghihi G, Keyvan S, Asilian A, Nouraei S, Behfar S, Nilforoushzadeh MA. Efficacy of autologous platelet-rich plasma combined with fractional ablative carbon dioxide resurfacing laser in treatment of facial atrophic acne scars: a split-face randomized clinical trial. Indian J Dermatol Venereol Leprol. 2016;82(2):162-8.
7. Abdel Aal AM, Ibrahim IM, Sami NA, Abdel Kareem IM. Evaluation of autologous platelet-rich plasma plus ablative carbon dioxide fractional laser in the treatment of acne scars. J Cosmet Laser Ther. 2018;20(2):106-13.
8. Gawdat HI, Hegazy RA, Fawzy MM, Fathy M. Autologous platelet rich plasma: topical versus intradermal after fractional ablative carbon dioxide laser treatment of atrophic acne scars. Dermatol Surg. 2014;40(2):152-61.

9. Nita AC, Orzan OA, Filipescu M, Jianu D. Fat graft, laser CO_2 and platelet-rich-plasma synergy in scars treatment. J Med Life. 2013;6(4):430-3.
10. Tenna S, Cogliandro A, Barone M, Panasiti V, Tirindelli M, Nobile C, et al. Comparative Study Using Autologous Fat Grafts Plus Platelet-Rich Plasma With or Without Fractional CO_2 Laser Resurfacing in Treatment of Acne Scars: Analysis of Outcomes and Satisfaction With FACE-Q. Aesth Plast Surg. 2017;4:661-6.
11. Sezgin B, Ozmen S. Fat grafting to the face with adjunctive microneedling: a simple technique with high patient satisfaction. Turk J Med Sci. 2018;48:592-601.
12. Hwang EJ. The efficacy and safety of new total combination techniques compared with classic sequential combination therapy with punch, fractional and long-pulsed Er-YAG laser for the treatment of acne scars. J Am Acad Dermatol. 2011;64(2) AB168: P3506.
13. Farkas JP, Richardson JA, Brown S, Hoopman JE, Kenkel JM. Effects of common laser treatments on hyaluronic acid fillers in a porcine model. Aesthet Surg J. 2008;28:503-11.

CHAPTER 27

Interesting Case Discussions

*Anil Ganjoo, Shehnaz Arsiwala,
Koushik Lahiri, Imran Majid, Niteen Dhepe*

CASE 1

Anil Ganjoo

A 25-year-old male due to get married shortly was psychologically disturbed due to his postacne scars. He also had hyperpigmentation following the resolution of his acne. The scars were grade 4 with boxcar, ice pick, and rolling scars **(Figs. 1A to D)**. The skin was type IV and was thus a challenge.

Solution

He was subjected to multiple procedural modalities including scar excision, subcision, and fractional CO_2 laser treatment followed by chemical peels. Initially deep scars were excised with a punch and closed using 5-0 Prolene® sutures. Once healing occurred, subcision was performed for the remaining depressed scars under local anesthesia. The patient was then treated with fractional CO_2 laser treatments at monthly intervals using energies ranging from 75 to 100 mJ with a distance of 1.5 mm between the spots. After three such treatments the scars improved considerably, but patient had a lot of postinflammatory hyperpigmentation (PIH). The patient was then treated with chemical peels using 50% glycolic acid every 2 weeks for three peels.

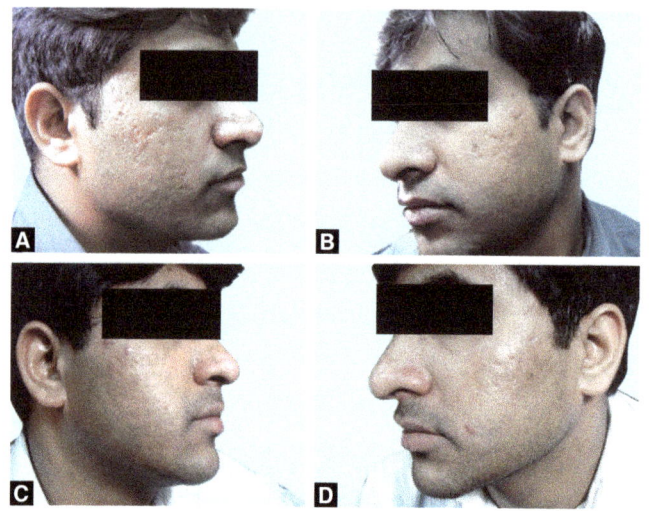

Figs. 1A to D: (A and B) Before treatment; (C and D) After treatment.

Results

The results were quite gratifying although the patient had to go through a number of procedures before the final outcome.

Comments

Most of the patients of acne scars need multiple procedures for significant improvement. We have to be particularly careful with darker skin types as they are prone to PIH. Each patient's scars need to be assessed properly before starting the treatment and a plan according to each scar needs to be put in place. One should start with surgical excision of very deep boxcar scars, chemical reconstruction of skin scars (CROSS) of ice pick scars and elliptical excision of deep linear scars. This should be followed by subcision for the rolling scars and the fractional laser sessions (I give four treatments at monthly intervals).

Finally the pigmentary and textural aberrations can be dealt with by appropriate peels.

CASE 2

Anil Ganjoo

A 50-year-old female with long-standing acne scars for three decades requested treatment. The scars were localized to the nose and were mostly rolling and boxcar type of scars, grade 3 **(Figs. 2A to D)**. The skin color was type III and therefore we could be a little more aggressive. The patient was taken up for spot CO_2 laser abrasion of the nose after proper counseling.

Solution

After infiltration of local anesthesia with 1% lignocaine, spot laser abrasion with a continuous wave CO_2 laser at a power of 7 watts was done over the nose.

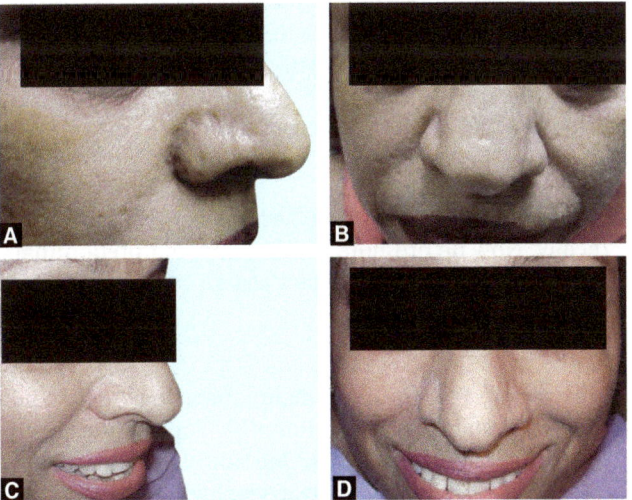

Figs. 2A to D: (A and B) Before treatment; (C and D) After treatment.

The area was dressed and dressings were repeated every day for the next 10 days. Once the dressing was off the patient was advised to stay indoors during the day and to avoid sun exposure for about 3 months until complete re-epithelialization occurred and the skin regained its original color.

Results

The outcome was very rewarding with most of the scars showing considerable improvement after this single sitting. The patient was very compliant and followed the postoperative instructions very religiously which went a long way in the satisfactory outcome.

Comments

Laser abrasion still holds good in postacne scars provided a proper selection of the patient is done and a strict postoperative care is taken both by the doctor and the patient. A single session can give significant results. The only problem is the long downtime associated with the continuous wave CO_2 laser.

CASE 3

Niteen Dhepe

A 26-year-old male with grade 3 acne for 8 years was treated medically. Now he presented with mixed but predominantly rolling acne scars and few ice pick scars.

Solution

We treated him with the 5-tier technique using the Ultrapulse Encore fractional CO_2 laser (Lumenis). Topical anesthesia is usually sufficient in most cases. One rule of thumb for the CO_2 laser is that the tissue should always be hydrated. Dry skin will lead to less penetration of the laser as water is the chromophore and more PIH. The elements of the 5-tier technique include the following:

Tier 1: Superficial fractional CO_2 laser for color match, Active FX 60 mJ, density 4, 60 W, two passes.

Tier 2: Scar shouldering around the edges of the scar to flatten the raised edges. The ablative mode of CO_2, most preferably high density (7 or 9 density) Active FX with spot size 1 or 2, 2 Hz is used on the edges of scars. Two rounds are given. The ablated tissue is wiped with wet gauze.

Tier 3: Deep fractional CO_2 laser (Deep FX 15-35 mJ and density 5%) is done for mid to deep dermal collagen induction. The entire face is treated that gives a global skin tightening effect and improves stretchability.

Tier 4: Very deep fractional CO_2 laser is done at the base of the scar. Typical parameters are SCAAR FX 60-80 mJ, 60 W, density 5%, and size 2-3 to match scar width. This acts as a form of vertical subcision and breaks the fibrous band that holds the scar base to the deep dermis or subcutis.

Tier 5: Subcision with the needle using the traditional technique.

The patient was treated three times that included subcision twice and shouldering once. Ultrapulse laser was used with typical parameters. The follow-up photo is after 2 weeks of shouldering **(Figs. 3A and B)**.

Results

The treatment is usually uneventful. A slight postinflammatory hypopigmentation is common on the shouldered area that fades in a couple of weeks. Moisturization, bleaching regimes, and sunscreen is the key to prevent hyperpigmentation, which can occur in darker skin types. The interval between sessions should be at least 6 weeks.

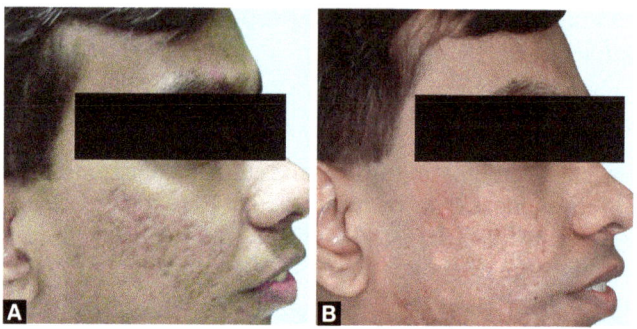

Figs. 3A and B: Scar shouldering done with Active FX 200 mJ 2 mm spot density 8 and 3 passes on edge of scar.

Comments

The 5-tier technique aims at collagen remodeling and textural modification at multiple levels in the skin. Stretchability of the scar along with depth is important parameter in selection of treatment parameters. Depth can be corrected by either stimulating collagen deposition in the dermis or resurfacing the epidermis or shouldering the edges of the scars or all of the three. Collagen remodeling in mid and deeper dermis beyond the scar margin results in skin tightening and hence improves stretchability of the scar. The 5-tier technique addresses these multiple mechanisms of scar improvement comprehensively.

CASE 4

Niteen Dhepe

A 19-year-old female presented with predominantly rolling scars on the cheeks. She was treated with the same technique for two sessions at 6-week intervals **(Figs. 4A and B)**.

Results

There was significant improvement with skin tightening.

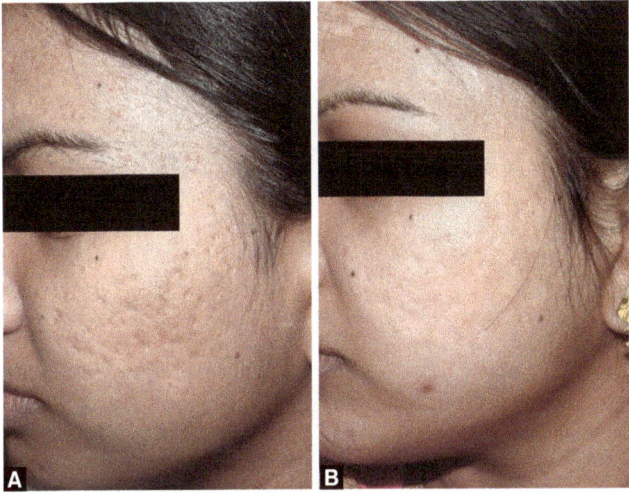

Figs. 4A and B: The 5-tier technique was used for rolling scars in a 19-year-old female. Note the skin tightening effect. The post photo is after 2 months after two sessions of this technique.

Comments

Rolling scars of treated adequately require fewer sessions to show significant results.

CASE 5

Niteen Dhepe

This 24-year-old patient had severe acne scarring and melasma.

Results

The post photo is 1 month after five sessions of the 5-tier technique **(Figs. 5A and B)**. The patient was on bleaching regime throughout. Subcision was done twice. Parameters were typical.

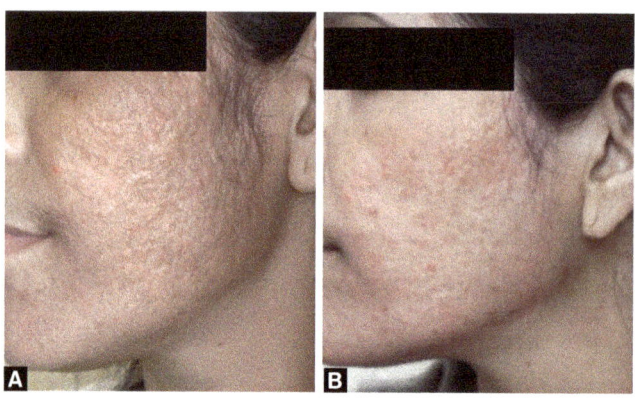

Figs. 5A and B: The 5-tier technique used for rolling scars. Note the skin tightening effect.
(*Source*: Lahiri K. Scar reduction: principles and approach. Textbook of Laser Dermatology. New Delhi: Jaypee Brothers Medical Publishers; 2016.)

CASE 6

Imran Majid

This case is being presented to highlight the importance of treating cases of postacne scars as early as possible. If the scars are treated in the early stages the results are definitely better. A 26-year-old female presented with grade 3 postacne scars on her face. She had few lesions of active acne as well as prominent scarring **(Figs. 6A to D)**.

Solution

The patient was put on oral isotretinoin 20 mg daily for control of active acne, with significant improvement after 1 month. A session of fractional CO_2 laser resurfacing was done. Low-dose isotretinoin 10 mg was continued in between the laser sessions. Laser treatment was repeated at 6-week intervals and a total of three sessions were performed.

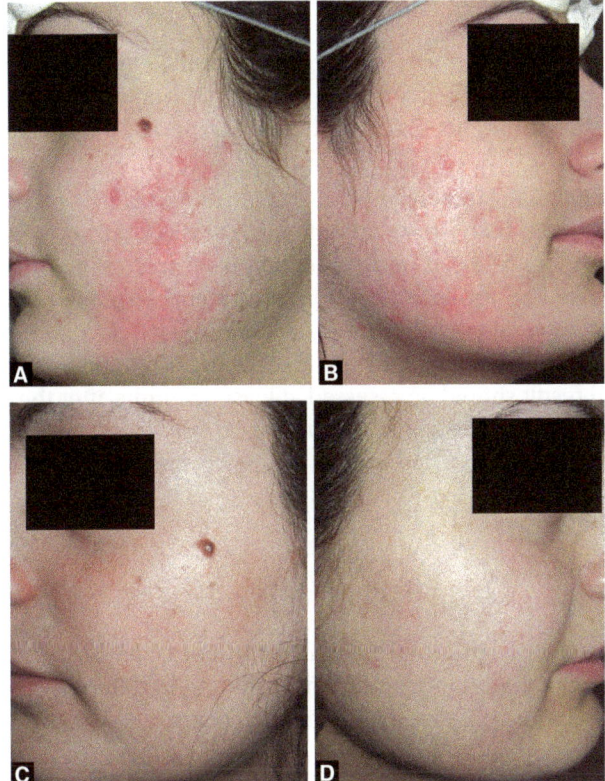

Figs. 6A to D: (A and B) Before treatment; (C and D) After treatment.

Results

The patient achieved a very good improvement in her scars and was happy with the results. The improvement in scars continued even after the active laser treatment was stopped and at 1 year of follow-up the scars were hardly visible at all. The patient did not receive any supplementary treatment with peels or topical treatment and whatever improvement was achieved was with fractional CO_2 laser resurfacing alone.

Comments

Treatment with fractional CO_2 laser should be started as early as possible after active acne is properly controlled with oral or topical treatments. Early treatment is expected to give better results.

Fractional laser resurfacing can be undertaken even while the patient is on isotretinoin therapy. This is contrary to what was being believed in the past that laser treatments should be avoided during isotretinoin treatment. Improvement in the scars and overall skin texture continue to take place over months after fractional laser resurfacing is stopped and the final result should be assessed at least 6 months after the last laser session. The take home message is that treatment of acne scars should be started as early as possible once the active acne has healed.

CASE 7

Imran Majid

This case highlights the importance of combining two procedures working at different levels and by different modes of action to synergize the therapeutic effect.

A 29-year-old male, working as an executive in a pharmaceutical company presented to us with grade 3 to 4 postacne scars on the forehead **(Figs. 7A and B)**.

The scars were mostly rolling and boxcar type and were involving the temples predominantly. Going by the depth of the scars, a single modality of treatment was unlikely to cause a good therapeutic effect in the patient. The patient was also reluctant to tolerate any downtime with any procedures on his face. We thus decided to combine subcision with microneedling in the patient as both the procedures are office-time procedures with little downtime.

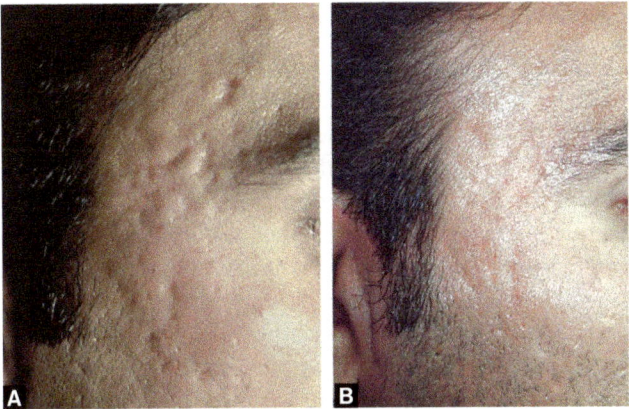

Figs. 7A and B: (A) Before treatment; (B) After treatment.

Solution

In the initial stage the scars were treated with subcision with a 16-gauge subcision needle. About 1 week after the subcision procedure, microneedling was performed with a dermaroller having 1.5 mm long needles. For most of the scars only one session of subcision was performed while it was repeated on some deeper scars just before the second microneedling session. In total, four sessions of microneedling were performed at 6-week intervals and the final assessment was performed 3 months after the last session.

Results

After just one session of subcision the patient could notice a significant reduction in scar depth and after combining it with four sessions of microneedling, a very satisfactory therapeutic effect was achieved. The overall cosmetic effect obtained was excellent and the patient was also quite satisfied with the results obtained. Moreover, no adverse effects were seen and there was no downtime associated with any of the procedures performed.

Comments

This particular case thus teaches us that subcision is a very simple surgical procedure that is easy to perform and needs no special or costly instruments. The procedure leads to a rapid reduction in scar depth and the base of the scar can then be treated with some other treatment modality like lasers or microneedling. Microneedling, which is also known as collagen induction therapy, is a safe office-time procedure with no downtime and no significant post-treatment sequelae. The procedure is popularly known as "poor man's laser". It is claimed to achieve almost similar therapeutic results as fractional laser resurfacing without the need for costly instruments. Combining two treatment options like subcision and microneedling, which act by two different mechanisms on the scar tissue, can lead to a synergistic effect as far as scar amelioration is concerned.

CASE 8

Koushik Lahiri

A 28-year-old male reported to us with acne scars on his face. The scars were mainly boxcar and rolling scars with a few ice pick scars and craters **(Figs. 8A and B)**.

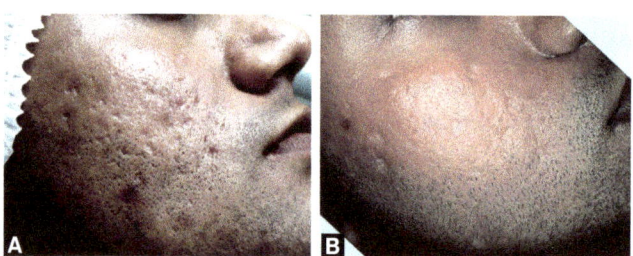

Figs. 8A and B: (A) Before treatment; (B) After treatment.

Solution

He was treated with the fractional Ultrapulse CO_2 laser (Lumenis). The setting of the machine was as follows: Deep FX: energy 5–20 mJ, density 5–10 mJ, pattern repetition rate 0.50 second, single pass, and full face coverage. The sessions were always preceded with subcision. Priming and maintenance treatment was with sunscreen and tretinoin (0.025%) at night. The interval between two sessions was 6 weeks.

Results

After four sessions the result was very encouraging. The patient took a total of six sessions.

Comments

Severe scarring requires multiple sittings to be effective. It is better to undertreat to avoid complications in darker skin types.

CASE 9

Koushık Lahırl

A 28-year-old sales person had grade 3–4 acne, with recurrent nodular lesions since his teen age. The scars were mainly deep boxcars and some ice pick scars (**Figs. 9A and B**).

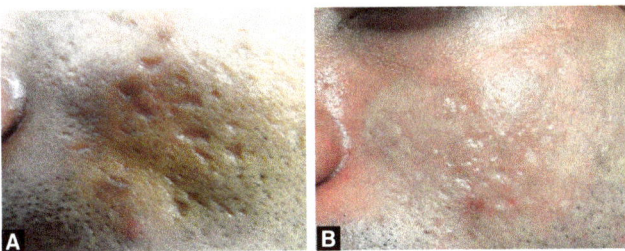

Figs. 9A and B: (A) Before treatment; (B) After treatment.

Solution

He was treated with five sessions of CO_2 fractional laser (Ultrapulse, Lumenis). All the sessions were preceded by subcision. The interval between two sessions was 6–8 weeks. The settings were as below:

Deep FX: Energy 10 mJ, density 10 mJ, pattern repetition rate 0.50 second, single pass, and full face coverage.

Active FX: Energy 100 mJ, Hertz rate 100 Hz, density 3, single pass, and full face coverage.

Results

The result after five sessions showed significant 80–90% improvement.

Comment

Combining subcision with fractional CO_2 laser gives excellent results, even with deep scars.

CASE 10

Koushik Lahiri

A 43-year-old lady presented with varioliform scars on the face following smallpox in childhood. The scars were mainly pigmented boxcar scars, similar to acne scars **(Figs. 10A and B)**.

Solution

She was treated with five sessions of fractional Ultrapulse CO_2 lasers. The settings were as follows: Deep FX: energy 10 mJ, density 5 mJ, pattern repetition rate 0.50 second, single pass, and full face coverage. In addition two sessions of Q-Switched neodymium-doped yttrium aluminum garnet (Nd:YAD) laser 1,064 nm was done to improve the pigmentation. Four sessions of easy phytic peels between the sessions were done. The sessions were not preceded by subcision.

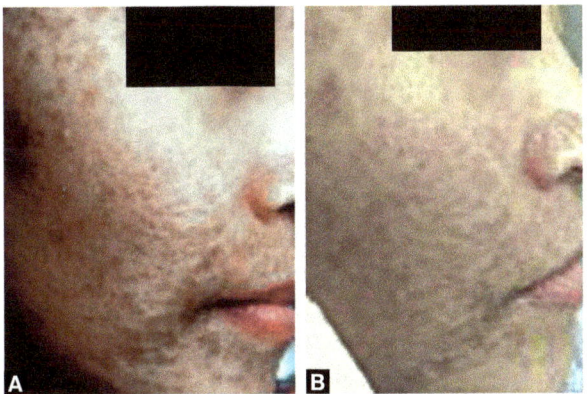

Figs. 10A and B: (A) Before treatment; (B) After treatment.

Results

After all the sessions the change was remarkable and her quality of life improved vastly.

Comments

Each modality of treatment has its advantages. Fractional CO_2 laser improves the atrophic scars, Q-switched Nd:YAG laser improves hyperpigmentation and chemical peels improve the surface texture and pigmentary abnormalities. Hence combination of treatment gives optimal results.

CASE 11

Shehnaz Arsiwala

A 24-year-old female, with skin type V, with grade 1 hyperpigmented scars wanted a quick resolution of her pigmentation as she was to get married shortly (**Figs. 11A and B**). The response to topical agents was slow.

Solution

Chemical peels were offered to hasten resolution after priming with sunscreens and topical adapalene at night.

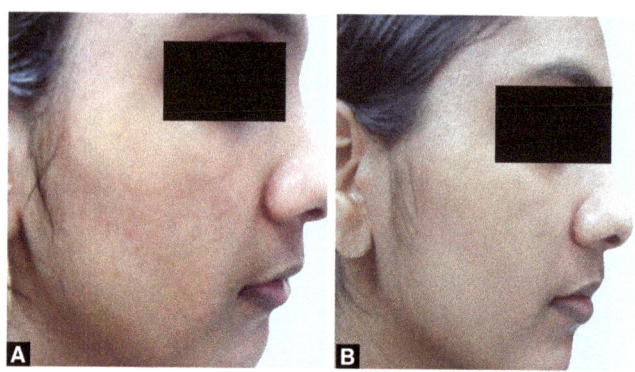

Figs. 11A to B: (A) Before treatment; (B) After treatment.

Results

Excellent response after three sessions of slow release easy phytic combination peels at 2 weekly intervals. Easy phytic peel contains a combination of glycolic acid, lactic acid, mandelic acid, and phytic acid.

Comments

In type V skin, aggressive peels can cause PIH. Hence initial peeling should be with gentle gel based peels. Salicylic-mandelic acid combination peel is another option.

CASE 12

Shehnaz Arsiwala

A 25-year-old female presented with mild to moderate acne scars grade 3 with type V skin **(Figs. 12A and B)**. She did not want any procedure with a prolonged downtime.

Solution

A combination of skin tightening with near-infrared laser at 3 J/cm^2 total 8 kJ followed by 7 × 7 mm long pulse erbium-doped yttrium aluminum garnet (Er:YAG) resurfacing at 1,000 mJ/p for three passes was carried out.

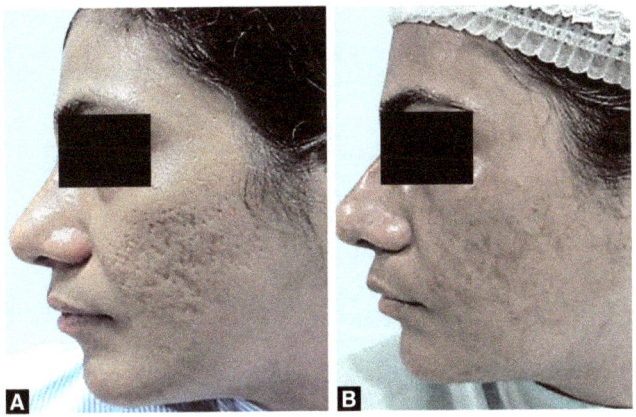

Figs. 12A and B: (A) Before treatment; (B) After treatment.

Results

Good improvement was observed after four sessions.

Comments

Patients with rolling scars and skin laxity show a significant response with skin tightening combined with a fractional resurfacing laser.

CASE 13

Shehnaz Arsiwala

A 23-year-old female with grade 2 scars with type IV skin presented for treatment of postacne scars **(Figs. 13A to C)**.

Solution

Treatment with a combination technique of one session of fractional CO_2 laser followed by four sessions of rotational Erbium Pixel laser.

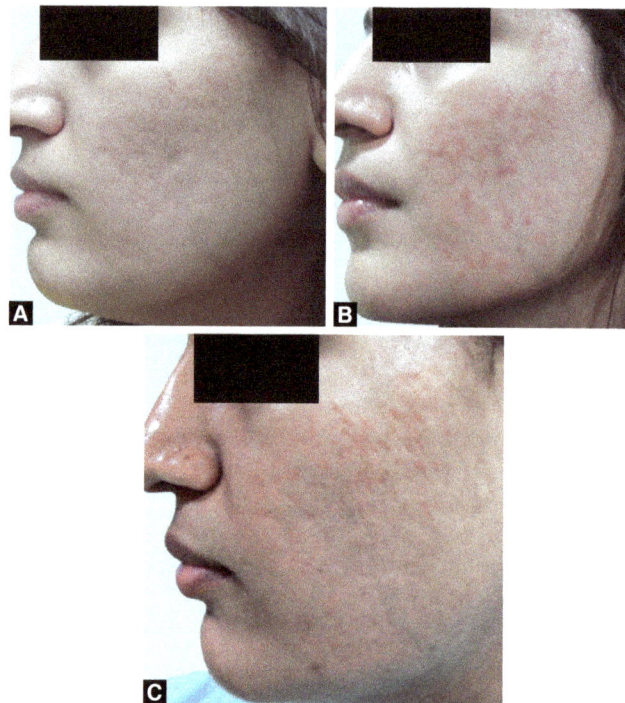

Figs. 13A and C: (A) Before treatment; (B) After one session; (C) Spontaneous reduction of erythema.

Results

Good improvement was observed after the treatment, but patient developed postlaser erythema.

Comments

Fractional CO_2 laser can cause temporary erythema, which eventually subsides.

CHAPTER 28

Algorithmic Approach to Acne Scars

Niti Khunger

PATIENT ASSESSMENT

History

- What is the duration of acne and appearance of acne scars?
- Is acne still active? Are breakouts occasional or regular?
- What treatment is being taken: topical and systemic?
- Have you taken isotretinoin? If yes when and for how long? Are you still on isotretinoin?
- Have any procedures being performed for acne scars previously? If yes which ones and what was the response?
- Do you have any irritation from any products applied on the skin?
- Are you using any products, scrubs, moisturizers, sunscreens or steroids on the skin?
- How does acne or any injury heal? Is there persistent redness or pigmentation?
- Is there history of excessive scarring or keloid formation?
- Give the patient a mirror and tell the patient to point out which scars are most bothersome.
- How distressed are you about the scars?
- What are the social and psychological problems you are facing with relationships, workplace, school, college, etc.?
- Is there any impending social function, job interview, marriage, etc.
- What is the improvement you expect?

Examination

- Examine the patient in direct and indirect light. Take photographs in three views, fontal right and left oblique and close-ups.
- See for the presence of active acne, type, and grade of acne.
- See for presence of hirsutism, hypertrichosis, telangiectasia, and signs of steroid abuse.
- Evaluate skin type of the patient. See degree of redness and pigmentation.
- Check for hypertrophic or keloid scars on the mandibular area, chest, back, shoulders, and upper arms.
- Evaluate the type of scars present and those which are predominantly seen—macular, atrophic, and hypertrophic.
- Grade the severity of scars.
- Assess the color. Stretch the scars to see if they disappear.
- Palpate the scars to see for thickness, fibrosis, atrophy or loss of underlying fat.
- Evaluate the psychological makeup of the patient. Is the distress proportional to the severity of the scars or is there excessive distress with minor scars.

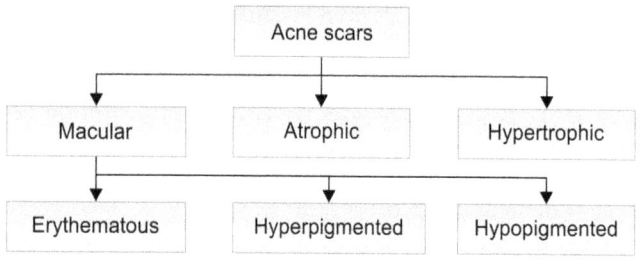

Flowchart 1: Broad classification of acne scars.

Flowchart 2: Management of erythematous scars.

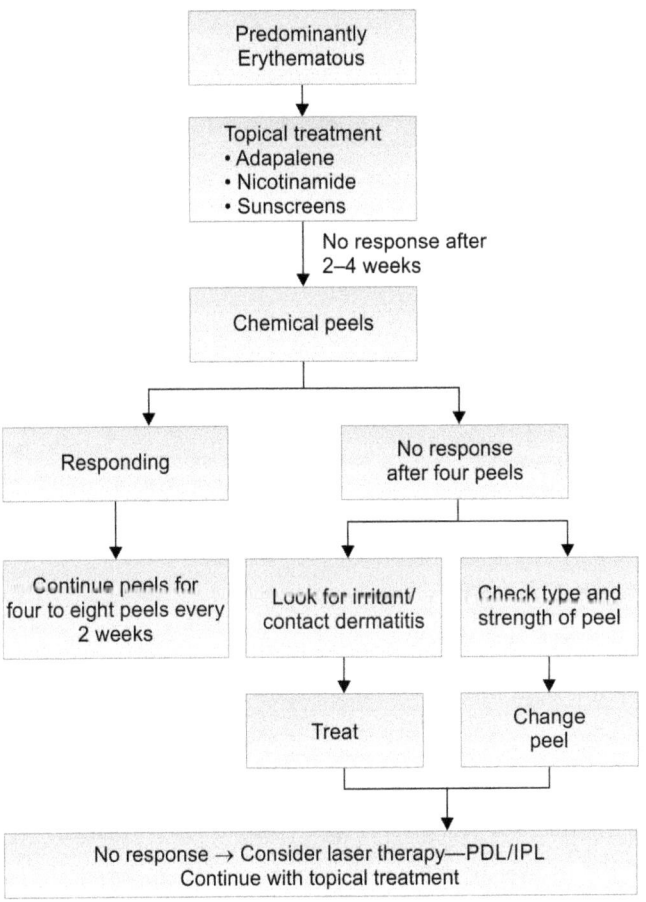

(IPL: intense pulsed light; PDL: pulsed dye laser)

Flowchart 3: Management of hyperpigmented scars.

```
                    Predominantly hyperpigmented
                                │
                         Topical treatment
                   Sunscreens topical hydroquinone,
                   kojic acid, azelaic acid, tretinoin,
                   adapalene and glycolic acid
              ┌─────────────┴─────────────┐
          Response                  No response in
              │                        2–4 weeks
              ▼                           ▼
      Continue treatment            Chemical peels
              ┌─────────────┬─────────────┐
          Response                  No response
              │                     in two peels
              ▼                           ▼
        Continue for             • Strict sunprotection
      six to eight peels         • Change topical treatment
              │                  • Look for irritant contact
              ▼                    dermatitis-treat
        Switch to topical        • Change peel
        treatment for
        maintenance                       │
                                          ▼
                                    No response
                                          │
                                          ▼
                              • Microdermabrasion/
                                dermabrasion/low fluence
                              • Q-switched Nd:YAG
                              • Continue with topical treatment
```

(Nd:YAG: neodymium-doped yttrium aluminum garnet)

Flowchart 4: Broad classification of atrophic scars.

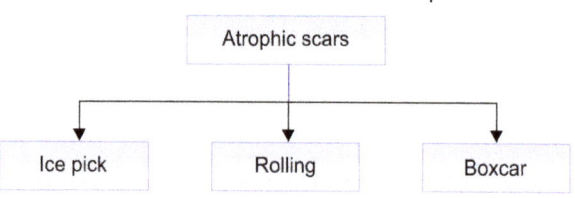

Algorithmic Approach to Acne Scars

Flowchart 5: Management of ice pick scars.

```
┌─────────────────────────────────┐
│         Ice pick scars          │
└─────────────────────────────────┘
                 ↓
┌─────────────────────────────────┐
│ • Priming agents for 2–4 weeks  │
│   – Sunscreens, topical hydroquinone, kojic acid, │
│     azelaic acid, tretinoin adapalene, glycolic acid │
└─────────────────────────────────┘
                 ↓
┌─────────────────────────────────┐
│ • CROSS technique combined with subcision │
│   – Three to four sessions at 2–4 weeks interval │
│   – Pinpoint $CO_2$ laser irradiation │
└─────────────────────────────────┘
                 ↓
┌─────────────────────────────────┐
│ • Follow-up with fractional ablative or │
│   nonablative laser             │
│   – Microneedling for further improvement │
│   – Chemical peels for texture improvement │
└─────────────────────────────────┘
```

(CROSS: chemical reconstruction of skin scars)

Flowchart 6: Management of rolling scars.

```
┌─────────────────────────────────┐
│        Rolling scars            │
│  (Disappear to a great extent   │
│    when skin is stretched)      │
└─────────────────────────────────┘
                 ↓
┌─────────────────────────────────┐
│  Subcision with microneedling   │
│  four sessions at monthly intervals │
└─────────────────────────────────┘
                 ↓
┌─────────────────────────────────┐
│          No response            │
└─────────────────────────────────┘
                 ↓
┌─────────────────────────────────┐
│ • Fractional ablative/nonablative laser │
│ • Fillers/fat transfer for quick response │
│ • Chemical peels for texture improvement │
└─────────────────────────────────┘
```

Flowchart 7: Management of boxcar scars.

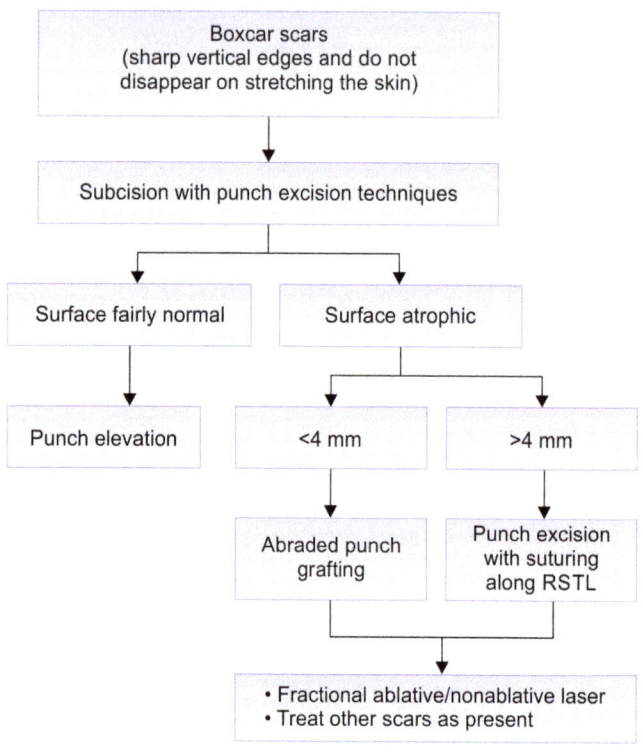

(RSTL: relaxed skin tension line)

Algorithmic Approach to Acne Scars

Flowchart 8: Management of linear scars.

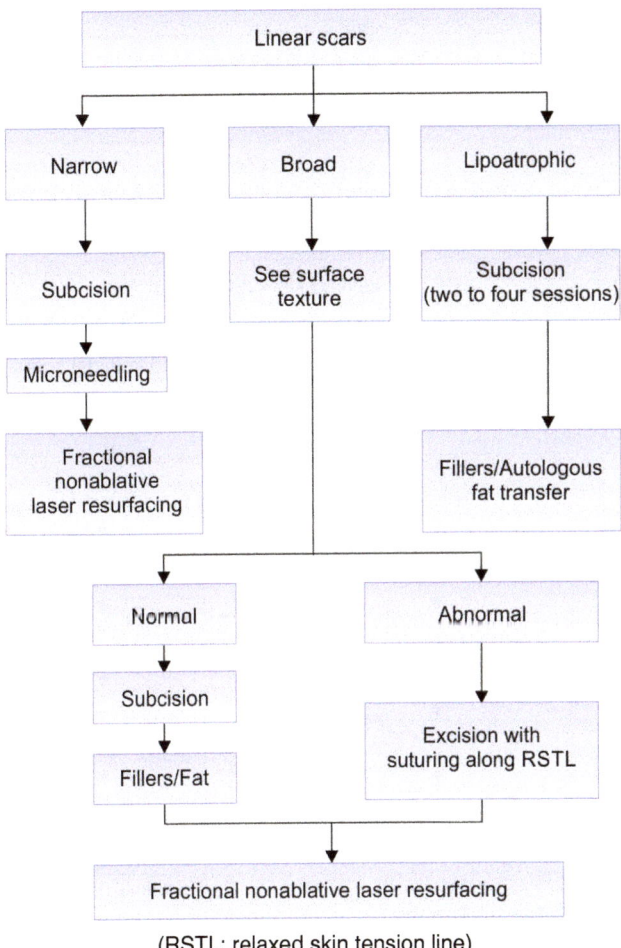

(RSTL: relaxed skin tension line)

Flowchart 9: Management of bridging scars.

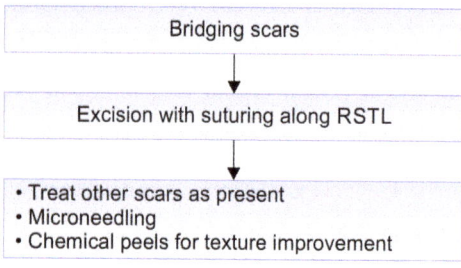

(RSTL: relaxed skin tension line)

Flowchart 10: Management of hypertrophic and keloidal scars.

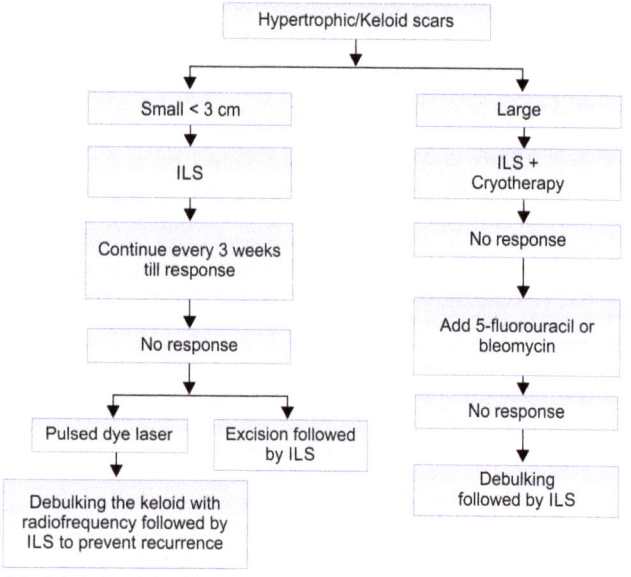

ILS—Intralesional steroids

Index

Page numbers followed by *b* refer to box, *f* refer to figure, *fc* refer to flowchart, and *t* refer to table.

A

Ablative fractional laser resurfacing 149
Ablative lasers 280
Acetic acid 67*f*
Acetone 85
Acne 11, 16, 17, 19, 28, 31, 49, 49*b*, 68*f*, 178, 238, 246
   active 67*f*, 138
      severe 269
   aggravation of 76
   comedonal 56
   control 270
      of active 241
   evaluation of 2
   excoriée 33, 52*f*, 65, 66
   flare 275, 289, 294
   fulminans 9
   hormonal 55
   hypermelanotic macules 160
   improvement of 75*f*
      active 68*f*
   lesions, inflamed 49
   moderate 52
   nodulocystic 53
   pathogenesis of 18, 18*f*, 19
   premenstrual flares of 8
   role of diet in 11
   severe 51, 251
   steroid-induced 49, 50*f*
   treatment of 1, 52, 249
   with isotretinoin, flare of 54
Acne scar 17, 18, 23, 31, 46, 57, 59, 62, 79, 144, 153*f*, 169-171, 182, 193*f*, 196, 253, 259, 263, 299, 304, 307, 308, 311, 319, 334, 350, 357
   appearance of 305*f*
   atrophic 33, 233*f*
   camouflage techniques for 311
   classification of 33, 358*fc*
   combination treatments for 329
   complications of 263, 281*t*
   deep 271
   distensible 226
   excision techniques for 105*t*
   fillers, newer 171
   grading of 42
   hyperpigmented 66
   hypertrophic 157
   imaging techniques for 304
   laser devices to treat 145*t*
   light devices to treat 145*t*
   makeup products for 314
   management of 263, 330
   minimally invasive techniques for 331*t*
   moderate 156*f*
   morphological types of 32*t*, 33
   newer laser technologies for 165
   pathophysiology of 16, 23
   peculiar features of 264*b*
   prevention of 48, 49, 49*b*

procedure for 271
severe 151*f*
stages of 268*b*
superficial 138
system 42
technique for 304
treatment of 45, 146, 263, 321
    mild-to-moderate 150
    types of 160*t*
types of 23*f*, 31, 32*f*, 91, 221, 324, 331

Acne vulgaris 1
  management of 3*t*
  pathogenesis of 19
Acneiform eruption 161, 288, 289, 294
  folliculitis 164*f*
Adapalene 4, 53, 272
  cream 203
Adipocyte 190, 197
Adrenaline 184
Allergic reactions 179, 288, 290
Allium cepa 248
Alpha hydroxy acid 59, 60, 142, 276, 332
Alpha-keto acid 60
Aluminum oxide 133
  crystals 134*f*
    microdermabrasion 133
Amoxicillin 6
Analgesics 283
Androgens, circulating 19
Anesthesia 94, 161, 188
  infiltration 242
  topical 234
  tumescent 190
Anetodermas 238
Angiogenesis 21
Anti-acne
  regimen 269
  therapy 4

Antibacterial agents 4
Antibiotics
  post-treatment 280
  topical 2, 4, 286
Anticoagulant therapy 175
Antifungal agents, topical 294
Anti-inflammatory agents 4, 286
  topical 332
Apoptosis, inhibitor of 22
Arbutin 295
Aseptic precautions 188
Aspiration, functional 324
Aspirin 93
Atrophic acne scars, mild-to-moderate 155
Atrophic scars
  classification of 360*fc*
  depressed 35
  M-shaped 45
  U-shaped 44
Atrophic shiny skin 298
Atrophy 75
Auricular nerve paresthesia 327
Autoimmune diseases 171
Autologous fat
  grafting 193*f*, 197
  one session of 225*f*
  transfer 182, 232*f*
    lumpy appearance after 225*f*
Autologous fibroblast 225, 226
Automated rollers 118
Azelaic acid 2, 5, 53, 295
Azithromycin 5, 6, 7

B

Bacterial colonization 18, 18*f*
Bacterial infection 161, 269, 292
  secondary 159, 275
Bacteriostatic agent 188

Bent insulin syringe 82*f*
Benzoyl peroxide 2-4, 52, 53
Beta-hydroxy acids 276
Biopsy punches, disposable 103
Bipolar microneedling
        radiofrequency 226
Bipolar radiofrequency 323
Bleaching
    agents, postprocedure 274
    regime 343, 345
Bleeding diathesis 175
Blindness, higher risk of 234
Blood
    cells 190
    dyscrasias 6
    oozing 286
    vessels 21
Body dismorphophobic disorder
        159, 331
Bovine collagen 169
Boxcar scars 25, 26*f*, 32*f*, 36, 37*f*,
        148, 158*f*, 212-214, 220,
        236, 331, 335, 341, 352
    atrophic 81
    complications of 218
    contraindications of 214
    deep 214*f*
    indications of 214
    limitations of 215
    management of 362*fc*
    multiple 219*f*
        punched-out 213*f*
    postprocedure care of 218
    precautions of 215
    preprocedure preparation of
        215
    superficial 148
    technique of 215
    therapy for 336
    treatment of 213
Boxcar with sharp vertical contours
        213*f*
Bradycardia 299
Breast
    cancer 8
    enlargement 8
Bridging scars, management of
        364*fc*
Brimonidine gel 318
Bruising 178, 288

C

Calcium hydroxylapatite 177, 236
Camouflage makeup 313
Candida 294
    infection 283
Carbon dioxide 145, 222, 231, 236
    laser
        fractional 149
        principle of fractional 147*f*
        resurfacing, fractional 296*f*
Carboxymethylcellulose 172
Cell
    death, programmed 195
    lysis 191
Cervical cancer 8
Chemical peels 3, 10, 65, 260, 276,
        280*b*, 281, 339, 353
    gel-based 323
    medium-depth 66, 236
    superficial 66, 71, 77, 295
Chest 29*f*
Chickenpox scars 93
Chronic disorder 1
Citric acid 67*f*
Clindamycin 4, 5, 53
Clostridium difficile infection 6
Cobblestone appearance 210
Collagen 21, 170, 171
    gene expression 60
    injections 171
    regeneration of 183

Combination techniques, advantages of 330
Comedogenesis 19
Comedonal acne, mild 52
Comedone 138
    extraction 3
Correct technique pinpoint frosting 84*f*
Cosmetic
    camouflage 312
    procedures 138
Cross-hatching technique 176*f*
Cryosurgery 276
Cryotherapy 57, 59, 62, 248, 249, 252
Crystal microdermabrasion machine 133, 134*f*
    principle of 134*f*
Cutaneous infestations 308
Cutibacterium acnes 1, 16, 17
Cyst 1
    drain eye of 57*f*
Cystic acne 26, 38, 287*f*
    treatment of 57*f*
Cystic lesions 27

D

Dapsone 2, 5, 53
Darker skin 219, 236
    complications in 257*t*
    problems in 264
    types 253, 299
        treatment for 257
Deafness 298
Dehydroepiandrosterone sulfate 2
Demarcation lines 297
Depigmented macules 34*f*
Dermabrasion 260, 276
Dermal chromophores 285
Dermal hyaluronic acid 60
Dermal injury 261
Dermal tissue, loss of 237
Dermapen 119
Dermaroller 119
    therapy 286
Dermastamp 118
Dermatitis 52
    contact 60
    irritant 312
Dermatoses, evolving 139
Dermatosurgical procedures 286
Dermoscopy 308
Diabetes 186
    mellitus, uncontrolled 139
Diamond microdermabrasion 136
    machines 137
    tips 136
Diamond peel 137*f*
Diarrhea 299
Digital photography 304
Diode laser 157
Distensible scars, moderate-to-severe 225
Diuresis 8
Dizziness 6, 8, 298, 299
Donor site selection 188
Dot peels 150
Doxycycline 5, 6
Drospirenone 7
Drowsiness 299
Drug reaction 7
Drugs, photosensitizing 271
Ductal corneocytes, inadequate separation of 19
Ductal hyperkeratosis 18, 18*f*
Ductal keratinocytes, hyperproliferation of 19
Dyschromias 254
Dyspnea 299

E

Echelle d'evaluation clinique des cicatrices d'acne scale 44
Ectropion
   development of 285
   formation 161
Eczema 139
Edema 124, 161, 162, 178, 288, 289, 336
Elastolysis, superficial 45
Electro-optical synergy 324
Elliptical excision 105
Emphasis 295
Energy based devices 258
Eosinophilia 7
Epidermal growth factor 20, 21f
Epidermal heating, uncontrolled 285
Epidermal keratinocytes 255
Epidermal melanin
   elimination of 295
   increased 255
Epidermal necrotic debris, microscopic 147
Epidermis, dermabrasion of 110f
Epithelial tracts 251
Erbium glass laser, fractional 243
Erbium pixel laser 355
Erbium:yttrium-aluminum-garnet 145, 265
   laser 145, 162f, 163f, 164f
      resurfacing 148
      sessions 153f, 158f
Erbium-doped yttrium aluminum garnet 331
   laser 222
      fractional 150
Erosions 138
   superficial 161
Erythema 49, 74f, 84f, 161, 162, 178, 276, 279f, 288, 289
   postlaser 356
   postmicroneedling 124f
   postprocedure 207, 290
   prolonged 237, 261, 283, 336
   reduction of 356f
   temporary 356
   transient 325, 336
Erythematous macular scars 158f, 160
Erythematous scars 331, 332
   management of 359fc
Erythromycin 5-7
Estrogen 7
Ethinylestradiol 7

F

Facial acne scar 46
Facial herpes simplex, history of 203
Facial makeup, color of 316
Facial modeling device 307
Fan technique 176f
Fat
   aspiration of 190f, 191f
   efficacy of 195
   future of 197
   grafting 197f
      donor sites for 189f
      instruments for 185f
      technique 188
      types of 183f
   harvesting 184, 188, 189
   injection 192
   placement 188, 192
   preparation 191
   processing 186, 188, 190
   reinjection 186
   survival of 195
   transfer 186, 237
      disadvantage of 187

Ferrous fumarate 7
Fibroblast 21
    growth factor, basic 20, 21*f*
    reactive 255
Fibronectin 21
Fibroplasia 21
Fibrous tissue 16
Fillers 169, 335
    adverse effects of 288
    injection techniques of 176*f*
    substances 173
Fitzpatrick skin 253, 254, 256
    phototypes 254
    type 260, 334
Flotation 105
Fluocinolone acetonide 295
Fluorouracil 160
Flutamide 7, 9
Focal postinflammatory erythema 292*f*
Focal pustular acne 275*f*
Food and drug administration 5
Fractional ablative
    lasers 281
    technologies 144
Fractional laser 254, 283
    ablation 126
    resurfacing 348
Fulminant acne 50
Fulminant hepatic necrosis 6

G

Gastrointestinal disturbances 6
Glabellar area 229*f*
Global acne qualitative scale 43
Glycolate hypersensitivity 60
Glycolic acid 3, 10, 59, 60, 70, 241, 272, 278, 354
Glycolic peels 276
    high-strength 277*f*

Graft
    elevation of 113*f*
    retention, minimal 196
Granuloma formation 237, 290, 298
Growth factor 124, 247
    beta, transforming 20
    insulin-like 22
    platelet-derived 21*f*, 247

H

Hair
    disorder 308
    follicles 238
Headache 8, 299
Healing, delayed 297
Hematoma 236
    formation 234
Herpes infection, active 138
Herpes labialis 81
Herpes simplex
    activation of 161
    active 66, 68*f*
    history of 271
    infection 175
        active 269
Hirsutism 8
Homecare dermarollers 118
Hormonal agents 7
Hormonal therapy 7, 55
Human dermal fibroblasts 20
Human immunodeficiency virus 172, 235
Hyaluronic acid 124, 170, 171, 180, 207, 237
    cross-linked 287
    derivatives 169
    filler 178*f*, 222, 235
Hyaluronidase 250*f*, 253, 258, 272
    injection 237
Hydroquinone 60, 241

Hyperandrogenism 8
Hyperpigmentation 51, 82, 113*f*, 276, 294
    postinflammatory 5, 51, 69, 76*f*, 88*f*, 99, 120, 163, 163*f*, 209*f*, 210, 218, 241, 243, 257, 296*f*, 321, 339
    risk of 271, 333
Hyperpigmented scars, management of 360*fc*
Hyperplastic epithelium 24
Hyperplastic papular scars 44
Hypersensitivity 6
    reactions 7
Hypertrophic scars 29*f*, 32, 38, 40*f*, 43, 45, 51, 61, 79, 148, 161, 164, 179, 246-248, 253, 256, 283
    and keloids, history of 69
    management of 364*fc*
    treatment of 60, 252
Hypodermic needle 222
Hypopigmentation 276, 295
    postinflammatory 163
    secondary 297
Hypopigmented macules 33
Hypoxia 195

I

Ice pick 36*f*, 201*f*
    acne scars 79, 85, 206*f*
Ice pick scar 26, 32*f*, 35, 42, 81, 93, 200, 201, 210, 331, 333, 351
    deep 32*f*, 202, 202*f*
    depth of 201, 203*f*
    management of 361*fc*
    mild superficial 202*f*
    moderate 202*f*
    treatment of 203
    typical 36*f*

V-shape epithelial tract of 201*f*
worsening of 209*f*, 298
Immunocompromised status, history of 159
Infection 76, 178, 290, 292
    active 214, 223
Infiltration anesthesia, discomfort of 234
Inflammation 19, 174, 178, 246
    active 214, 223
    phase of 20, 21
    reduce 258
    secondary 18*f*
Inflammatory acne 5, 19, 269
Inflammatory disease
    chronic 16
    multifactorial chronic 11
Inflammatory disorder 1
Inflammatory infiltrate 269
Inflammatory lesions, active 81
Inflammatory mediators destroy 26
Inflammatory papules 57
Injectable fillers 287
Instruments 131, 104
Insulated needles 323*f*
Insulated wire electrode 240
Intense pulsed light 160, 359
    devices 157
    treatment 161*b*
Intralesional corticosteroids 57
Intralesional radiofrequency 239, 242*f*, 244*f*, 249
Intralesional steroids 104, 105, 248, 250, 364
Intralesional triamcinolone acetonide 250*f*
Intra-treatment vigilance 273
Iontophoresis 59, 62
Iris scissors 104
Irritation 290

Ischemia 187, 195
Isotretinoin 9, 10, 54, 249, 271, 327
   therapy 10

J

Jasmonic acid 67f
Jessner's solution 65
   modified 70
Jewelers forceps 104

K

Keloid 27, 79, 138, 179, 246, 248, 252, 297
   acne scars 313
   formation 297
   frequency of 255
   risk of 256
   scars 39, 40f, 43, 51, 164, 248, 253, 261
      management of 364fc
   tendency 81, 269
   treatment of 60, 249
Keratinocyte growth factor 21f
Kojic acid 241, 278, 295

L

Labile melanocyte responses 255
Lactic acid 67f, 70, 354
Laser
   abrasion 342
   beam 203f
   complications of 161b
   devices 144, 258
   energy, melanin absorption of 285
   exfoliation, post-fractional resurfacing 284f
   parameters, selecting appropriate 274
   resurfacing 280
   therapy, contraindications of 159b
   treatment 254, 346
Lens
   contact 72
   reflex camera, single 305
Lesions
   healing 269
   nodulocystic 57
   removal of pigmented 254
Levomefolate 7
Light devices 144
Light-emitting diode 118
Lightening agents 272
Lignocaine 106, 184, 188
Linear acne scars 228, 231f
   lipoatrophic 230f
Linear atrophic scars, narrow 229f
Linear scars 26f, 37, 38f, 229f, 231
   hypopigmented 231
   management of 363fc
   narrow 232
   subtypes of 228
   treatment of 228
      of narrow 231
Linear threading technique 176f
Lipoatrophic acne scars 174f, 228
Lipoatrophic linear scars 229, 232f
Lipoatrophic scars 29f, 38, 39f
Lipoatrophy 223f
Lipografting, technique of 184f
Liposuction cannula 185f
Local anesthesia 106, 234, 339
   infiltration of 341
   lignocaine 104
Lumenis 342
Lumpiness 290
   formation 298
Lupus
   drug induced 7
   erythematosus 139
Luteinizing hormone 2

M

Macular acne scars 67f, 152f
Macular atrophic scars 42
Macular erythematous acne scars 66
Macular scars 33, 332
Macules acne scars, hyperpigmented 65
Magnesium oxide 133
Makeup 317
    fixing 317
    setting 317
Mandelic acid 3, 10, 53, 59, 60, 69, 70, 277, 332, 354
    peel 70
Matrix metalloproteinases 20, 53, 61
Maturation, phase of 20
Medical therapy 52
Melanocytes 295
Melanosomes, larger 255
Melasma 259
Menarche 8
Menstrual irregularities 8
Mesosolutions 323
Metallic crystals 136
Metalloprotein, tissue inhibitor of 21f
Metalloproteinases, tissue inhibitor of 247
Methyl alcohol 81
Microdermabrasion 130, 275, 281
    advantages of 142
    causes 131
    crystals 131, 132, 136
    diamond tips suitable for 137f
    effective 142
    erythema after desired endpoint of 141f
    machine 132, 137f
        types of 133
    tips 136, 137f
Microfat 197
Microneedle 115, 128, 280, 281
    after three sessions of 126f
    delivery systems 119
    endpoint of 122f
    instrument 117f
    principle of 116
    radiofrequency 239, 288, 321, 322, 322f, 331, 333
        fractional 321
        treatment 324f
Microthermal zones, density of 259
Milia 161, 178, 275, 294
Minipunch grafting 202
Minocycline 5-7
Mitogen-activated protein 247
    kinases 20
Moisturization 315, 343
Molluscum contagiosum 68
Mometasone 295
Monocytes 21f
Monopolar radiofrequency 323
Monotherapy 67f
Multifactorial disorder 1
Myocardial contraction 278
Myocardial infarction 8

N

Nail disorder 308
Nanofat 197
Nasolabial fold, lipoatrophic in 230f
Needle
    abrade 115
    holder 104
    selection 94
Negative pressure 141

Neodymium:yttrium aluminum garnet 331, 332
Neodymium-doped yttrium aluminum garnet 254, 352, 360
  laser 155
Neutral pH balance 135
Nicotinamide 53
Nodular keloids 297
Nodular lesions 351
Nodules 1
Nokor needle 93, 95f, 235
Nonablative fractional *erbium* glass laser 154
Nonablative laser 154, 239, 281, 285
  fractional 156f
Noninsulated needles 323f
Nonsurgical conservative therapy 248
Norethindrone acetate 7
Norgestimate 7
Normal skin 146

O

Obesity 2
Office procedure, simple 127
Oily cysts 195
Onion extract 61
Oral antibiotics 159
Oral contraceptive pills, combined 7
Oral zinc 11

P

Pain 178, 292, 336
  management 283
  mild 326
Papillary dermis 141, 154
Papular acne scars 239f, 244f
  hypopigmented 239f
Papular postacne scar, typical 229f
Papular scars 28f, 39, 41f, 238, 240, 240f, 243
Papules 1
  raised 32f
  visible 237
Papulopustular acne 244f
Peel
  combination 70
  complications 278
  superficial 69
  timing of 69
Peeling agent 69, 276, 278
Peeling area, open wounds on 68
Percutaneous collagen induction 231
Persistent edema 276
Persistent erythema 161, 162f, 226
  edema 275
Persistent erythematous macules 34f
Persistent hyperpigmented macules 35f
  scars 51, 332
Persistent keloids 250f
Petechiae 163
Phenol peels 236, 269
  deep 261
Phenolization 57
Photodynamic therapy 11, 57
Photorejuvenation 254
Photosensitivity 6
Photothermolysis
  fractional 146
  principle of selective 146
Phytic acid 354
Pigment 6, 68f
Pigmentary disorders, prevalence of 255
Pilosebaceous follicle 19, 53
  obstruction of 18, 18f

Platelet-rich plasma 195, 289, 323, 329, 331, 334
Polyacrylamides 172
Polycystic ovarian syndrome 2, 55
Poly-L-lactic acid 235
Polymorphonucleocyte 18, 18f, 21f
Poor skin texture 333
Postablative laser skin
    dermabrasion 81
    resurfacing 81
Postacne scars 339, 346
    linear 237
    treatment of 355
Post-carbon dioxide laser
    immediate post 293f
    resolution 293f
Postprocedure care 87, 99, 109, 123, 126
Povidone-iodine 104
Prednisolone, low-dose 9
Pregnancy 60
Progesterone 7
Proliferation, phase of 20, 21
Prophylaxis 294
Propionibacterium acnes 1, 17
Pros and cons 114
Proteoglycan 21
Pruritis 294
Pseudotumor cerebri 7
Psoriasis 139, 269, 308
    active 159
Psychosocial distress 312
Pulsed dye laser 154, 160, 248, 359
Punch closure 107
Punch elevation 105, 107
    principles of 108f
Punch excision 114, 217f, 286
    and grafting 105
    at recipient site 110f
    complications of 112
    of donor grafts 110f
    techniques 103, 104, 114, 219, 220
Punch flotation 217, 286
Punch grafting 107, 109f, 112f, 286
    abraded 107, 110f
    cobblestoning following 113f
Purpura, delayed 161
Pustules 1
Pyruvic acid 60, 61, 70

Q

Quantitative scale 44

R

Radiofrequency
    devices 254
    fractional 321
    machine 240, 242
        wire electrode of 241f
Reactions, irritant 52
Reflectance confocal microscopy 308
Relaxed skin tension 236
    line 104, 251, 362, 363
Remodeling, phase of 20
Renal failure 186
Retinoic acid 60, 142
    receptors 4
Retinoid 2, 60, 253, 272
    dermatitis 4, 53b
    topical 4, 52, 224, 241
Ribonucleic acid 22
Right peel, strength of 273
Ring scars 111, 111f
Rolling acne scars 227
Rolling scar 25f, 36, 37f, 221, 223f, 331, 333, 346f
    complications of 226
    contraindications of 223

deep 32f
depressed 93
indications of 223
instruments of 222
limitations of 223
management of 361fc
postprocedure care of 226
precautions of 224
treatment of 221, 223
Rosacea, active 138

S

Salicylic acid 2, 3, 5, 10, 53, 67f, 69, 70, 276, 298, 332
    peels 54f, 56f, 74f, 267
Salicylic peels 269
Salicylic-Mandelic acid peels 75f, 278
    flare after 279f
Scalp rollers 118
Scar 16, 238, 250, 252, 257, 312, 350
    after stretching skin, effacement of 240f
    atrophic 32, 44, 66, 143, 306f, 333, 353
        mild superficial 65, 66
    bigger 176
    bottom of 212
    bridging 27f, 41, 41f, 246, 251, 251f
    broader 237
    clinical acne-related 46
    cobblestoning and ring 220f
    correction, principle of 170
    counting 42
    deep 212, 214
    depressed 35, 219, 339
    development of 248
    distribution of 265
    edges of 343
    elevated 38, 112f
    excision of 233f
    hyperpigmented 331, 332
    in acne 228
    ineffective for 267
    intervention, stage of 268
    irregular depressed 212
    marking of 113f
    mild 265
    narrow 237
    permanent hypopigmented 256
    predominant 265
    revision techniques 286
    right 217
    severe 264, 265
    shallow depressed 173f
    shouldering 344f
    size, smaller 176
    skin 251
    tissue 195
    treatment of 177, 196
    types of 160, 221, 230, 265, 331
        medical makeup for 313
    wide 177
    worsening of 89f, 282, 298
Sebaceous duct, hyperkeratinization of 19
Sebaceous secretion 18f
Sensitive skin 332
    types 277
Serial puncture technique 176f
Sex hormone-binding globulin 7
Shallow rolling scar 32f
Shallow scars 212, 213
Shamban acne scale 45t
Shamban scale 45
Silicon
    based products 248
    gel 61, 249
    implants 170
    sheets 249

Sinus tracts 41
Skin 131
    ablation, partial 141
    atrophy 250
    cleansing 315
    color 253
    contact, amounts of 132
    dry sensitive 266
    dryness of 283, 342
    injury 282
    irritation 76
    lightening agent 203, 332
    needling 115, 309
    phototypes 253
    products, deep 170
    smooth 313
    stretching 28*f*
    suture 6-0 prolene 104
    texture 236
    tightening 254, 344
    tightness of 283
    tumors, malignant 138
    type 198, 253, 265
Skin scar 150
    chemical reconstruction of 72, 79, 89, 125, 201, 205, 206*f*, 214, 222, 231, 268, 329-331, 340, 361
    technique 79
        chemical reconstruction of 77*f*, 79*f*, 81*f*, 87, 88*f*, 100, 160, 208*f*, 209*f*, 210
Smallpox 352
Sodium
    bicarbonate 133
        microdermabrasion crystals 135
    chloride 133
Soft tissue augmentation 237
Spirit 81, 104
Spironolactone 7, 8
Staphylococcus aureus 10
Stem cells 190
Stereoimage optical topometer 307
Sterile
    abscesses 288
    hypodermic needle 93
Steri-strips 104
Steroid
    mild topical 62
    potent 290
    superpotent 50*f*
    topical 249, 266
Stratum corneum 60, 62, 147
Stretch test 222*f*
Stromal vascular fraction 195
Subcision 91, 106, 197, 231*f*
    adequate 224
    after four sessions of 225*f*
    danger areas of 98*f*, 98*t*
    modified 92*f*
    principle of 92*f*
Subcutaneous incision less surgery 91
Subcutaneous tissue 212
    loss of 237
Sulfamethoxazole 6
Sun control 271
Sun protection, adequate 236
Sunscreens 59, 224
Surgical glue 104
Surgical marking pen 104
Surgical scar 93
    revision techniques 263
Surgical therapy 55
Systemic antibiotics 1, 5, 57

T

Tattoo removal 254
Tazarotene 4, 272
Test patch 272

Tetracyclines 5
Thermal injury, columns of 146
Tinnitus 6, 298
Tissue
    connective 286
    destruction, excessive 243
Tools 314
Topical nicotinamide 5
Topical retinoic acid 60
Toxic dose 188
Toxicity 298
Traditional glycolic peels 277
Traditional laser 258
Traditional liposuction 196
Traditional subcision 95*f*
Tram-track appearance 127
Tranexamic acid 124
Transitory reactions 288
Transplanted fat, zones of 195*f*
Traumatic scars, depressed linear 93
Tretinoin 4, 142, 272
    binding 4
    iontophoresis 62
Triamcinolone acetonide 237, 249
Trichloroacetic acid 65, 79, 80, 81*f*, 125, 160, 205, 222
    peels 279*f*
Trimethoprim 6
Triple laser technique, combination 336
Tumescent anesthesia, amounts of 186
Tumescent fluid 188

U

Ulcers 138
Ultrapulse laser 343
Ultrasound, high frequency 305
Ultraviolet
    A 271
    B 271
Unrealistic expectations 174, 269

V

Vaginal candidiasis 6
Varicella scars 118
Vascular endothelial growth factor 247
Viral warts 68
Vitamin
    C 124, 295
        topical 142
    D level 2
    E 93
Vitiligo 159
    unstable 269

W

Warts 138
Wooden toothpick, sharpened 82*f*
Wound 138
    healing, phases of 20, 21*f*

EU GSPR Authorised Reprsentative
Logos Europe, 9 rue Nicolas Poussin
1700, La Rochelle, France
Phone: +33 (0) 6 67 93 73 78
E-mail: contact@logoseurope.eu

www.ingramcontent.com/pod-product-compliance
Ingram Content Group UK Ltd.
Pitfield, Milton Keynes, MK11 3LW, UK
UKHW021827140426
5217IPUK00016B/1234